EPIDEMIOLOGY IN HEALTH SERVICES MANAGEMENT

G. E. Alan Dever, Ph.D., M.T.

Director
Health Services Analysis, Inc.
Stone Mountain, Georgia
and
Director of Clinical Epidemiology and Biostatistics
Mercer University School of Medicine
Macon, Georgia

With the special assistance of
François Champagne, Ph.D.
University of Montreal

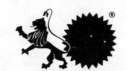

AN ASPEN PUBLICATION®
Aspen Publishers, Inc.
Rockville, Maryland
Royal Tunbridge Wells
1984

Library of Congress Cataloging in Publication Data

Dever, G. E. Alan
Epidemiology in health services management.

"An Aspen publication."
Includes bibliographical references and index.
1. Epidemiology.   2. Health services administration.
3. Health planning.   I. Champagne, Francois.   II. Title.
[DNLM: 1. Epidemiology.   2. Health policy.   3. Health
services—Organization and administration.   W 84.1 D4912]
RA651.D48   1984   614.4   83-19675
ISBN: 0-89443-850-6

Publisher: John Marozsan
Editor-in-Chief: Michael Brown
Executive Managing Editor: Margot Raphael
Editorial Services: Eileen Higgins
Printing and Manufacturing: Debbie Collins

Library of Congress Catalog Card Number: 83-19675
ISBN: 0-89443-850-6

Printed in the United States of America

*To Georgie,
Tammy, and Jamie-
for their powerful
inspiration*

Table of Contents

Preface

The basic premise of this book is that hospitals and other health-related organizations require the basic tools of epidemiology to make sound health policy decisions based on epidemiological evidence. They must know and understand the epidemiology of disease and how it relates to the utilization of services.

To do this, they also must understand the principles and methods peculiar to epidemiology and allied disciplines that must be applied to the policy and management areas of the health institution. These many aspects of epidemiology in health services management are discussed here in detail (see Table 1).

This book is oriented to and permeated with concern for prevention and wellness, adapting a holistic approach to health care. Health care organizations also should be concerned about disease prevention and health promotion, for therein lies the greatest potential for improving the population's status of health—a basic but often forgotten value to the health care industry.

Prevention is a basic and multidimensional element of care and therefore must be an integral part of the institutional approach to health service management. This also is where the best possibility for expansion of services exists.

This book also is designed to supply health care managers with the perspective and basic tools of epidemiology so they can participate effectively in a sound health policymaking process and contribute to improvement in the population's health level.

It should be noted that the use of the term "disease" is broadened throughout the text to encompass such other health problems as motor vehicle and all other accidents, homicide, and suicide, all of which are included in epidemiological statistics as major causal factors in deaths and other conditions that have an impact on health.

The author assumes full responsibility for the accuracy of all mathematical equations, calculations, tables, etc. Readers who detect any errors are asked to write to the author (care of Aspen Systems Corporation) so corrections can be made in subsequent editions. p, 127

G.E. Alan Dever, Ph.D., M.T.

Table 1

The Contributions of Epidemiology to Health Services Management

Management		The Planning Process	Contributions of Epidemiology	Chapters Reviewing These Contributions
Functional Approach	Process Approach			

Planning	Technical	Identification of needs and problems	• Descriptive Epidemiology:
			  • Person
			  • Place
			  • Time
			• Description of health problems in terms of mortality, morbidity, and risk factors
			• Demography
			• Analysis of etiology (risk factors)
				1,2,3
				
				4, 5, 6, 7, 8, 9, 10, 11, 12

	Administrative and Political	Establishment of priorities	Estimation of: • Magnitude of loss • Amenability to prevention or reduction • Epidemiological Measurement	3, 4, 5, 10
		Setting of objectives	• Quantified objectives • Feasibility	3, 4, 5, 10
		Implementation of activities to attain objectives	• Generation of alternatives • Cost-benefit analysis	1, 2, 3, 4, 5, 10, 11, 12

Organizing
Directing
Coordinating

Controlling

Technical

Mobilization and
coordination of resources

Evaluation

● Monitoring of program
● Marketing

4, 5, 10

● Clinical trials
● Outcome assessment

4, 8, 10

Acknowledgments

This book represents the culmination of several years work with several key people. In particular, Francois Champagne worked one year with me on a Fellowship from the University of Montreal, Canada. He had a major role in the writing of this book. The text has many distinct qualities that only Francois was able to impart. Probably the most important aspect, however, is our friendship, which grew during the writing. I have a lasting respect for him and for his extensive ability. There are several chapters to which only Francois was able to provide his unique perspective.

I especially want to thank James Alley, M.D., Director of Public Health in Georgia who saw the need for utilizing these methods and techniques and who gave many of us opportunities to work in our special areas. I thank William Bristol, M.D., Dean of Mercer Medical School who provided the resources and immense support for the completion of this project.

Many others also helped greatly. I wish to thank Judy Morris for her support. She is both a friend and a superb typist. Nancy Jean Smith is to be thanked and recognized for her typing of certain key chapters of the manuscript. Also, I wish to thank Becky McQueen, Chuck Benson, Bryan Darling, Butch Ferguson and Tom Wade for their research assistance and support. Many thanks to Aspen, in particular, Mike Brown, Eileen Higgins, and Kevin Blanc for their encouragement and patience.

Chapter 1

Epidemiology: Focus on Prevention

IMPROVEMENT IN HEALTH STATUS

As pointed out in *Healthy People: the Surgeon General's Report on Health Promotion and Disease Prevention (1979)*, "If our nation is to improve the health of its citizens, it must reorder its present priorities in health care to put greater emphasis on the prevention of disease and the promotion of health."[1] All providers have to join in this effort by broadening their comprehension of their patients' health problems and by extending their activities into their community or target populations.

The concepts of disease prevention and health promotion not only encompass the tenets expressed in *Healthy People* but also must reflect their application to the management of care services. The disease prevention and health promotion framework adopted in this book suggests a need for a broader consideration of a patient who presents health problems. As Blum points out:

> The ecologic paradigm suggest that all human support services should be integrated at the point of primary care, an entry point for those with hurts or problems of any sort. Manifestations in one sphere may be caused by stresses in the others (even accidents are mostly not accidental). Simple problems are handled directly. More extensive ones are carried past any crisis aspects and then receive attention in order to interrupt the forces, whether they be family, occupation, employment, housing, infections, or whatever that underlie the presenting conditions. When indicated, search is directed to the aggravating, predisposing or risk factors which underlie the presence of the so-called proximal causes.[2]

Furthermore, health care providers need to extend their services into the community in an effort to reach not only the patients who initiate contact but also all others who might be at risk from their environment, life style, or heredity (biology). Providers should be committed to the health of the community as a whole and of its individual members and to involving them in programs before they become sick.[3]

EXPANSION OF SERVICES

Prevention and health promotion also represent a way of dealing with changes in the field and with expanding services. Many changes are affecting the industry. Health care costs have been rising steadily while hospital occupancy rates and average length of stay have been going down. At the same time, survival rates for many chronic diseases have increased and the population of those 65 and older has grown. These last two trends point to the obviously increasing need for secondary and tertiary prevention. Primary prevention represents an opportunity for providers to cope with these and other changes.

Obviously, the entire burden of improving the practice of disease prevention and health promotion cannot be carried by the institution nor the medical professional generally. The health promotion market must be widened, however, so that people slowly but surely will become motivated to take more responsibility for their own health.

In any case, changes are occurring and although health care providers may have no control over them, they can anticipate them and plan for them. For example, they can manage their services creatively and effectively in gearing them to the needs of their target communities. That is what this book is all about.

A FRAMEWORK FOR HEALTH CONCEPTS

To be able to look at associations between risk factors and states of health and disease, an overall framework or conceptualization of health and its determinants is needed. This framework must be broad, comprehensive, and manageable from the viewpoint of policy. It also must accommodate two epidemiological models— those involved with multiple cause/multiple effect factors and those associated with risk factors, as opposed to a more traditional limited emphasis on strict causality.

The Traditional Model

The traditional epidemiologic model of disease has three components: agent, host, and environment (Figure 1-1). Agents of disease include infectious organisms, physical agents, allergens, chemical agents, and dietary excesses and deficiencies. Host factors are intrinsic elements influencing the individual's sus-

Figure 1-1 The Traditional (Ecological) Model

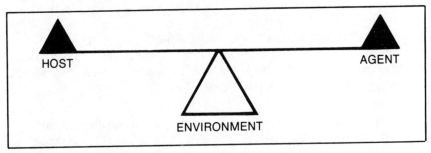

Source: Reprinted from *Community Health Analysis* by G.E. Alan Dever with permission of Aspen Systems Corporation, ©1980, p. 11.

ceptibility to the agent. Environmental factors are extrinsic entities influencing exposure to the agent. Factors in each of these categories interact to produce disease. A change in any of the three will alter an existing equilibrium to increase or decrease the frequency of disease.

The model in Figure 1-1 was developed when infectious diseases were the main, if not sole, preoccupation of epidemiologists. Infectious organisms were accorded a status separate from other factors and were identified as agents. With the shift in disease patterns and in the focus of epidemiological studies, new models were developed by stretching the traditional one, deemphasizing agent, and broadening host and environmental factors.

This stretching does not alter the fact, however, that the traditional framework was developed under the assumption of a single cause/single effect model. Host and environmental factors simply influence the exposure and susceptibility of the individual but do not correspond adequately to present comprehension of most noninfectious diseases.

Some writers talk about the "human host as a causative factor" and "environmental causative factors."[4] However, the author believes it is much simpler and more appropriate to adopt a framework that is broader, more comprehensive, and more fitting to a multiple cause/multiple effect view of health and disease. This multidimensional framework allows health care executives to approach the management of services from a broader epidemiological perspective.

A Program for the 80s and 90s

A plan for the 80s and 90s was developed in 1973 when Laframboise proposed a conceptual framework for analysis of the health field.[5] This framework, later described as the "health field concept" in a Canadian governmental working paper[6] that became the basis for that country's policy, holds that health is determined by a variety of factors falling into four primary divisions: life style, environment, health care organization, and human biology (Figure 1-2) (each of which is discussed in Chapter 3).

In 1974, Blum proposed an "environment of health" model (Figure 1-3), later retitled the "Force Field and Well-Being Paradigms of Health." In 1976, Dever, building on the Laframboise and Lalonde model, labeled it "An Epidemiological Model for Health Policy Analysis" (Figure 1-4).

> Blum suggests that the width of the four inputs contributing to health indicate assumptions about their relative importance. The four inputs relate to and affect one another by means of an encompassing wheel containing population, cultural systems, mental health, ecological balance, and natural resources. On the other hand, the assumptions of Lalonde and Dever are that the four inputs are weighted equally and must be in balance for health to occur. The important question to answer is, How do these four inputs operate when analyzed for specific diseases; or, alternatively, how do these four inputs operate when no disease exists (that is, a state of wellness)? The analysis of risk factors for disease categories within the framework of Dever's epidemiological model for policy analysis provides results similar to those hypothesized by Blum.[7]

As stated, an overall framework or conceptualization of health is needed for examining and studying the relationship between risk factors and states of health and disease. The ultimate purpose of such an exercise is to preserve and restore health. The underlying framework should force the investigator or analyst to consider all factors coming into play in the preservation and restoration of health.

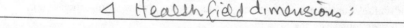

Figure 1-2 The Health Field Concept

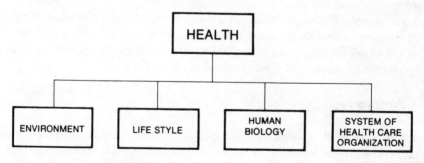

Source: Reprinted from *A New Perspective on the Health of Canadians* by Marc Lalonde with permission of the Office of the Canadian Minister of National Health and Welfare, April 1974, 31.

Figure 1-3 The Force Field and Well-Being Paradigms of Health

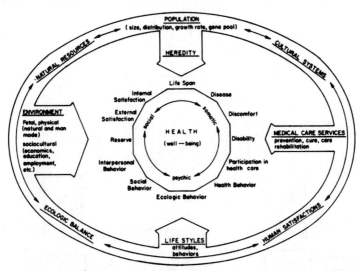

The width of the four large input-to-health arrows indicates assumptions about the relative importance of the inputs to health. The four inputs are shown as relating to and affecting one another by means of an encompassing matrix that could be called the "environment" of the health system.

Source: Reprinted from *Planning for Health* (2nd. ed.) by Henrik L. Blum with permission of Human Sciences Press, ©1981, 5.

As Kerr puts it:

> I would agree that the mechanistic or reductionistic view of health and disease should be supplemented by this broader psychobiological view of man who, starting with his aliquot of genes, enters a life of complex internal and external transactions that are as yet only vaguely understood . . . . The need for a theoretical framework that does not require all noxious agents to be physical, chemical, or biological and that leaves room for such complex deleterious influences on health as noise pollution, jet fatigue, occupational stress, domestic violence, inadequate parenting, and sexual strife is readily apparent.[8]

The health field concept is such a framework, allowing the broad psychosociobiological analysis of any state of health or disease. It is a comprehensive structure that forces the equal examination of life style, environmental, and biological elements as well as health care organization factors. The model also is ideally suited to the elaboration of preventive measures. The United States government adopted this model in the "Prevention Profile" annexed to *Health, United States, 1980.*[9]

Figure 1-4 An Epidemiological Model for Health Policy Analysis

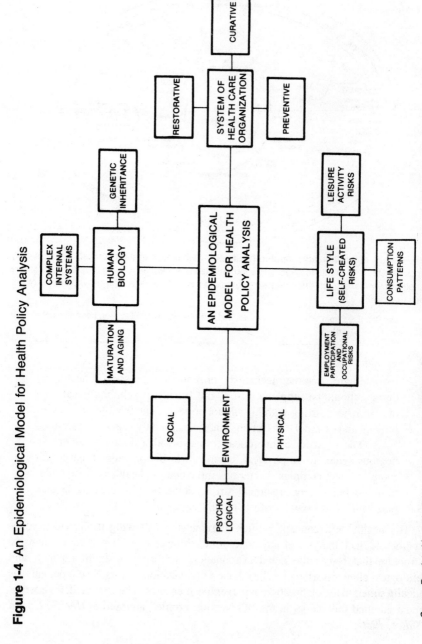

Source: Reprinted from "An Epidemiological Model for Health Policy Analysis" by G.E. Alan Dever, *Social Indicators Research 2,* ©1976, 455.

LIFE STAGES, DISEASE PATTERNS, PREDICTABILITY

An example of applying the four components of the health field concept to life stage patterns in health promotion and disease prevention is *Passages: Predictable Mortality through the Life Stages.*[10] This 1980 document demonstrates the need for increased emphasis on prevention if the major cripplers and killers in society are to be overcome. By analyzing social, psychological, and epidemiological patterns by life stages, it suggests a major role for health services management in the area of health promotion.

Passages shows that the development of people's attitudes toward life assumes that a particular event (death, injury, or disease) always will happen to the other person and at any point during life, in a most random manner. The fact is, these events have a high probability of occurring to everyone or anyone, and the life stages at which they occur are predictable.

A brief overview of mortality patterns from *Passages* underscores the concept that poor health habits early in life contribute to poor health later. Heart attack is an excellent example. It appears in early adulthood (20 to 29 years), as the ninth or tenth most frequent disease. In the next life stage, young adulthood (30 to 44), heart attack moves up to rank first for white males and fourth or sixth for the other groups. By middle adulthood (45 to 59), it is first for white males and females and black males and second for black females. It continues to be a major problem throughout the final two life stages. As this demonstrates, patterns of mortality begun in the early life stages are predictable in the later phases.

Whether or not a person will experience a particular event during a particular life stage is dependent upon several factors: life style, environment, biology, and health care system. No one dies from the major cripplers and killers because there is *not* sufficient knowledge about their causes. Society has the ability to reduce substantially and, in some instances, to eradicate the major cripplers and killers at each life stage but this comes about only through concerted action in all elements of the health field. Preventive and curative action, as well as health promotion, are needed. Furthermore, all these activities should be geared toward the population at risk. As is shown later, epidemiology offers methods and techniques to health service managers to identify such populations and to cope with the issues.

PREVENTION AND HEALTH PROMOTION

Three general levels of prevention are:

1. primary, the inhibition of the development of a disease before it occurs
2. secondary, the early detection and treatment of disease
3. tertiary, the rehabilitation or restoration of effective functioning.

Primary Prevention

In the prepathogenesis period, prevention consists of measures designed to promote optimum general health and of specific protective elements (Figure 1-5). The latter include immunization, environmental sanitation, and protection against accidents and occupational hazards. This is prevention in its conventional sense. These measures have proved very effective in reducing mortality and morbidity from infectious diseases. General health promotion measures incorporate life style, environmental, and biological factors. This area may contribute the most to furthering reductions in mortality and morbidity.

"Health can be delivered only in a small part; it must largely be lived."[11]

Secondary Prevention

Secondary prevention consists mostly of the early diagnosis and treatment of diseases through such measures as screening and periodic health examinations. The early detection of cancer, hypertension, venereal diseases, and other such treatable illnesses is the aim of secondary prevention. For certain diseases, such as arthritis or other morbid conditions associated with the aging process, secondary prevention might consist of limiting the disability—preventing further complications or sequelae.

Tertiary Prevention

Where disease already has occurred and has left residual damage, tertiary prevention is the avoidance of complete disability after anatomical and physiologi-

---

Figure 1-5 Application of Preventive Measures in Disease

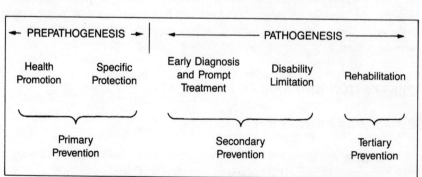

Source: Reprinted from *Preventive Medicine for the Doctor in His Community* by H.R. Leavell and E.G. Clark with permission of McGraw-Hill Book Company, ©1965, 20.

cal changes are more or less stabilized. The aim is to restore an affected individual to a satisfying and self-sufficient life.

Figure 1-6 delineates some diseases as a "continuum for preventability." The shading represents the possibility of preventing diseases or conditions by applying known intervention methods. The darkest area, at the left end of the shaded bar, indicates conditions that can be prevented unequivocally. In the center are some conditions where drastic, sizable, or at least some reductions in risk could be achieved. The lightest area, at the right, illustrates conditions where no progress in reducing risks can be expected until breakthroughs in knowledge are made.

AN APPLICATION: STRATEGIES FOR PREVENTION

An example of putting together the health field concept, *Passages*, and levels of prevention is outlined in Exhibits 1-1, 1-2, and 1-3. The three specific diseases are osteoporosis, COPD (chronic obstructive pulmonary disease—e.g., lung cancer, emphysema, and asthma), and hypertension/stroke. In each example the life stage is middle adulthood (ages 30 to 44); the risk factors are life style, environment, biology, and the health care delivery system; and the levels of prevention are primary, secondary, and tertiary.

This approach outlines strategies for prevention/intervention for each level of prevention and for each broad category of risk factors. This application serves two specific purposes:

1. Professionals involved in patient care can determine quickly where their resources should be concentrated to potentially prevent (and certainly intervene) in the disease process.

Figure 1-6 A Continuum for Preventability

Absolutely preventable				No known prevention
Smallpox	Lung and other cancers	Congenital anomalies	Suicide	Brain tumors
Measles	of the respiratory	Infant mortality	Homicide	Rheumatoid arthritis
Poliomyelitis	system	Cardiovascular disease		
	Asbestosis	Stroke		
	Dental caries	Trauma from accidents		
	Cancer of cervix	Cancer of bladder		
		Pneumonia and influenza		

Note: The order and placement of the diseases and conditions listed are intended only to be illustrative.

Source: U.S. Department of Health and Human Services, *Health, United States, 1980* (Washington, D.C.: U.S. Government Printing Office, 1980).

Exhibit 1-1 Strategies for Preventing Osteoporosis in Young
Adults (30 to 44 Years)

	Life Style	Environment	Biology	Delivery System

Primary Prevention	Exercise
	Diet
	Nutrition
	Vitamin and
	  mineral
	  supplementation
		Fluoride water
		supplementation
			Hormones
			Calcium
			Vitamin D
			Fluoride
			Endometrial
			  biopsy if
			  indicated
				Patient education re:
				  high risk
				  hysterectomy
				  diet
				  exercise

Secondary Prevention	Exercise
	Diet
	Changes secondary
	to arthritis;
	compression Spinal
	fractures hip, wrist
		Safe environment
		Family counseling
			Screening for
			  causes not
			  related to
			  aging
			Hormones
			Calcium
			Vitamin D
			Fluoride
			Endometrial
			  biopsy if
			  indicated
			Physical therapy
				Access to care
				Payment for care:
				  medications
				  medical
				  appointments

Tertiary Prevention	Prevention of
	  immobility
	Debilitation
	Disposition
		Accident-proof
		  home
		Provision of places
		  to use a walker
		Family support
			Hip pinning
			High suspicion
			  of fractures
			Physical therapy
				Access to care
				Payment for care

2. Health services managers should be able to realize the vast potential for using it in managing the institution.

Specifically, the primary prevention level—no matter what the element of the health field concept—should promote ideas for health marketing and disease prevention. Such an analysis by life stage, elements of the health field concept, and prevention levels has unlimited value when applied to the various disease categories. The use of this approach is to be encouraged to further the principles of epidemiology in managing health services.

The application of these 3 levels of prevention to the proposed framework of health by life stage requires a basic understanding of what epidemiology is and what it encompasses. Health service managers are familiar with some of these aspects but this approach has had limited use. The rest of this chapter therefore provides an overview of the shift in disease patterns and the changing nature of

Exhibit 1-2 Strategies for Preventing Pulmonary Disease in Young Adults (30 to 44 Years)

	Life Style	*Environment*	*Biology*	*Delivery System*
Primary Prevention	No smoking Exposures from hobbies, i.e., welding, woodworking Nutrition	Workplace surveillance Obedience to work regulations Air pollution Allergens	Family history and risks re asthma, lung disease, exposures Respirator use at work if indicated	Research in occupational health, extrapolation of findings to others for early prevention or diagnosis Occupational history to identify high risk
Secondary Prevention	Cessation of smoking Self-protection during hobbies Personal adjustment to problems with breathing Nutrition	Occupational regulations set re findings of surveillance above Job change if necessary Avoidance of city, pollen, cigarette smoke, cotton dust Air conditioning Family counseling	Early treatment of infections Screening for TB Bronchodilators Immunizations: flu, pneumococcus Screening: chest x-rays, pulmonary function tests, blood gases Treatment: respiratory therapy	Patient education Payment for care medications Access to care and therapy
Tertiary Prevention	Cessation of smoking Debilitation Chronic care, home or institution Dependency Nutrition	One-story house Ban on matches around oxygen Avoidance of exacerbating situations Family support	Oxygen Tracheotomy Lung cancer Chest x-rays	Medications and respiratory therapy; special precautions Access to care, home or institution Payment for care

epidemiology—its aims, types, and method of investigation. Only basic aspects are covered; exhaustive treatment is dealt with in later chapters.

A SHIFT IN DISEASE PATTERNS

The turning point for infectious and chronic diseases in the United States occurred about 1925 (Figure 1-7). Collectively, deaths from infectious diseases

Exhibit 1-3 Strategies for Preventing Hypertension or Stroke in Young Adults (30 to 44 Years)

	Life Style	Environment	Biology	Delivery System

Primary Prevention	Stress reduction
	Diet low in salt,
	  fat, calories
	Exercise
	No smoking
	Vitamins
		Awareness of job
		  and
		  environmental
		  stresses
		Lead
			Risks re sex,
			  family
			  history, lipid
			  levels
			Aspirin
				Patient education:
				  How to take own
				  blood pressure

Secondary Prevention	Stress management
	Diet low in salt,
	  fat, calories
	Exercise
	Halt to smoking
	Life style
	  adjustment re
	  medication and
	  medical
	  appointments
	Vitamins
		Job change if
		  necessary
		Family counseling
			Medications:
			  compliance
			  side effects
				Patient education:
				  relaxation
				  techniques
				Evaluation for
				  secondary causes

Tertiary Prevention	Stress reduction
	Diet
	Mild exercise
	Halt to smoking
	Adjustment to
	  dependency:
	  walker, etc.
	Disposition
	Vitamins
		Safety:
		  one-story house
		  care
		  space for
		  walker,
		    wheelchair
		Family support
			Compliance
			  with and
			  education re
			  medications
			Physical therapy
			Speech therapy
				Patient education re
				  complications,
				  i.e., Myocardial
				  infarction,
				  cerebrovascular
				  accident, renal
				  failure
				Emergency medical
				  technicians
				Coronary care units
				Access to delivery
				  system and
				  therapy
				Payment for care
				Screening for rest of
				  family

declined from about 650 per 100,000 population in 1900 to about 20 per 100,000 in 1970 (a drop of 96 percent). A major epidemic of influenza in 1918 peaked the death rate at 850 per 100,000. Chronic diseases, on the other hand, collectively accounted for about 350 deaths per 100,000 population in 1900 and increased to about 690 per 100,000 in 1970 (a jump of 97 percent). However, from 1970 to 1980 there has been a 5.6 percent decrease.

Figure 1-7 Infectious and Chronic Disease Death Rates, 1900–1970

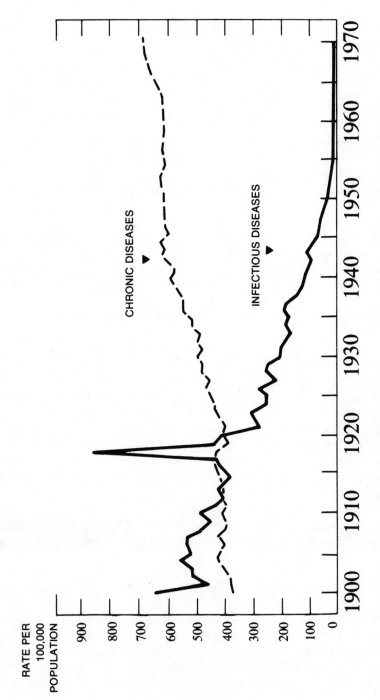

Source: Reprinted from *Dynamics of Health and Disease* by C.L. Marshall and D. Pearson with permission of Appleton-Century Crofts, Inc., ©1972, 131.

This transition—not unlike a demographic transition—represents a shift in disease patterns. The reason is to be found in a societal shift from an agrarian to an industrialized society. Diseases afflicting a given segment of a culture vary with the social and physical conditions characterizing society at the time. Thus, at the turn of the century, the nation's roots were based on a life style that was agricultural in nature; with the advent of industrialization, those societal roots changed, producing the shift in disease patterns.

The agrarian society generated a cycle of events that is portrayed in the infectious disease model (Figure 1-8). That era reflected high fertility, with needs that were basic: food, shelter, and clothing. Thus, in 1900, 52 percent of the population was under 21 years of age and 3 percent was over 65. (This type of population pyramid is typical of today's inner cities and developing countries where the infectious disease model still is applicable.)

The results were devastating: with no specific treatment, parasitic and infectious diseases and malnutrition contributed to high infant and preschool mortality. In fact, 34 percent of all deaths occurred between birth and 5 years of age. In that agrarian culture, high fertility compensated for high mortality. Large families also were essential for harvesting food from the land.

Industrialization produced drastic changes in disease patterns, as demonstrated by the chronic disease model (Figure 1-9). Because of its changing values, contemporary society can induce certain kinds of diseases; deleterious social, physical, emotional, and environmental ways of life have resulted from affluence, changing values, and increased leisure time.

This overall societal change produced low fertility: by 1970 those under 20 years of age had decreased to 40 percent of the population, those over 65 had increased to 8 percent. Consequently, the diseases of an older age group began to plague the country. With increases in chronic diseases and in the overall mortality level, 51 percent of all deaths were among those 65 and older. In 1970, as well as in 1980, the big three—heart disease, cancer, and stroke—accounted for more than 60 percent of all deaths.

With this shift, epidemiologists started to study not only infectious diseases but also chronic ones. As a result most textbooks now define epidemiology as the study of the distribution and determinants of diseases in human populations.

EPIDEMIOLOGY OF HEALTH

The evolution of health care in the 1970s produced some interesting ideas. For instance, the traditional concerns of legislation—cost containment, accessibility, availability, quality, continuity, and acceptability—gained increased emphasis in the pursuit of health. The more significant aspects of health care of the 1970s that continued into the 1980s and could be expected in the 1990s are the concerns with

Figure 1-8 Cycle of Disease Patterns, Infectious Disease Model (1900)

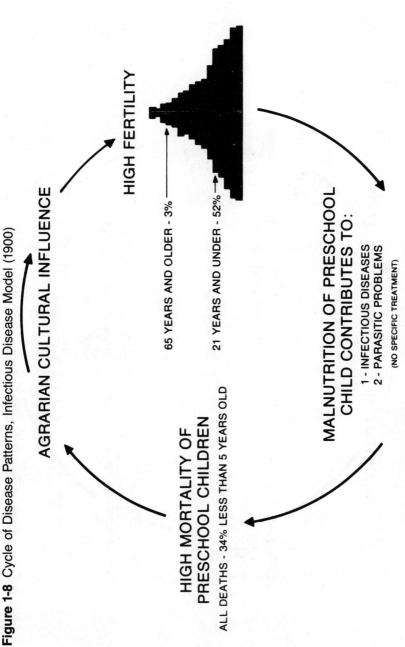

AGRARIAN CULTURAL INFLUENCE

HIGH FERTILITY

65 YEARS AND OLDER - 3%

21 YEARS AND UNDER - 52%

MALNUTRITION OF PRESCHOOL
CHILD CONTRIBUTES TO:

1 - INFECTIOUS DISEASES
2 - PARASITIC PROBLEMS

(NO SPECIFIC TREATMENT)

HIGH MORTALITY OF
PRESCHOOL CHILDREN

ALL DEATHS - 34% LESS THAN 5 YEARS OLD

Source: Reprinted from "The Pursuit of Health" by G.E. Alan Dever with permission of *Social Indicators Research 4*, ©1977, 485.

Figure 1-9 Cycle of Disease Patterns, Chronic Disease Model (1970)

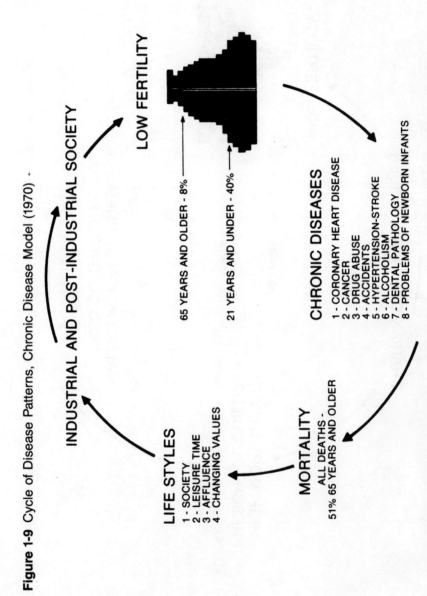

INDUSTRIAL AND POST-INDUSTRIAL SOCIETY

LOW FERTILITY

65 YEARS AND OLDER - 8%

21 YEARS AND UNDER - 40%

CHRONIC DISEASES

1 - CORONARY HEART DISEASE
2 - CANCER
3 - DRUG ABUSE
4 - ACCIDENTS
5 - HYPERTENSION-STROKE
6 - ALCOHOLISM
7 - DENTAL PATHOLOGY
8 - PROBLEMS OF NEWBORN INFANTS

LIFE STYLES

1 - SOCIETY
2 - LEISURE TIME
3 - AFFLUENCE
4 - CHANGING VALUES

MORTALITY

ALL DEATHS -
51% 65 YEARS AND OLDER

Source: Reprinted from "The Pursuit of Health" by G.E. Alan Dever with permission of *Social Indicators Research 4,* ©1977, 486.

holism, wellness, and self-responsibility. These facets of being healthy reflect personal awareness of self-actualization in physical activity, nutrition, stress management, and overall individual life styling.

The result was the development of holistic health centers, wellness resource centers, health spas and resorts, and a more aware population concerned about its physical and mental condition. Jogging, tennis, basketball, bicycling, vitamins, health foods, and coping skills became part of the public's needs. The emphasis obviously is not on illness but on health and wellness, extending even to a plateau of high-level wellness.

This is what community health care is and what it is expected to be in the decades ahead. Indeed, the task is to create the space where people may be transformed so that wellness becomes a typical part of their lives. This is a major area in which institutions can become involved and can promote their health services in disease prevention. Institutions can have an impact on and serve the population utilizing a prevention-oriented approach.

Redefinitions of epidemiology reflect this change of focus from disease to health: "Epidemiology is now concerned with health and all illness in population groups and with the factors—including health services—which affect them"[12] and "the science concerned with the occurrence, distribution, and determinants which affect them."[13]

The distinctive characteristic of epidemiology is that it is concerned with health in populations and groups, while clinical disciplines are concerned with ill health in individuals. Epidemiology always has been a method of analysis for community health. Because of this, epidemiology may be defined as "the provision of preventive and curative services using modern epidemiologic technics in assessing health needs of population groups, the setting of priorities, and the assessment of results achieved."[14] Similarly, it is proposed here that epidemiology be used as a basic method in the management of health services.

AIMS, TYPES, AND METHODS OF EPIDEMIOLOGY

Aims

Epidemiology has three main aims:

1. to study the occurrence, distribution, and progression of disease problems and, more generally, to describe the health status of human populations so as to provide a basis for the planning, evaluation, and management of health promoting and restoring systems
2. to provide data that will contribute to the understanding of the etiology of health and disease
3. to promote the utilization of the epidemiological concepts to the management of health services.

Exhibit 1-4 illustrates the three main aims of epidemiology in relation to their associated type of strategies and methods. Traditionally, Aims 1 and 2 foster the general principle of epidemiological investigation. However, Aim 3 shows that the descriptive, analytical, and experimental types have application to managing health services. These applications range from service area disease-specific studies to determine market penetration to utilizing market analysis (marketing) and demographic trends to promote health education and disease prevention.

This new approach is a must for health service managers in an era of growing interest in self-care and reduced reliance on institutional care. They must use these

Exhibit 1-4 Aims, Types, and Methods of Epidemiologic Investigations

Aims	Types	Methods
1. To study the occurrence, distribution, size, and progression of health and disease in human populations	Descriptive	Analysis of morbidity and mortality data, collected either • routinely or • by special studies
2. To provide data that will contribute to the understanding of the etiology of health and disease	Descriptive	Same as above; such descriptive analyses help formulate hypotheses on the etiology of health and disease
	Analytic	Retrospective/case-control studies Prospective/cohort studies Cross-sectional/survey/longitudinal studies
	Experimental	Clinical/controlled studies
3. To promote the utilization of the epidemiological concepts to the management of health services	Descriptive	Description of morbidity and mortality data: by service area, by diagnosis-related groups (DRGs)
	Analytic	Determination of patient flow by disease category (DRGs); determination of disease-specific rates; market penetration and market segmentation (age-specific rates)
	Experimental	Identification of potential new health markets, of research areas for expansion, and of demographic trends

techniques to identify new markets and to know what type of services to expand. For instance, the pharmacy at the institution not only could dispense the traditional drugs but also expand to include vitamins, minerals, and other health promotion items. The hospital also could provide antigravity rooms, weight-lifting rooms, and jogging or walking tracks in the halls. There is an unlimited potential for institutions in this new era of health promotion.

Types and Methods

The three types of epidemiological strategies involve a variety of associated methods:

1. Descriptive epidemiology is concerned with the occurrence, distribution, size, and progression of health and disease in the population.
2. Analytic epidemiology may involve three main types of studies: retrospective, prospective, and cross-sectional. In a retrospective or case-control study, the epidemiologist collects data back in time (retrospectively) from two comparable groups of individuals, one with a specific disease or condition and one without, to identify any history or exposure to one or more factors of interest (precursor characteristics). A prospective, cohort, or longitudinal study involves the opposite process. It starts with a group of people (a cohort) characterized by some factor of interest (precursor characteristic) and follows them forward (prospectively) in time (longitudinally) to determine the incidence (i.e., observe the subsequent development) of some disease or condition. A cross-sectional or prevalence study involves the collection of data from a defined specific population at one time.
3. Experimental epidemiology also is concerned with testing etiological factors, but it involves manipulation (or control) of them as well as the controlled (usually random) assignment of individuals to experimental and control groups. It consists of the evaluation of the effects of introducing, eliminating, or otherwise modifying the hypothesized (suspected) factors on the occurrence or progression of some state of health or disease. Such experiments usually are referred to as "clinical" or "controlled" trials and are used mostly in the evaluation of new treatments, drugs, or services.

THE CONCEPT OF CAUSALITY IN EPIDEMIOLOGY

Epidemiology is concerned with finding associations between states of health and disease and factors associated with them in a population. Association refers to the relationship that may exist between the occurrence of one thing and of another. Three possible relationships between these two things are:

1. a positive association (tending to occur together)
2. a negative association (tending not to occur together)
3. no association (occurring independently).

A positive association could be either wrong or right. It could be wrong by chance or by some kind of error (bias). If it is right, it could be a causal relationship, in which one causes the other; or it could be noncausal (associative), in which something else causes them both.

Over the past 100 years, three generalized causal models have directed epidemiological studies. The models are related intrinsically related to the concepts of health, of health measurement, and certainly of the shift in disease patterns.

3 CAUSAL MODELS

Single Cause/Single Effect Model

The first and simplest epidemiologic causal model is the single cause/single effect pattern (Figure 1-10). A single cause is sufficient to produce an observed effect. This model is quite logical but operates only rarely. Epidemiologists used this approach in the late 1800s and early 1900s when infectious diseases were predominant and a single bacterium or virus was sufficient to produce disease.

Multiple Cause/Single Effect Model

A second, more complex model is the multiple cause/single effect pattern (Figure 1-11). An obvious extension of the single cause/single effect model, this approach is valid where disease patterns are in a transitory state—in communities or areas where infectious diseases are declining and chronic diseases are increasing. Thus, such chronic patterns as heart disease, cancer, stroke, and motor vehicle accidents may be analyzed using the multiple cause/single effect model. It also may be used with some infectious illnesses such as Legionnaire's disease.

Multiple Cause/Multiple Effect Model

The third model of causality, multiple cause/multiple effect, is extremely complex, indicating that several causes produce many observed effects (Figure

---

Figure 1-10 Single Cause/Single Effect Model

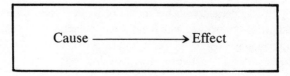

Cause ──────────→ Effect

Figure 1-11 Multiple Cause/Single Effect Model

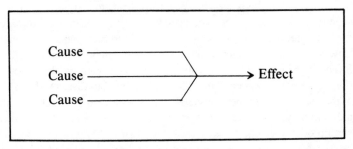

1-12). This model closely embraces the health concepts of holism and wellness and is quite applicable to the disease patterns of the 1980s. For instance, air pollution, smoking, and specific forms of radiation (causes) may produce lung cancer, emphysema, and bronchitis (effects).

Traditional Criteria for Determining Causality

With the acceptance of the germ theory in the 19th century, epidemiologists were concerned mainly with determining which diseases were caused by which germs, using a single cause/single effect causal model.

Robert Koch, the noted German bacteriologist and physician (1843-1910), in Koch's Postulates developed some simple rules to determine causality: "First, the organism is always found with the disease . . . , second, the organism is not found with any other disease . . . ; the 'regular' and 'exclusive' presence of the organism proves a causal relationship."[15] Thus, the germ had to be a necessary and sufficient cause of the particular disease. The illness could not happen without the germ, and its presence was all that was necessary for getting the disease.

Most epidemiology textbooks now use five basic criteria to determine causative associative relationships:

Figure 1-12 Multiple Cause/Multiple Effect Model

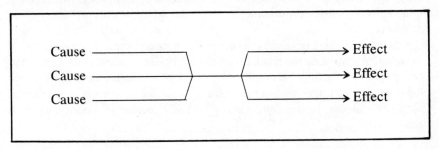

CAUSATIVE ASSOCIATION CRITERIA?

1. Temporal relationship: If A causes B, logically A should occur first.
2. Specificity: With high specificity, a cause leads to a single effect; with low specificity, a cause may be associated with multiple effects. In the latter case, for example, cigarette smoking can cause both lung cancer and bronchitis. Low socioeconomic status can be associated with both illness and disability.
3. Strength or intensity: This involves the association or the degree of correlation between the cause and the effect. For infectious diseases the association of the pathogen with the illness process usually is high. For chronic diseases the association is a statistical or probabilistic association, allowing for a certain degree of uncertainty, as in the relationship of exercise and diet to lower rates of coronary heart disease. The three causal models are not quite logical in dealing with this problem, requiring statistical probability tests and broader concepts of health.
4. Consistency: When the same type of association consistently turns up in research studies of different designs, the chances are that it is real and likely to be causative.
5. Coherence: A supposed causal relationship should make sense in the light of existing biological facts. Contrary evidence suggests, however, that this point should not be heavily weighted, especially in the case of sugar consumption related to such conditions as cancer and hypoglycemia.

Expanded Concept of Causality: Risk

Those five judgmental criteria are applicable and effective in the single cause/ single effect model. Chronic disease epidemiology and the holistic approach, however, correspond much more often to the other models, mainly to the multiple cause/multiple effect one. For this reason, epidemiologists often use an expanded and less rigorous concept of causality based on the odds (risks, chances) of the occurrence of one thing (a state of health or disease) associated with (following) the occurrence of another (a risk factor).

Under this expanded concept of causality, drinking alcohol can lead to automobile accidents although it is neither necessary nor sufficient as a cause. However it tremendously increases the odds of having an accident and therefore is a risk factor. In the multiple cause/multiple effect model of epidemiologic investigation of noninfectious diseases, drinking is one of the definitive causes of automobile accidents.

Similarly, smoking no doubt is a cause of lung cancer, without being necessary or sufficient. Everyone has heard of individuals having smoked all their lives and being "perfectly healthy" at age 90. All that can be said is that those persons beat the odds. The fact remains that the probability—or the proportion of time in the long run—of developing lung cancer is much greater in smokers than in nonsmokers.

In chronic disease epidemiology, most causal factors are similar to smoking: without being either necessary or sufficient, by themselves, they are contributory within a multiple cause/multiple effect model. As Austin and Werner put it so succinctly:

1. When, if you have "it" and the "disease" is *more* likely to occur, and
2. When you take "it" away, the "disease" is *less* likely to occur, then
3. "It" is considered a cause of the disease.[16]

SUMMARY

The application of epidemiology to health services management is a relatively new approach to the effective and efficient delivery of care. This chapter provides the focus and direction for that link between epidemiology and health services management. The concepts of disease prevention and health promotion as they are linked to the new framework suggests ways of improving individuals' physical and mental status and expanding the use of services. Institutions may create new dimensions to their delivery of services to reflect the challenge of health promotion and prevention. It is suggested that the concept of improving health status be changed from a disease-oriented perspective to a health-oriented perspective.

Of particular importance among the methods of epidemiology is the expanded concept of risk in relationship to disease. This introductory chapter sets the stage for the theme of this book: the application of health promotion and disease prevention techniques, as viewed by epidemiology, to the management of health services.

The dimensions of health—life style, environment, biology, and the delivery system of care—and their application to the management of services must be considered if the health status of population and patients is to continue to improve.

NOTES

1. U.S. Department of Health and Human Services, *Healthy People: the Surgeon General's Report on Health Promotion and Disease Prevention* (Washington, D.C.: U.S. Government Printing Office, 1979).

2. Henrik L. Blum, "Does Health Planning Work Anywhere, and If So, Why?" *American Journal of Health Planning*, 3, no. 3 (July 1978): 44.

3. Sidney L. Kark, *Epidemiology and Community Medicine* (New York: Appleton-Century-Crofts, Inc., 1974), 325.

4. H.R. Leavell and E.G. Clark, *Preventive Medicine for the Doctor in His Community* (New York: McGraw-Hill Book Company, 1965), 684.

5. H.L. Laframboise, "Health Policy: Breaking the Problem Down in More Manageable Segments," *Canadian Medical Association Journal*, 108 (February 3, 1973), 388-393.

6. Marc Lalonde, *A New Perspective on the Health of Canadians* (Ottawa: Office of the Canadian Minister of National Health and Welfare, 1974).

7. G.E. Alan Dever, *Community Health Analysis* (Rockville, Md.: Aspen Systems Corporation, 1980), Chap. 10.

8. L. White Kerr, "Contemporary Epidemiology," *International Journal of Epidemiology* 3, no. 4 (1974): 295-96.

9. U.S. Department of Health and Human Services, *Health, United States, 1980*, Annex: "Prevention Profile" (Washington, D.C.: U.S. Government Printing Office, 1980), 268-69.

10. G.E. Alan Dever, *Passages: Predictable Mortality through the Life Stages* (Atlanta: Georgia Department of Health and Human Resources, Division of Public Health, Health Services Analysis, Inc., September 1980), 299.

11. Aaron Wildavsky, "Can Health Be Planned?" (Lecture delivered at the University of Chicago, April 23, 1976).

12. Roy M. Acheson, "Epidemiology—Uses and Method," in *A Handbook of Community Medicine* ed. A.M. Nelson (Bristol, England: John Wright and Sons, 1975), 21.

13. J.H. Abramson, "Letters to the Editor," *American Journal of Epidemiology* 109, no. 1 (1979): 100.

14. W. Latham, "Community Medicine: Success or Failure?" *The New England Journal of Medicine* 295 (1976): 18-23.

15. Robert Koch, Ueber bakteriologische Forschug. Verbandlungen des x. Internationalen Medicinischen Congresses Berlin, 4-9 August 1890. 35-47 (Berlin: Hirschwald), quoted in M. Susser, *Causal Thinking in the Health Sciences: Concepts and Strategies in Epidemiology* (New York: Oxford University Press, 1973), 22-23.

16. D.F. Austin and S.B. Werner, *Epidemiology for the Health Sciences* (Springfield, Ill.: Charles C Thomas, Publisher, 1974), 43.

Chapter 2

Epidemiology and Health Policy

HEALTH POLICY PLANNING

Before the use of epidemiology in the management of health services is examined, it is necessary to take a more macroscopic view of its contributions to the health care system and its role in health policy.

Policy planning is a process aimed at attaining deliberate or intended social change.[1] It deals with society's value structure, or what society considers to be important. Planning at this level is normative, idealistic, or future creative, dealing with what ought to be. It is defined by Hyman as goal-oriented planning or new-system creating.[2] Emphasis is placed both on desired ends and on the means of achieving them. Bailey defines a policy analysis model as involving ". . . a careful, logical analysis of a complex of different problems at the policy level . . . for the purpose of making all assumptions more explicit, recognizing constraints more clearly, drawing conclusions from the assumptions in a more reliable manner, and so on."[3]

Several models may be used, including the following:

- Technical models, aimed at providing scientific understanding of behavior, for example, the population dynamics of diseases, and at forecasting possible outcomes of intervention with goals of optimum health. Demographic and manpower models fall in this category.
- Systems models, dealing with interactions among technical models.
- Information system models, dealing with the flow of information for decision making.[4]

Health policy planning consists primarily in developing medium- and long-term goals and criteria.[5] Health policy is determined by many factors: political, historical, cultural, economic, scientific, and technological, as well as epidemiological.[6]

As noted in Chapter 1, epidemiology has three main aims: to study the occurrence, distribution, size, and progression of health and disease in human populations; to contribute to the comprehension of the etiology of health and disease; and to promote the utilization of epidemiological concepts in the management of health services. These aims relate to and, in fact, become intertwined in the pursuit of health policy's ultimate goal: the promotion and preservation of the population's health.

As also was discussed, disease patterns switched over time from infectious to noninfectious chronic ailments. The greatest potential for the promotion and preservation of the public's health still lies in prevention. As it had for infectious diseases, epidemiology contributes most importantly to understanding the causes and means of preventing noninfectious ailments.

Ford describes three stages in the control of a disease: the popular, the scientific, and the application phases.[7] The popular phase consists of the gathering of knowledge "from its early roots in folk wisdom and common-sense observation." The scientific phase is the transformation of this common-sense knowledge into scientific understanding. The application phase translates this scientific understanding into effective prevention.

Descriptive epidemiology parallels the popular phase while analytic and experimental (as well as descriptive) epidemiology contributes to the scientific understanding of disease. In the application phase, the epidemiological data are translated into meaningful and natural public policy decisions. This is what Gordis calls the "societal responsibility" of epidemiologists,[8] and this is where they are in the handling of most leading causes of death. Epidemiological research already has identified the major risk factors in heart diseases, in most cancers, in cerebrovascular diseases, and in most other leading causes of death.[9] This knowledge, however, has yet to be translated fully into health policy.

The fact that health policy is determined by many factors other than epidemiology partially explains the nonapplication of epidemiological knowledge. In addition, as Ford points out, the major decision makers of health policy (namely, average citizens, physicians, health care managers, and public health experts) have different and distinct points of view on health and illness.[10]

Epidemiology and public health involve knowledge and consideration of both a numerator (number of cases, deaths, services, and so forth) and a denominator (the general population from which the numerator is taken). Average citizens are aware that they are part of the denominator but have only limited knowledge of the numerator or the extent of the populace.

In contrast, physicians are centered on, and value, the individual patient-doctor relationship. Physicians know quite a bit about the numerator but little about the denominator. Finally, health care managers usually are very much aware of the general population but too often in economic terms rather than by concern for unmet needs, prevention of illness, and health maintenance and promotion.

There are no easy pathways to society's goal of health for all. However, the widespread adoption of the epidemiological perspective may facilitate a reduction in the impact of the major cripplers and killers. Gordis writes: "In the last analysis, these [policy] decisions are societal and as active and concerned members of society, each of us should be a participant in this process and should not abdicate this community responsibility."[11]

The epidemiologist-public health expert should become more vocal and more involved in policy making. As many authors advocate, physician training should incorporate a widened epidemiological perspective in considering patients' health.[12, 13, 14, 15] The average citizen also must become involved through greater awareness of the determinants of health and illness and through increased participation in the formulation of policy.

Health care management should become population based. Health organizations must be aware of the needs and problems of the population they are serving. They also must get involved in the maintenance and promotion of the public's health.

EPIDEMIOLOGICAL MODELS FOR HEALTH POLICY

If epidemiology is used as a guide, health policy then will be based on the primacy of prevention.[16] Health policy should lead to the development of programs to prevent the major causes of death and disability. The following chapters explain how this is done through strategic and operational planning. An overall comprehension or framework of health, inherently prevention oriented, is a prerequisite, however, for the development of such preventive action. Three models reflect health and illness in such a way and promote an epidemiological approach to health policymaking: the health field concept, Rutstein's sentinel health events, and the Canadian health protection packages.

The Health Field Concept

Chapter 1 indicated how the traditional model of disease causation (agent-host-environment) was inadequate for the epidemiological analysis of today's noninfectious diseases. To replace it, the "health field" concept model was developed. This is broader, more comprehensive, and fits much better with a multiple cause/multiple effect view of health and disease and certainly to the expanded concepts of risk.

Although this conceptualization of health in four primary divisions (life style, environment, human biology, and system of health care organization) was proposed initially as a disease-causation model,[17] it became popular when applied to health policy in Canada.[18, 19] This epidemiological model provides a more balanced approach to the development of health policy when compared with the limiting, traditional divisions of prevention, diagnosis, therapy, and rehabilitation, or with public health, mental health, and clinical medicine.[20] Figures 1-2, 1-3, and 1-4 (in Chapter 1) show the primary divisions of this epidemiological model for health policy analysis.

Life Style

Life styles or, more accurately, self-created risks, may be divided into three elements: leisure activity risks, consumption patterns, and employment participation and occupational risks. This division of the epidemiological model involves the aggregation of decisions by individuals affecting their health and over which they have more or less control.[21] Bad or incorrect decisions result in destructive modes of health that contribute to an increased level of illness or premature death.

Leisure Activity Risks: Some self-imposed destructive modes are the result of leisure activity risks. For instance, lack of recreation is strongly associated with hypertension and coronary heart disease. Lack of exercise aggravates coronary heart disease, leads to obesity, and results in a total lack of physical fitness.

Consumption Patterns: Another kind of self-imposed risk involves consumption patterns. These include:

- overeating, leading to obesity and subsequent consequences
- cholesterol intake, contributing to heart disease
- alcohol addiction, leading to cirrhosis of the liver
- alcohol consumption, leading to motor vehicle accidents
- cigarette smoking, causing chronic obstructive pulmonary disease (chronic bronchitis, emphysema), lung cancer, and aggravating heart disease
- drug dependency and social drug use, leading to suicide, homicide, malnutrition, accidents, social withdrawal, and acute anxiety attacks
- abundant glucose (sugar) intake, contributing to dental caries, obesity, and hyperglycemia with its concomitant problems.

Employment/Occupational Risks: Destructive life styles resulting from employment participation and occupational risks are equally significant but far more difficult to identify. Work pressures lead to stresses, anxieties, and tensions that, in turn, may cause peptic ulcers and hypertension. Other habits (admittedly difficult to categorize) such as careless driving, lead to accidents, while sexual promiscuity can result in syphilis or gonorrhea.[22]

Environment

The environment in the epidemiological model is defined as events external to the body over which the individual has little or no control. This element may be subdivided into physical, social, and psychological dimensions.[23]

The Physical Dimension: In a physical environment, certain hazards show a close relationship to the use of energy (oil) by an expanding population. Per capita energy consumption is increasing concomitantly with the population and the standard of living. Thus, health hazards stemming from air, noise, and water pollution almost assuredly will also increase steadily. The resulting diseases and problems include hearing loss, infectious diseases, gastroenteritis, cancer, emphysema, and bronchitis. In limited cases, ionizing and ultraviolet radiation have health implications in terms of skin cancer and genetic mutation.[24]

The Social and Psychological Dimensions: These divisions of environmental health encompass major factors involving behavior modification, perceptional problems, and interpersonal relationships. For example, crowding, isolation, rapid and accelerated rates of change, and social interchange may contribute to homicide, suicide, decisional stress, and environmental overstimulation.[25, 26]

These environmental conditions create risks that are a far greater threat to health than any present inadequacy of the system of medical care organization.[27] The resulting health problems will be resolved only by imposing standards and controls on the responsible agencies and industries.

It is interesting to note that before the emergence of the germ theory of disease, the environmental determinant of health long had been considered the most important. Hippocrates discusses the influence of environmental factors and living conditions at the onset of illness in a book that may well have been the first epidemiological or, for that matter, medical treatise: *On Airs, Waters, and Places*.[28] More specifically, Hippocrates talks of the effects on health of the seasons, of the "warm and cold winds," of the water, and of the soil.

Human Biology

This element, focusing on the human body, is concerned with humans' basic biologic and organic makeup as individuals. Thus, a person's genetic inheritance creates genetic disorders, congenital malformations, and mental retardation. The maturation and aging process is a contributing factor in arthritis, diabetes, atherosclerosis, and cancer. Obvious disorders of the skeletal, muscular, cardiovascular, endocrine, and digestive systems are subcomponents of complex internal systems.

Disease categories involving human biology must be weighted in accordance with the other divisions of the epidemiological model. Genetic counseling of parents whose children may have Tay-Sachs disease is a step in the right direction.

If the problems resulting from the human biology of man can be overcome, it should be possible to save many lives, decrease misery, and reduce the cost of treatment services. This is an obligation to humanity.

System of Medical Care Organization

The final division of the epidemiological model is the system of medical care organization. This may be subdivided into three elements: curative, restorative, and preventive. The system itself consists of the availability, quality, and quantity of resources to provide health care. Its restorative elements include hospital, nursing home, and ambulance services. Its curative elements involve medical drugs, dental treatments, and medical professionals. The system has very limited preventive elements.

Efforts and expenditures to improve health in the United States have been directed almost totally toward the system of medical care organization. Yet the morbidity and mortality disease patterns of today are deeply entrenched in the three other divisions of the epidemiological model. The huge sums spent for restoring and curing could be used far more effectively if they could be earmarked for prevention of disease. Rather than concentrate on the failures of the system of medical care organization, it would be more advantageous to promote the positive points of the three other divisions—life style, environment, and human biology.

Advantages of the Model

The combination of the four divisions—system of medical care organization, life style, environment, and human biology—into an epidemiological model for health policy analysis has many advantages. Lalonde cites these:

1. This model raises Life Style, Environment, and Human Biology to a level of categorical importance equal to that of the System of Medical Care Organization.

2. The model is comprehensive. Any health problem can be traced to one or a combination of the four divisions.

3. The model allows a system of analysis by which a disease or pattern may be examined under the four divisions in order to assess relative significance and interaction (i.e., what percentage or proportion of Life Style, Environment, Human Biology, and System of Medical Care Organization contributes to suicide?).

4. This model permits further subdivision of the four major factors: for example, Environment is subdivided into physical, social, and psychological.

5. This model provides a new perspective on health that creates a recognition and exploration of previously neglected fields.[29]

Applications of the Model to Health Policy

The application of this model involves four steps:

1. the selection of diseases that are of high risk and that contribute substantially to overall mortality and morbidity

2. the proportionate allocation of the contributing factors of the disease to the four elements of the epidemiological model

3. the proportionate allocation of total health expenditures to the four elements of the epidemiological model

4. the determination of the difference in proportions between (2) and (3).

This is essentially what the Canadian government did, as a basis for its federal health policy, as Lalonde writes in *A New Perspective on the Health of Canadians.* For illustration, the use of the model in studying disease patterns in Georgia and in the United States can be examined. The application to Georgia is the result of a previous study by the author.

The top 13 causes of mortality were selected for analysis (Step 1). Table 2-1 shows the percentage distribution of deaths by age group and cause. Heart disease, cancer, and stroke ranked first, second, and third, respectively, with high-risk groups concentrated in ages over 55. Deaths resulting from automobile and other accidents were concentrated in the 15-to-34 age group. Two other causes, homicide and suicide, showed concentrations of high risk in the 15-34 and the 35-54 groups, respectively. Thus, the major cripplers and killers of Georgians were represented in multiple age groups in terms of high risk and in multiple etiologies in terms of determining preventive measures for the diseases.

As Step 2, the contributing factors of each cause were allocated proportionately to the four components of the epidemiological model. Table 2-2 shows that the major contributing factors are strongly rooted in life style, environment, and human biology. It also indicates that the system of medical care organization has limited impact with respect to disease prevention.

Table 2-1 Deaths by Age Group for Selected Causes

Georgia 1973

Cause of Mortality	Total, All Causes	% of Total Deaths	Percentage Distribution by Age Group									
			Under One	1-4	5-14	15-24	25-34	35-44	45-54	55-64	65-74	75+
TOTAL, ALL AGES	43,910	100.0	3.7	0.8	1.1	3.2	3.4	5.1	10.6	18.4	22.2	30.5
Diseases of the heart	14,922	34.0	0.1	0.1	0.1	0.2	0.7	2.8	9.6	20.3	28.2	37.8
Cancer	6,532	14.9	0.1	0.4	0.8	1.0	1.6	4.6	14.5	26.8	28.1	22.2
Cerebrovascular	5,897	13.4	0.0	0.1	0.1	0.4	0.8	2.3	6.2	14.1	25.9	50.1
Motor vehicle accidents	1,847	4.2	0.9	3.4	8.0	28.2	17.5	11.9	10.4	9.4	6.7	3.7
All other accidents	1,657	3.8	4.6	5.3	7.5	14.5	12.6	10.6	12.3	11.5	8.6	12.6
Influenza and pneumonia	1,648	3.8	11.6	2.2	0.8	1.6	2.1	4.7	8.4	11.4	18.9	38.2
Diseases of the respiratory system	1,179	2.7	2.4	0.9	0.6	0.8	2.0	2.6	9.4	22.6	30.4	28.2
Diseases of the arteries, veins, and capillaries	1,120	2.6	0.2	0	0.1	0.1	0.2	2.1	4.3	12.2	23.7	57.1
Homicides	985	2.2	0.5	0.7	1.3	22.8	26.9	21.2	13.0	9.2	2.9	1.3
Birth injuries and other diseases of early infancy	834	1.9	99.8	0.2	0	0	0	0	0	0	0	0
Diabetes mellitus	772	1.8	0	0	0.1	0.5	1.9	3.5	11.0	22.0	34.5	26.4
Suicides	630	1.4	—	—	0.8	15.6	17.0	19.0	22.1	14.4	7.8	3.3
Congenital anomalies	351	0.8	66.4	10.0	6.3	4.0	3.1	3.4	1.4	2.3	2.3	0.9

Source: Reprinted from "An Epidemiological Model for Health Policy Analysis" by G.E. Alan Dever with permission of *Social Indicators Research,* © 1976, 2, 460–461.

Table 2-2 An Epidemiological Model for Health Policy Evaluation

Georgia 1973

Percent Distribution of Total Deaths*	Cause of Mortality	Percentage Allocation of Mortality to the Epidemiological Model**			
		System of Medical Care Organization	Life Style	Environment	Human Biology
34.0	Diseases of the heart	12	54	9	28
14.9	Cancer	10	37	24	29
13.4	Cerebrovascular	7	50	22	21
4.2	Motor vehicle accidents	12	69	18	1
3.8	All other accidents	14	51	31	4
3.8	Influenza and pneumonia	18	23	20	39
2.7	Diseases of the respiratory system	13	40	24	24
2.6	Diseases of the arteries, veins, and capillaries	18	49	8	26
2.2	Homicides	—	66	30	5
1.9	Birth injuries and other diseases of early infancy	27	30	15	28
1.8	Diabetes mellitus	6	26	—	68
1.4	Suicides	3	60	35	2
0.8	Congenital anomalies	6	9	6	79
	Percent Allocation: Average	11	43	19	27

*1973.
**Because of rounding, may not add to 100 percent.

Source: Reprinted from "An Epidemiological Model for Health Policy Analysis" by G.E. Alan Dever with permission of *Social Indicators Research,* © 1976, *2,* 462.

In Table 2-2, the allocations to the four categories were achieved by polling 40 professionals and paraprofessionals to determine what factors of life style, environment, human biology, and system of health care organization they felt contributed to each cause of mortality listed. The 40 responses were then summed and averaged to determine the potential impact of the four factors on each cause. It is recommended that any agency using this model form a similar group of professionals for this task. Although the analysis in Table 2-2 is subjective and, in most instances, judgmental, it does agree with a majority of the medical literature.[30, 31, 32]

Step 2, then, allows programmatic areas dealing with specific mortality causes to set priorities and to decide upon health policy. This type of analysis may reveal gaps in the delivery of health services. A reduction of mortality will occur only if the health program is proportionately directed toward each element of the epidemiological model.

A total of $29.2 billion was spent for health by the federal government in 1974.[33] This amount was estimated to increase to $35.0 billion and $37.7 billion for 1975 and 1976, respectively. Table 2-3 shows the distribution of federal outlays for health activities by category. In that form, the table provides little information in terms of the proposed epidemiological model for health policy analysis. Therefore, Table 2-4 was prepared to correspond to the four elements of the epidemiological model (Step 3). Over the three years, the majority of federal expenditures—an average of 90.6 percent—was allocated to the system of medical care organization (Table 2-5). The elements of human biology, environment, and life style accounted for an average of 6.9 percent, 1.5 percent, and 1.2 percent, respectively.

Table 2-3 Federal Outlays for Medical and Health-Related Activities

(in millions of dollars)

Health Programs	Outlays		
	1974 Actual	1975 Estimate	1976 Estimate
Development of health resources, total	$ 4,383	$ 5,242	$ 5,362
Health research	2,085	2,424	2,512
Training and education	1,146	1,324	1,145
Construction	761	967	1,108
Improving organization and delivery	392	527	596
Provision of hospital and medical services, total	23,918	28,783	31,348
Direct federal services	4,797	5,390	5,828
Indirect services	19,120	23,393	25,520
Prevention and control of health problems, total	888	1,019	989
Disease prevention and control	419	458	405
Environmental control	90	129	137
Consumer protection	378	432	446
Total: Health Programs	29,189	35,044	37,699

Note: Fiscal data were not available at the time of this study for Georgia so U.S. figures are used.

Source: Adapted from Office of Management and Budget, *Budget of the United States Government, Federal Health Programs, Special Analysis K,* 1976, p. 169.

Table 2-4 Allocation of Federal Expenditures under Epidemiological Model for Health Policy Analysis

1974, 1975, and 1976

Elements of the Epidemiological Model for Health Policy Analysis	Federal Outlay (in millions)		
	1974 Actual	1975 Estimate	1976 Estimate
Total federal health expenditures	$29,189	$35,044	$37,699
Systems of medical care organization	26,216	31,601	34,197
Training and education	1,146	1,324	1,145
Construction of health care facilities	761	967	1,108
Improving organization and delivery	392	527	596
Provision of hospital and medical services	23,918	28,783	31,348
Direct federal services	4,797	5,390	5,828
Indirect services	19,120	23,383	25,520
Percent of total federal health expenditures	89.8%	90.1%	90.7%
Life style	420	458	405
Disease prevention and control	420	458	405
Percent of total federal health expenditures	1.4%	1.3%	1.1%
Environment	468	561	583
Environmental control	90	129	137
Consumer safety	378	432	446
Percent of total federal health expenditures	1.6%	1.6%	1.5%
Human biology	2,085	2,424	2,512
Health research	2,085	2,424	2,512
Percent of total federal health expenditures	7.1%	6.9%	6.7%

Source: Reprinted from "An Epidemiological Model for Health Care Analysis" by G.E. Alan Dever with permission of *Social Indicators Research 2,* © 1976, 454.

Finally (Step 4), Table 2-5 compares Tables 2-2 and 2-4. It shows a vastly disproportionate amount of money allocated for the system of medical care organization, despite the fact that the means for reducing mortality and morbidity are rooted deeply in life style, environment, and human biology elements and that only minimal reductions in mortality and morbidity can be expected from the system.

A refreshing and creative use of the epidemiological model for health policy analysis has been outlined by the Centers for Disease Control.[34] Building on

Table 2-5 Comparison of Federal Expenditures to Allocation of Mortality under Epidemiological Model for Health Policy Analysis

Epidemiological Model for Health Policy Analysis	Federal Health Expenditures 1974–1976 (%)	Allocation of Mortality to the Epidemiological Model (%)
System of medical care organization	90.6	11
Life style	1.2	43
Environment	1.5	19
Human biology	6.9	27
Total	100.2*	100

*Because of rounding, does not add to 100.0 percent.

Source: Reprinted from "An Epidemiological Model for Health Policy Analysis" by G.E. Alan Dever with permission of *Social Indicators Research 2*, © 1976, 465.

Dever's model design, the center analyzed the top ten causes of death by race and sex in terms of years of potential life lost (before age 75 and before age 65) and of total mortality of one-plus years of age. It used the data in Table 2-2 as the basis for the proportional allocation of the contributing factors of premature mortality to the four elements of the epidemiological model.

The results for the ten leading causes of death among the total population of one-plus years of age, ranked by number of years of life lost before age 65 (United States, 1975), are given in Table 2-6. Figure 2-1 presents that table's data graphically, showing differences when total mortality (one-plus years of age) and years of life lost (before age 75) are used as different points of departure. For the years of life lost before age 65, it is evident that life style and environment (53.1 percent and 21.7 percent, respectively) are significant factors contributing to premature mortality for the total United States population (Table 2-6). In contrast, the contributions from human biology and the medical care system are substantially lower.

Both of these applications seem to point to a conclusion that should affect health policy profoundly. Unless health policy is shifted dramatically from current procedures for reducing mortality and morbidity, there will be little or no change in disease patterns. In fact, with the population aging there well might be major increases in mortality and morbidity.

It is clear that present policies do not support methods most likely to improve health status. If, however, the epidemiological model is applied to health status

Table 2-6 Allocation of Premature Mortality Factors to the
Epidemiological Model

United States, 1975

Ten Leading Causes of Death	Years of Life < 65 Lost	%	Health System*	Life Style*	Environ- ment*	Human Biology*
Cancer	1,802,820	17.5	10	37	24	29
Heart disease	1,769,180	17.2	12	54	9	28
Motor vehicle accidents	1,424,823	13.8	12	69	18	1
All other accidents	1,166,793	11.3	14	51	31	4
Homicide	621,846	6.0	0	66	30	5
Suicide	583,751	5.7	3	60	35	2
Cerebrovascular disease	352,524	3.4	7	50	22	21
Cirrhosis of the liver	320,457	3.1	3	70	9	18
Influenza and pneumonia	206,673	2.0	18	23	20	39
Diabetes	118,119	1.1	6	26	0	68
% Allocation— Average			9.8	53.1	21.7	16.8

Note: In the U.S. Centers for Disease Control report, the years of potential life lost were determined by computing the mean age of death for each cause, subtracting that number from either 65 or 75, and multiplying the difference by total number of cause-specific deaths. This was calculated for deaths of one-plus years.

*Percentages are based on Table 2-2.

Source: Reprinted from "Ten Leading Causes of Death in the United States, 1975," U.S. Department of Health, Education and Welfare, Public Health Service, Centers for Disease Control and Georgia Bureau of State Services, Health Analysis and Planning for Preventive Services, 1978, 46.

(disease specific), it will provide a basic framework for specifying goals and objectives. This will lead to recommendations for public and private institutions' programming actions at state and area levels to improve health status. The goals developed would relate to both health status and health system, the latter type describing the desired system and giving considerable attention to services for promoting health and preventing disease.

Figure 2-1 Allocation of Mortality Factors to the Four Elements of the Health Field

United States, 1975

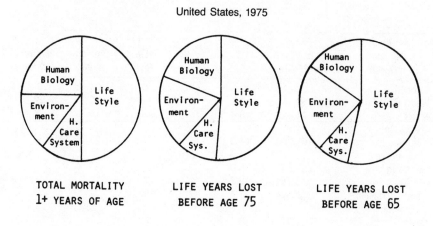

Source: Reprinted from "Ten Leading Causes of Death in the U.S., 1975," U.S. Department of Health, Education, and Welfare, Public Health Service, Centers for Disease Control and Georgia Bureau of State Services, Health Analysis and Planning for Preventive Services, 1978, 35.

The 'Sentinel' Health Events

A second application of the epidemiological approach to health policy is outlined by Rutstein and colleagues.[35,36] Although their model is intended to measure the quality of medical care, it is essentially a guide to the formulation of health policy.

They present a list of conditions that they term sentinel health events—warning signals that the quality of care may need to be improved. They assume that if the health care system had functioned satisfactorily, three basic types of conditions—unnecessary disease, unnecessary disability, and unnecessary untimely death—would have been prevented or managed. Moreover, they indicate whether each of these was preventable or treatable (or both).

Table 2-7 lists some of these sentinel health events. For example, cholera is a preventable, unnecessary disease; unnecessary, untimely death from it can be avoided through both prevention and treatment. Although the incidence of appendicitis cannot be controlled, unnecessary untimely death from it can be avoided by treatment. Similarly, many or most maternal deaths could be avoided through preventive care.

Table 2-7 Sentinel Health Events*

Condition	Unnecessary Disease[1]	Unnecessary Disability[1]	Unnecessary Untimely Death[1]	Notes[2]
Cholera	P		P T	
Typhoid fever	P		P T	
Botulism	P		P	
Tuberculosis (all forms)			T	
Silicotuberculosis	P	P	P T	P—Occupational
Plague			T	
Diphtheria	P		P T	
Rubella	P	P	P T	Disability in off-spring
Congenital syphilis	P	P	P T	
Major complications of syphilis	P T	P T	P T	
Gonococcal infections			T	
Malignant neoplasm of lip	P		P T	P—Pipe smoking and sun exposure
Malignant neoplasm of larynx	P		P T	P—Cigar and cigarette smoking
Malignant neoplasm of trachea, bronchus, and lung	P		P	P—Cigarette smoking and occupational exposure
Malignant neoplasm of bladder	P		P	P—Aniline dyes and cigarettes
Malignant neoplasm of eye		T	T	Genetic—screening and treatment
Thyroid carcinoma	P		P	P—Radiation exposure
Endemic goiter	P			Iodine deficiency
Nutritional deficiencies	P	P T	P T	Not associated with neoplasia and malabsorption
Pernicious anemia		T	T	
Pulmonary heart disease	P	P	P	P—Occupational and environmental exposure
Chronic bronchitis, emphysema	P	P	P	P—Occupational and environmental exposure
Appendicitis			T	
All maternal deaths			P	

*This listing is intended only as an illustration.

1. P denotes prevention; T denotes treatment.

2. The symbols P or T in the notes indicate that the prevention or treatment is limited to the circumstances described.

Source: Reprinted from "Measuring the Quality of Medical Care: A Clinical Method," by David D. Rutstein, M.D., William Berenberg, M.D., Thomas C. Chalmers, M.D., Charles G. Child III, M.D., Alfred P. Fishman, M.D., and Edward B. Perrin, Ph.D., with permission of *The New England Journal of Medicine,* ©1976, *294:* 585.

Rutstein et al. regard the occurrence of any of these diseases, disabilities, and untimely deaths as a warning, signaling a need to improve the quality of care and that something is wrong somewhere in the health care system. If the previous model is combined with this one, a sentinel event is a warning that something is amiss in the health field. It is an indicator of a need for a change or improvement in one or more of the health field components. In the words of those authors, this listing of sentinel health events "can be used to determine the level of health of the general population and the effects of economic, political, and other environmental factors upon it." [37] It can be added that the combination of a health field approach and the sentinel model can greatly benefit the formulation of health policy.

The Health Protection Packages

In this third application of the epidemiological approach and techniques in the formulation of health policy, a Canadian task force in 1980 reported on periodic health examinations. [38] The panel identified nearly 100 major disabling and/or killing conditions and unhealthy states and behaviors affecting Canadians as being potentially preventable. It explained: "Such states and behaviours are those that, when discovered, indicate that a person is at a degree of risk for a subsequent disease or disorder." [39]

Each of these potentially preventable conditions was studied extensively in reviewing the world literature and in assessing the scientific evidence, mostly epidemiologic, on the benefits of early detection or prevention. For each of the conditions then judged preventable, recommendations were developed on the procedure and frequency of the desirable specific test or maneuver. These individual maneuvers then were grouped into packages of examinations to be carried out at specific ages. The result was a proposal for a lifetime program of periodic health assessments or health protection packages for all Canadians.

The most interesting aspect of this model lies in the use of the epidemiological approach to arrive at a highly concrete, selective, and efficient health policy. Instead of the conventional, routine, nondirected method, this series of health protection packages provides a selective approach to prevention, health maintenance, and health promotion. The task force commented:

> This will help health professionals and the health service system to concentrate on the identification and early management of conditions that are potentially preventable. This selective approach restricts detection manoeuvres to those for which there is evidence of benefit through casefinding or screening. [40]

One of these health protection packages (for women and men aged 16 to 44 years) is reproduced in Table 2-8.

Table 2-8 Health Protection Package

(for Women and Men Aged 16 to 44 Years)

Target Condition	Maneuver	Optimal Frequency of Maneuver	Remarks
Poliomyelitis	Immunization	Booster at 16	Only persons in good health should be immunized. In certain circumstances (e.g., for persons with immunodeficiency), it is better to use inactivated poliomyelitis vaccine (Salk) instead of oral vaccine (Sabin). The vaccine is contraindicated in certain conditions. Immunization of pregnant women is not contraindicated if protection is required.
Tetanus and Diphtheria	Immunization	Booster every 10 years (optional for diphtheria)	Only persons in good health should be immunized.
Alcoholism Smoking Motor Vehicle Accidents	Elicit information on patient's history; counseling; provide effective contraceptive services to alcoholic sexually active women; control underlying medical conditions	At first encounter and at regular and appropriate intervals thereafter	Research priority: to establish the effectiveness of counseling
Family dysfunction; marital and sexual problems	Elicit history; counsel	Appropriate intervals based upon clinical judgment	Research priority: to determine the effectiveness of preventive maneuvers
Hearing impairment	Elicit history and conduct clinical examination	During visits for other reasons	Research priority: to determine the value of early detection and of the detection strategies available

Table 2-8 continued

Target Condition	Maneuver	Optimal Frequency of Maneuver	Remarks
Hypertension	Blood pressure measurement	At least every 5 years	At every visit made for other reasons
Dental caries Periodontal diseases Oral cancer	Oral examination, plus roentgenography if indicated; encourage daily oral hygiene	Annually	Research priority: particularly to establish the optimal frequency of examination
Rubella	Immunization of women at risk	Once	If immunization has not been carried out before, and provided the woman is not pregnant and will avoid becoming pregnant for the next 3 months
Cancer of the cervix	Papanicolaou smear	When first sexually active, but recheck within a year, then every 3 years to age 35 and every 5 years thereafter	For subjects at high risk: annual smears, particularly when early age of onset of sexual activity and multiplicity of sexual partners. Research priority: to determine the optimal age and frequency for taking smears
Muscular dystrophy	Determination of serum creatine phosphokinase concentration	Frequent testing may be required since there may be an overlap between values in carriers and in unaffected women	For female relatives of muscular dystrophy patients
Immunizable conditions related to international travel	Immunization; prophylaxis	Varies with different conditions	

Table 2-8 continued

Target Condition	Maneuver	Optimal Frequency of Maneuver	Remarks
Tuberculosis	Tuberculin sensitivity testing; immunization with bacille Calmette-Guerin vaccine and chemoprophylaxis as necessary	On the basis of clinical judgment	For persons exposed to the disease through their work, in contact with infected people, or living in communities with a high infection rate
Gonorrhea	Smears of cervix and/or urethra; cultures of cervical and/or urethral secretions and of first-voided urine	At appropriate intervals on the basis of clinical judgment	Pregnant women should be tested; incidence higher in persons with history of multiple sexual partners
Syphilis	Serologic testing	At appropriate intervals on the basis of clinical judgment	Pregnant women should be tested; incidence higher in persons with history of multiple sexual partners
Thalassemia	Elicit history; laboratory screening; counsel	Once	For Asian, African, and Mediterranean persons of parenting age who, having first been informed that no assistance is available to the carrier, still want to be screened. Research priority: to determine the effectiveness of preventive maneuvers
Iron-deficiency anemia and malnutrition	History taking; determination of serum protein and hemoglobin concentrations; measurement of height and weight	At appropriate intervals on the basis of clinical judgment	Women in low socioeconomic circumstances; Indians and Inuit; food faddists

Table 2-8 continued

Target Condition	Maneuver	Optimal Frequency of Maneuver	Remarks
Cancer of the skin	Inspection; counseling	At appropriate intervals on the basis of clinical judgment	High-risk groups: persons who work outdoors or are in contact with polycyclic aromatic hydrocarbons
Tay-Sachs disease	Measurement of resistance of serum hexosaminidase to heat inactivation	As part of premarital screening	High-risk groups: Ashkenazi Jews; aminocentesis can confirm diagnosis if expectant parents are known carriers
Cancer of the bladder	Cytologic analysis of urine	On the basis of clinical judgment	High-risk groups: occupationally exposed to bladder carcinogens, and smokers

Source: Reprinted from *Periodic Health Examination Monograph,* Report of a Task Force to the Conference of Deputy Ministers of Health with permission of Health and Welfare Canada, 1980, 114-115.

SUMMARY

This chapter has examined the role of epidemiology in health policy. It has argued that the adoption of the epidemiological perspective by all involved in health policymaking—including health care managers—would lead to a reduction in today's major cripplers and killers.

This impact on the population's health will come through careful analysis of prevalent health problems. This analysis should be supported by an inherently prevention-oriented conceptualization (or framework) of health and illness. Three examples or models of such an approach were reviewed.

NOTES

1. Henrik L. Blum, *Planning for Health* (2d. ed.) (New York: Human Sciences Press, Inc., 1981), 5.

2. H.H. Hyman, *Health Planning—A Systematic Approach* (Rockville, Md.: Aspen Systems Corporation, 1975), 67.

3. N.T.J. Bailey, "Systems Modeling in Health Planning," in *Systems Aspects of Health Planning*, ed., N.T.J. Bailey and M. Thompson (Amsterdam: North-Holland Publishing Company, 1975), 9.

4. Ibid.

5. World Health Organization, *Application of Systems Analysis to Health Management*, Report of a WHO Comité Experte—Technical Report Series No. 596 (Geneva: World Health Organization, 1976), 27.

6. M. Jenicek, *Introduction à l'épidémiologie* (St. Hyacinthe, Quebec: Edisern, 1976), 372-373.

7. A.B. Ford, "Epidemiological Priorities as a Basis for Health Policy," *Bulletin of the New York Academy of Medicine* 54, no. 1 (January 1978): 10-22.

8. L. Gordis, "Challenges to Epidemiology in the Coming Decade," *American Journal of Epidemiology* 112, no. 2 (1980): 319.

9. Milton Terris, "Epidemiology as a Guide to Health Policy," *Annual Review of Public Health, 1980,* 1, 323-44.

10. Ford, "Epidemiological Priorities," 10-13.

11. Gordis, "Challenges," 319.

12. K.L. White, "Teaching Epidemiologic Concepts as the Scientific Basis for Understanding Problems of Organizing and Evaluating Health Services," *International Journal of Health Services* 2, no. 4 (1972): 525-29.

13. M. Jenicek and R.H. Fletcher, "Epidemiology for Canadian Medical Students—Desirable Attitudes, Knowledge, and Skills," *International Journal of Epidemiology* 6, no. 1 (1977): 69-72.

14. C.W. Blair, "Teaching Community Diagnosis to Medical Students," *Journal of Community Health* 6, no. 1 (Fall 1980): 54-64.

15. M.A. Faghih, "Epidemiology and the Training of Physicians," *International Journal of Epidemiology* 6, no. 4 (1977): 331-33.

16. Terris, "Epidemiology as a Guide," 334.

17. Henrik L. Blum et al., *Notes on Comprehensive Planning for Health* (San Francisco: American Public Health Association, Western Regional Office, 1968).

18. H.L. Laframboise, "Health Policy: Breaking the Problem Down in More Manageable Segments," *Canadian Medical Association Journal 108* (February 3, 1973): 388-393.

19. Marc Lalonde, *A New Perspective on the Health of Canadians* (Ottawa: Health and Welfare Canada, 1974), 76.

20. Laframboise, "Health Policy," 388.

21. Lalonde, "A New Perspective," 76.

22. Minister of Industry, Trade, and Commerce, *Perspective Canada: A Compendium of Social Statistics* (Ottawa: Statistics Canada, 1974), 321.

23. G.E. Alan Dever, "Dimensions of Environmental Health" (Paper presented at the Annual Convention of the Georgia Public Health Association, Macon, Ga., 1974), 11.

24. U.S. Department of Health, Education, and Welfare, "Man's Health and the Environment—Some Research Needs," in *Report of the Task Force on Research Planning in Environmental Health Sciences* (Washington, D.C.: U.S. Government Printing Office, March 10, 1970), 258.

25. J.B. Cullingworth, ed., *Problems of an Urban Society,* vol. 3: *Planning for Change* (Toronto: University of Toronto Press, 1973), 195.

26. Alvin Toffler, *Future Shock* (New York: Random House Inc., 1970), 562.

27. E.P. Eckholm, *The Picture of Health—Environmental Sources of Disease* (New York: W.W. Norton & Company, Inc., 1977).

28. C.E.R. Lloyd, *Hippocratic Writings* (Hammondsworth, England: Penguin Books, 1978), 32.

29. Lalonde, "A New Perspective," 76.

30. C.L. Erhardt and Joyce E. Berlin, eds., *Mortality and Morbidity in the U.S.,* Vital and Health Statistics Monographs, American Public Health Association (Cambridge, Mass.: Harvard University Press, 1974), 289.

31. J.M. Hunter, ed., *The Geography of Health and Disease,* Papers of the First Carolina Geographical Symposium (Chapel Hill, N.C.: University of North Carolina, 1974), 193.

32. A.M. Lillefeld and A.J. Gifford, eds., *Chronic Diseases and Public Health* (Baltimore: The Johns Hopkins Press, 1966), 846.

33. Office of Management and Budget, *Special Analyses, Budget of the United States Government, Federal Health Programs, Special Analysis K,* 1976, 169-196.

34. *Ten Leading Causes of Death in the United States* (Washington, D.C.: U.S. Department of Health, Education, and Welfare, Public Health Service, Centers for Disease Control), Atlanta: Bureau of State Services, Health Analysis and Planning for Preventive Services, 1978, 70.

35. D.D. Rutstein et al., "Measuring the Quality of Medical Care—A Clinical Method," *The New England Journal of Medicine* 294, no. 11 (March 11, 1976): 582-588.

36. D.D. Rutstein, *Blueprint for Medical Care* (Boston: The MIT Press, 1974), 161-224.

37. D.D. Rutstein et al., *op. cit.,* 582.

38. Health and Welfare Canada, *The Periodic Health Examination Monograph,* Report of a Task Force to the Conference of Deputy Ministers of Health (Ottawa: Health and Welfare Canada, 1980).

39. Ibid., 15.

40. Ibid., 96.

Chapter 3

Epidemiology in Health Services Management

USES OF EPIDEMIOLOGY

Epidemiology is a discipline which has evolved relatively specialized methods for investigating disease causation and bringing to bear, according to the needs of the moment, specific knowledge and special skills from many other sciences. With some justice, epidemiology has been called a method rather than an independent science.[1]

Epidemiologic principles and methods can be applied to a wide range of problems in many fields. These principles and methods relate to the description of human populations, to the investigation of the processes underlying their present state, to the interpretation and analysis of such information, and to the uses to which these data can be put. In the health field, epidemiology has three main uses: etiological, clinical, and administrative.

Etiological Use

"Classical" epidemiology is concerned primarily with the search for causes of health and disease. In cooperation with the other medical sciences, such as biochemistry, physiology, microbiology, and pathology, epidemiology contributes to the understanding of the natural history of diseases and of their determinants and deterrents. As discussed in Chapter 1, an expanded and multifactorial conceptualization of causality allows epidemiologists to determine risk factors; that is, to estimate individuals' risks and chances of developing some state of health or disease.

Clinical Use

In a clinical setting, epidemiology is used, in the words of Morris, to help complete the picture there and to aid in the clarification of clinical syndromes.[2] As the International Epidemiological Association puts it:

A [medical] student's understanding of anatomy, physiology, and biochemistry will be seriously deficient if he does not appreciate the variability of physical, physiological, biochemical, immunological, and other attributes in the general population and understand that it is rarely possible to draw a clear line between the normal and the pathological. In the clinical disciplines, knowledge of prevalence, etiology, and prognosis derived from epidemiological research has obvious implications for the diagnosis and management of individual patients and of their families.[3]

Administrative Use

Epidemiology can and should be used for purposes of health services management. It contributes to the making of a community diagnosis of the presence, nature, and distribution of health and disease. It provides a means of monitoring the health of a population as well as charting changes over time and among places.

Through the use of epidemiological principles and methods, health service managers can determine which diseases are of major importance in their population. Furthermore, using the causal data available from classical epidemiologists, they can identify individuals at risk—their potential market or target population. Epidemiology thus supplies many of the facts needed for the management and planning of health services and for their evaluation.

HEALTH SERVICES MANAGEMENT

The provision of health care to populations necessitates some form of collective, organized action. It involves the coordination of interrelated parts of an organization to achieve the objectives embodied in providing care.[4] Management is the process that oversees the production of services—in this case, health.

The 'Functional' Approach

Although everyone has some kind of idea of what managers do, the management process always has been hard to circumscribe. Most management textbooks, and most classical organizational theorists, have adopted a functional approach to defining the process. They examine the work of managers in terms of functions, or areas of activity.

Unfortunately, there is lack of agreement on listing those functions. Furthermore, their conceptualization usually is ambiguous. In any case, five functions seem to be mentioned consistently: planning, organizing, directing, coordinating, and controlling. From a comprehensive literature review of functional authors, Lorgest describes these as follows:[5]

Planning

The primary management function is planning. In essence, planning means to decide in advance what is to be done. It charts a course of action for the future. The aim of planning is to achieve a coordinated and consistent set of operations aimed at desired objectives.

Organizing

Organizing can be defined as relating people and things to each other in such a way that they are combined into a unit capable of being directed toward organizational objectives. The basic objective of the organizing function is the development of a framework called the formal organizational structure.

Directing

Once plans are made and an organization is created to put them into effect, the next logical function of management is to stimulate the effort needed to perform the required work. This is done through the directing function, including order giving, supervising, leading, motivating, and communicating.

Coordinating

Coordinating is the act of assembling and synchronizing people and activities so that they function harmoniously in the attainment of organization objectives.

Controlling

Controlling can be defined as the regulation of activities in accordance with the requirements of plans. It consists of measuring and correcting activities of people and things in an organization to assure that objectives and plans are accomplished.

The Process Approach

Another, more realistic way of looking at management is to subdivide it into component processes. Levin identifies three types of processes that, together, comprise the area of management's concerns: the technical, the administrative, and the political.[6]

The technical process specifies the actions that will be accomplished. The administrative process enables the actions to be taken and is concerned with the methods of carrying them out. The political process involves doing whatever is necessary to achieve the objectives of the organization by mobilizing support for the actions. Progress toward an action blends the necessary objective or technical evidence with the equally essential administrative and political elements.[7]

The process-oriented approach to the analysis of management has several advantages:

- It reflects the dynamic and political nature of management much more than does the functional approach. Managers are involved continually in a negotiation process with the organization's internal and external influencers.[8] Recognition of this political aspect is essential if the orientation of the management and planning of health services is to be influenced successfully.

- It also allows the examination of any level of management, from a country's government to the smallest organization. At any level, organized action results from a blend of the technical, administrative, and political processes.

- It is consistent with a comprehensive, systemic analysis of a given action. Managing and planning for health programs or institutions without full consideration of their interdependencies with other parts of society ignores the fact that the programs or facilities are part of a larger system.

Epidemiology and Decision Making

Whatever approach is adopted, what ties together the functions or the subprocesses is decision making, the essence of management. Furthermore, decisions always will be made on the basis of some "information."

Those who occupy management positions within any system function, at least in intention, as receivers and perceivers of information or signals from the environment, as decoders of this information, as deciders of courses of action, and as composers and transmitters of messages designed to influence others in the system to act according to these decisions.[9]

This information might be "hard" (formal) or "soft" (more or less subjective). In either case, the managers will process some kind of information on which their decisions will be based. The courses of action they determine from those decisions are translated into some organized action. The use of epidemiology in health services management is to supply some of this "hard" information as a basis for decision making.

The rest of this chapter explains how an expanded comprehensive planning process provides a framework for managerial decision making. The management process, examined from either the functional or the process approach, can be seen operating within that overall planning framework. It is through that planning process that the contributions of epidemiology to health services management are analyzed.

THE PLANNING PROCESS

In its usual, everyday meaning, planning refers to the design of a desired future and of effective ways of bringing it about.[10] The contention here, however, is that planning can be considered in a much broader perspective so as to incorporate policymaking at the societal level as well as program management in an organizational setting.

Planning is the guidance of change within a social system,[11] the process by which present decisions are related to future desired results.[12] It aims to enrich decision making. Its fundamental purposes are to extend the depth of understanding and to broaden the vision of those responsible for decision making at any level. Defined in this way, planning is an action-oriented process by which the institution adapts to changes in both its internal constituency and its external environment.

As stated previously, decision making is the essence of management. It takes place in an arena of uncertainty. As organizational theorists have demonstrated convincingly, the decision-making process rarely corresponds to the classical, rational model. To the contrary, it essentially is a process of "short-run adaptive reactions,"[13] "satisficing" instead of "maximizing,"[14] a "muddling through,"[15] or "disjointed incrementalism."[16] Decision making is highly "reactive-adaptive."

> It is the paradox of decision making that effective action is born of reaction. Only when organizations as open systems take in information from the environment and react to changing conditions can they act on that same environment to reduce uncertainty and increase discretionary flexibility.[17]

Planning, as conceived of here, is a process of collecting this information from the environment and putting it to use in the development and elaboration of the organization's actions and activities. For a health-related institution, epidemiology provides a method, within the planning process, of collecting this information and guiding the implementation of the activities or programs.

Levels of Planning

This analysis is based on the concept of three levels of planning: normative or policy planning, strategic or comprehensive planning, and tactical/operational or program planning. Figure 3-1 illustrates the interrelation of these three planning levels. Chapter 2 already has dealt with policy planning so the focus here turns

Figure 3-1 A Paradigm for Planning

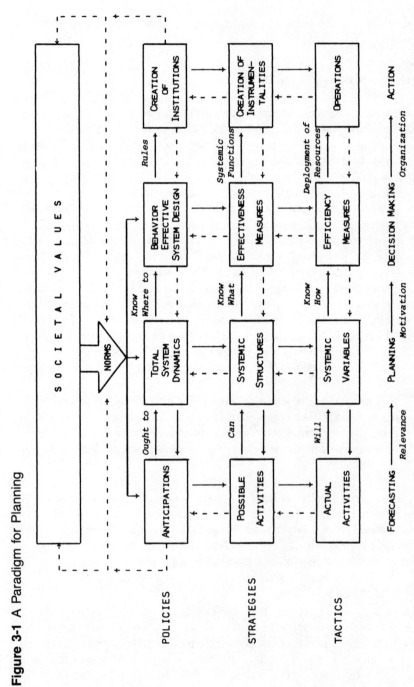

Source: Adapted from *Technological Planning and Social Futures* by Erich Jantsch with permission of Associated Business Programmes, London, ©1972, 16.

more particularly to strategic and tactical planning, with which health managers are more directly concerned. (Further material on policy planning is available from other sources.[18, 19])

Strategic Planning

Strategic planning provides a general framework for organizational action. This process is aimed at establishing the entity's principal objectives and priorities. At the strategic level, long-range goals are established and possible means of achieving them are considered.

As indicated in Figure 3-1, strategic planning deals with the examination of possible activities to carry out the anticipations of society. Specific system structures are established, hopefully effective outcome indicators are defined, and instrumentalities or means to operationalize institutions are created. The emphasis is on predicting the future behavior of external variables and the formulation of alternative courses of action in light of expected events.[20]

Operational Planning

This final level consists of developing the detailed plans for carrying out the strategies (or some of those considered priorities) that were developed at the previous planning level. Operational planning describes an iterative process in which expectations about when, where, and how activities will occur are set and in which results are monitored, measured, and redirected when deviations from the expressed targets are detected.

The important point is that the operational plan must be implemented. To be capable of being implemented, it must fit within the operational (production) framework of the organization and it must influence how its resources are assigned. "The acid test for the success of health planning is its ability to influence the allocation of resources so that what is planned for comes to pass."[21]

Planning for Health

Planning, at whatever level, is not carried out in a vacuum. To the contrary, at all points it is permeated by social values and by the prevalent paradigm or framework of health. This is illustrated in Figures 3-2 and 3-3.

Figure 3-2, the traditional planning model for medical care, pays no attention to societal values. "Norms" and "Anticipations" depend only upon the technological ability to accomplish something. Furthermore, the conception of health system activities ignores life style and environmental "aspects" of health and disease.

In contrast, Figure 3-3, based on the holistic (ecological) framework of health described previously, indicates that people value a high quality of life, an opportunity for a productive being, wellness, and freedom from sickness. The associ-

Figure 3-2 The Traditional Planning Model for Medical Care

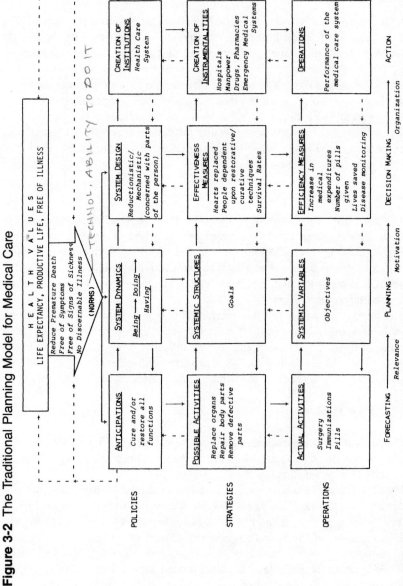

Source: Adapted from *Technological Planning and Social Futures* by Erich Jantsch with permission of Associated Business Programmes, London, ©1972, 16.

Figure 3-3 A Planning Model for Wellness and Holistic Health

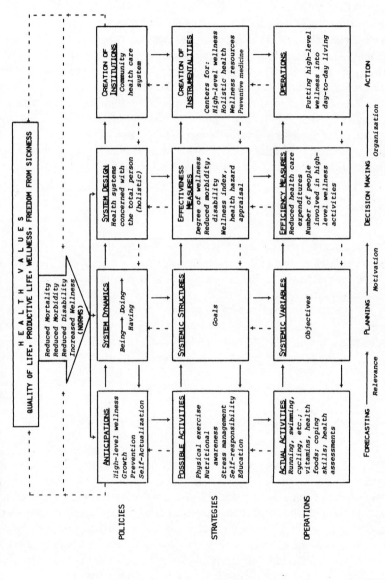

Source: Adapted from *Technological Planning and Social Futures* by Erich Jantsch with permission of Associated Business Programmes, London, ©1972, 16.

ated norms of reduced morbidity, disability, and mortality, and of increased levels of wellness become expectations in the model. At the policy level, anticipations of high-level wellness proceed dynamically through appropriate functions toward being and the achievement of a healthier society. This holistic design leads to the creation of an institution called a community health care system.

In the second phase of planning, strategies that closely parallel the policy phase are determined. For example, anticipations of a healthier society evolve to strategies of physical exercise, nutritional awareness, stress management, and self-responsibility. At that operational phase of the planning process, the activities become running, swimming, cycling, consuming healthful foods and vitamins, and developing coping skills. These put high-level wellness into day-to-day living and point up the need for individuals' responsibility and authority in the management of their health. Development of a health care system reflecting these values generates greater potential to meet the needs of society.

Steps in the Planning Process

The planning process consists of a series of steps, as illustrated in Figure 3-4. These are not in an immutable order but are followed in a more or less systematic way. The planning process is inherently cyclical and continual.

The first two steps, the identification of needs and problems and the establishment of priorities, are preliminary to program planning. This part of strategic planning allows determination of priorities among the different problems and, consequently, provides justifications for the actions or programs. In other words, health program planning must take place within a larger strategic planning process.[22]

PLANNING AND HEALTH SERVICES MANAGEMENT

Table 3-1 illustrates the correspondence between the planning process just described and management. The first four steps correspond to the narrowly defined planning functions of management. The fifth, mobilization and coordination of resources, involves the organizing, directing, and coordinating of managerial functions; the last step, evaluation, refers to the controlling function. From a process approach, the technical aspect refers to the first and last steps of (cyclical) planning—the identification of needs and the evaluation. The administrative and political processes operate concurrently within the other parts.

This correspondence paves the way for analysis of epidemiology's contributions to health services management through the various planning steps.

Figure 3-4 Steps in Health Program Planning

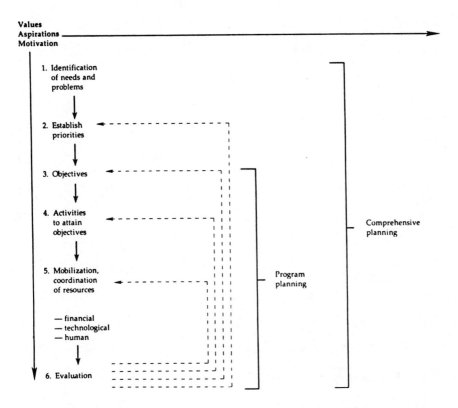

Source: Adapted from "Eléments et étapes d'élaboration d'un programme de santé communautaire" by R. Pineault with permission of *Union Médicale du Canada* 105, no. 8, ©1976, 1208–1214, as reprinted in "Program Planning in a Small Community Health Care Setting" by Carol Clemenhagen and Francois Champagne with permission of *Health Care Management Review* 7, no. 1 (Winter 1982), ©1982, 50.

Step 1. Identification of Needs and Problems

The Concept of Need

The concepts of need and of target populations are central to any level of health planning. The process starts with the identification of a population's needs for health services. What is meant by health needs, however, is subject to much debate

Table 3-1 How Planning and Management Correspond

The Planning Process	Management	
	The Functional Approach	The Process Approach
1. Identify needs and problems		Technical
2. Establish priorities	Planning	
3. Set objectives		Administrative and Political
4. Specify activities to attain objectives		
5. Mobilize and coordinate resources	Organizing Directing Coordinating	
6. Evaluation	Controlling	Technical

in the literature on health planning, medical care organization, and health care sociology.

Donabedian briefly defines need as "some disturbance in health and well-being."[23] What constitutes a "disturbance," however, is far from straightforward. Such a disturbance is always a perception and its assessment depends upon who is doing the perceiving. As Donabedian himself suggests, there are at least two perspectives on need: that of the client and that of the provider.[24] Many more conflicting perspectives are likely since the definition of needs is conditioned by value judgments and by the comprehension or framework of health within which the description is found. No undue emphasis is placed here on the semantics of the concept of needs. Several authors already have provided more than adequate discussion.[25, 26, 27]

Needs Assessment Approaches[28]

As can be expected, approaches vary in complexity, cost, time necessary for completion, and relative effectiveness.[29] Three functions characterize needs assessment approaches: compilation (collecting data from already existing sources), development (producing new information), and integration (synthesizing information originating from inside and outside the system boundaries).[30]

Table 3-2 Needs Assessment Approaches and Methods

Approach	Method	Information Processing Function	Measurement Expertise Needed	Time and Resources Needed
Indicator approach				
Health indicators	Analysis of statistics on life expectancy, morbidity, mortality, and disability	Compilation	Moderate to high	Moderate
Social indicators	Analysis of social statistics related to health and health care utilization	Compilation	Moderate to high	Moderate
Extrapolation/ assumption	Need extrapolations based on epidemiological data from reference population	Compilation and integration	Moderate	Minimal
Survey approach	Analysis of service utilization or rates under treatment	Compilation	Moderate	Moderate
	Survey sample of labor and service facilities	Compilation and development	Moderate	Moderate
	Survey sample of general population	Development	High	Extensive
	Survey sample of service or provider population	Development	High	Moderate
Consensus-reaching approach	Community forum	Integration	Low	Moderate
	Nominal group	Development	Moderate	Minimal
	Key informants	Development	Moderate	Minimal
	Delphi technique	Development and integration	Moderate	Moderate
	Community impressions	Development, compilation, and integration	Moderate	Minimal

Sources: Adapted from "Need Identification and Program Planning in the Community Context" by L.M. Siegel, C.C. Attkisson, and L.G. Carson in *Evaluation of Human Service Programs,* ed. C.C. Attkisson, with permission of Academic Press, Inc., ©1978, p. 226; from *Guide to Health Needs Assessment: A Critique of Available Sources of Health Care Information* by L.W. Chambers, C.A. Woodward, and C. Dok with permission of the Canadian Public Health Association, ©1980, p. 32, and from *Determining Health Needs* by Robin E. MacStravic with permission of Health Administration Press, ©1978, p. 268, as reprinted in "Program Planning in a Small Community Health Care Setting" by Carol Clemenhagen and Francois Champagne with permission of *Health Care Management Review,* 7, no. 1 (Winter 1982), ©1982, 47–55.

Table 3-2 provides a summary of the needs assessment methods documented in the literature based on the indicator approach, the survey approach, and the consensus-reaching approach.

Indicator Approaches: There are three of these: health, social, and extrapolation/assumption. Since needs for care are based on the health status of the population, indicators used to measure that factor can measure needs as well. Such health indicators are developed through analysis of morbidity, mortality, and, more recently, disability data. Sources of this information include hospital admission and discharge reports; notifiable disease statistics; maternal, neonatal, and infant mortality statistics; life expectancy tables; and disability indexes for specific populations.[31]

Social indicators are relevant to health needs because they correlate with utilization of care.[32] As with health indicators, need is inferred from measurements of the social condition of the population. Social indicators generally are used only as rough pointers, since the relationship between social factors and health may be tenuous.[33] Sources of information for construction of social indicators include statistics on age, sex, education, ethnic background, housing, employment, and food consumption.

The extrapolation/assumption method applies epidemiological data on the prevalence and incidence of diseases and certain health conditions in a smaller reference population. The purpose is to estimate expected health needs associated with these same conditions in a larger population. The quality of the estimates depends on the validity of the rates calculated for the reference population and on their applicability to the study population.

Survey Approaches: There are four elements here: analysis of utilization, rates under treatment, labor and service facilities, and sample surveys.

The analysis-of-utilization method of assessment examines need in terms of the demand for services. Demand is measured by the types and amounts of services actually utilized. In its narrowest interpretations, this method assumes that no need exists that does not result in utilization of services and that those used totally meet the need expressed.[34]

More broadly, this analysis compares utilization among income, ethnic, or other groups. One reason for this comparison is to gain insight into possible barriers to service that may affect particular segments of the population.

The rates-under-treatment method looks specifically at instances of service utilization. For example, a survey of service encounters, e.g., clinic visits, during a specified time period may be undertaken. Data such as client characteristics, services received, health status, transportation problems, and waiting times may be collected in specially designed encounter forms or abstracted from agency records. Information is obtained through the organization providing services.[35]

Needs assessment is based on the characteristics documented in the encounter survey. This measure of need is biased toward heavy service users.

The method involving labor and service facilities is based on the assumption that individuals receiving care do in fact need it. The number of service providers and facilities in the setting under study is compared with the volume of known service utilization. The extent to which providers and facilities cannot cope with existing utilization represents the degree of need.[36] Need is extrapolated from the supply of health personnel and service facilities.

Sample surveys of the general population assess needs by collecting data on health problems, disability, and needs perception directly from respondents, often in their own homes. An alternative approach consists of interviewing service users at the point of utilization. This method collects information from a group that has had at least some contact with health services. It differs from the rates-under-treatment method in that the service agency is not involved directly. Like the rates-under-treatment method, this one misses nonusers. A survey of persons involved in providing services would collect data on their perceptions of client needs. These opinions would, of course, reflect the professional perspective.[37]

Consensus-Reaching Approaches: This segment involves five factors: community forum, the nominal group, key informants, the Delphi technique, and community impressions.

The consensus-reaching approach focuses on means by which lay and professional views of health care needs can be assessed in participative group discussions. The community forum is an open meeting to which all members are invited to present views on their area's needs. This is justified as a supplement to more thorough methods and is used to verify findings and build a "supportive consensus."[38]

The nominal group process consists of a very structured, multiphased meeting of individuals who are closely associated with the problem area being assessed. For example, a small target group (seven to ten individuals) of health care consumers and facility administrators and staff members may meet to define the nature of health care needs in the community.

A preset, orderly procedure is followed so that ideas are defined individually and independently at first, then enumerated and clarified in the group through a round-robin process. The group then rates these ideas by secret ballot. The result is a rank ordering of needs defined by the group.[39]

In the key informant method, interviews are conducted with community residents or local workers having extensive firsthand experience in the area under study. Interview questions relate to existing services and demographic characteristics of the community. The data collected are aggregated to obtain an overall picture of the community from the key informants' perspectives.[40]

The Delphi technique has been defined as a "method for systematic solicitation and collection of judgments on a particular topic through a set of carefully designed sequential questionnaires interspersed with feedback of opinions derived from earlier responses."[41] This technique collects and refines judgments from experts through a reiterative process. It ultimately produces a collective agreement as to the nature and range of existing community health care needs or a prediction of future wants. Opinions usually are submitted anonymously. The nature of the topic being investigated affects how the Delphi process is organized. Variations in question structure, rules governing aggregation of judgments, and the interaction of respondents, among other things, determine its specific form.[42]

The community impressions method integrates information collected in interviews with small groups of key informants with an as-wide-as-possible range of existing indicator, utilization, or survey data. The scenario of needs developed in this manner then is validated through the community forum process.[43]

Health Services Management and Needs Identification

There obviously is considerable controversy surrounding the concept of needs, a condition intensified by the many different approaches to their assessment. Nevertheless, health services management requires—and even presupposes—a pragmatic look at the identification of needs and problems. Health service managers must determine which services should be offered, and to whom.

The first four steps of the planning process (Table 3-1, supra) respond to these two basic questions. The first planning step, regardless of the different meanings of the concept of need, boils down to a description of the population surrounding the organization, of its health problems, and of its utilization of health services; analyses of the possible etiology or factors involved in such health problems; and identification of the resources present in the community to address such factors.

This gives an overall picture of health needs by identifying some type of gap, service potential, or market opportunity. Figure 3-5 illustrates the components of this first planning step.

Description of the Population: The description of the population to be served by the organization is essential to the planning and management of health care. This population should be analyzed by demographic, socioeconomic, and geographic attributes. (This is discussed in Chapter 9, on demography, and in Chapter 10, on marketing.)

Description of Health Problems: As noted earlier, three major approaches to needs assessment are the indicator, the survey, and the consensus-reaching approaches. There is no doubt that a combination of approaches, taking account of the purposes of a given needs assessment, is more productive and adequate than any single method. The contribution of epidemiology to health services management, however, is examined here primarily as to the indicator approach, which is

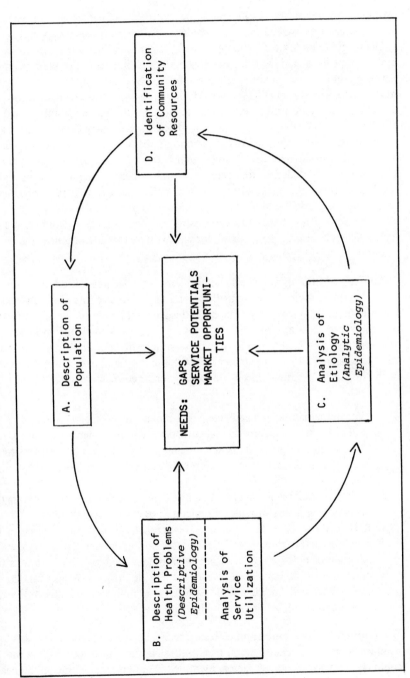

Figure 3-5 Identification of Health Needs and Problems

A. Description of Population

B. Description of Health Problems *(Descriptive Epidemiology)*

Analysis of Service Utilization

C. Analysis of Etiology *(Analytic Epidemiology)*

D. Identification of Community Resources

NEEDS: GAPS
SERVICE POTENTIALS
MARKET OPPORTUNI-
TIES

essentially the descriptive-epidemiologic approach. (Chapter 8 also examines service utilization, which can be considered part of the survey approach.)

Using epidemiological principles, methods, and techniques, health service managers need to analyze three main categories of indicators, or phenomena, to get a picture of the health problems of the population under consideration: mortality, morbidity, and risk factors. Morbidity includes disease, discomfort, and disability, both acute and chronic. Risk factors relate to elements within each of the four dimensions of the health field concept noted previously (biology, life style, environment, and health care organization). For example, data on the smoking or dietary habits of the population might contribute to the identification of need for a given service. Included in this category are the "health maintenance needs" or needs for "services presumed to benefit people who are well by improving or protecting their good health."[44]

Such an analysis of health problems using data on mortality, morbidity, and risk factors is what descriptive epidemiology is about. (This is examined in detail in Chapters 4, 5, 6, 7, and 8.)

Analysis of Etiology: Once some problems have been identified, it is useful to try to determine their source or, as Blum puts it, the "prime forces which causally underlie them."[45] As noted in Chapter 1, these causal forces can be approximated or understood through "risk factors." Using data and knowledge from analytic epidemiology, the health problem, expressed in terms of mortality or morbidity, can be translated into its precursory risk factor in one or all of the four dimensions of the health field. This approach is useful for three main reasons:

1. "The immediate search and analysis of precursor risk factors to major causes of ill health reveal that certain precursors are common to many conditions."[46] This fact allows grouping problems into more manageable segments rather than trying to develop or expand a program directed at each morbid condition identified as a problem.
2. It gives a direction for intervention: the risk factor becomes the problem that needs solving; this provides a concrete possibility of intervention.
3. It is likely to provide for a more comprehensive and global view of the problems and of the possibilities of intervention through using an extended ecologic or holistic model of health. Problems and possible solutions that otherwise would have been considered outside the boundaries of the health care sector can be identified. Similarly, it indicates the possibilities of cooperation with other community agencies.

Identification of Community Resources: The last component of this first planning step is the identification of all other community resources that are, or could be, addressing the risk factors identified. These might include public health agencies, hospitals, schools, or community groups. This can be done in a summary manner or by marketing techniques (described in Chapter 10).

Needs: Gaps and Market Opportunities

From the demographic evaluation of the population and the epidemiologic description and analysis of mortality, morbidity, and risk factor data there should emerge a clear picture of the area's health problems. Similarly, the analysis of service utilization and the identification of other community resources indicate which of these problems the institution could address. This constitutes the input into the second step of the planning process, the setting of priorities.

Step 2. Determination of Priorities

Once problems that the organization could address are identified, health service managers must determine which ones are most important and therefore call for the most attention in planning and allocating resources.[47]

Many criteria, including some highly political ones, come into play in the determination of priorities. One source lists the following factors: "time horizon, scope, and range of problems, range of interested parties, degree of uncertainty, degree of complexity, degree of consensus."[48] Epidemiology also has an important role to play in helping decision makers (health service managers) rationalize priorities. Anderson comments: "Because health needs at any time exceed the resources available, choices must be made. The community physician (epidemiologist) has the function of providing the evidence which is to guide the political and policy choices about alternatives, particularly in the second and third stages of planning."[49]

Epidemiology's contribution to the determination of priorities is based on a fairly simple notion: the health problems that are most important are those that cause the greatest loss and are most amenable to prevention and amelioration.[50] Two sets of epidemiologic criteria can be used in this second planning step: (1) the magnitude of the loss, and (2) the amenability of loss to prevention or reduction.[51]

Magnitude of the Loss

Epidemiologic techniques can be used to estimate loss of life because of a given cause of mortality or, similarly, time lost because of morbidity. The relative importance of risk factors can be assessed through the use of epidemiologic concepts, such as attributable risk, absolute risk, excess risk, and relative risk. (All of these are reviewed in Chapter 4.) .

Amenability to Prevention or Reduction

The second set of criteria that epidemiology can contribute to the determination of priorities is the sensitivity of the problem to a health program, or the "readiness with which the disease may be prevented or its adverse effects minimized."[52] This amenability or sensitivity can be determined in any of the following ways:[53]

- normatively, using experts' judgment and consensus
- empirically, based on the experience of other regions, states, or countries
- operationally, using some type of cost-benefit analysis—the lower the cost of a program in achieving a predetermined objective, the more amenable or sensitive it is to prevention or reduction.

(Chapter 4 briefly examines cost-benefit analysis and epidemiology's role in it.)

Step 3. Setting Objectives

Once priorities are determined, program planning can take place for each group of problems or risk factors. The planning of each program starts with setting its objectives. Epidemiology's contribution in this step is mostly in expressing the objectives in a quantified way (using incidence or prevalence rates). Epidemiology also can contribute information on the feasible range of reduction of incidence or prevalence, again through the use of the various risk ratios.

Step 4. Activities To Attain Objectives

For the objectives to be met (and therefore for the "need" previously identified), they now must be translated operationally into activities or services. This also involves the prediction, identification, and allocation of resources that will be needed to produce the services required.

This fourth planning step starts with the generation of ideas for possible ways of achieving the objectives. Once again, the framework adopted by the health service manager crucially influences the generation of activities and services. Similarly, the analysis of risk factors performed in Step 1, using the four dimensions or inputs to health, can and should be of much help and creative inspiration in developing alternatives.

Once alternatives are generated, they should be evaluated using cost-benefit analysis, comparing the benefits expected from each alternative with the cost and risks of adopting it.

1 biology
2 life style
3 envir.
4 hlthcare org.

Step 5. Mobilization, Coordination of Resources

The activities to achieve the objectives have been chosen, and the appropriate resources have been determined and allocated. This fifth step of the planning cycle is the actual delivery of the services. This is where most of the traditional management functions operate and dominate (see Table 3-1, supra). The contribution of epidemiology is minimal, being limited to the collection of data that can be used to monitor the program and its effects and, subsequently, to evaluate it more formally.

Situations also may arise in which "a definite form of service cannot be determined from the beginning" and in which epidemiology can be used to "design and conduct experiments and pilot implementations to guide subsequent decisions."[54]

Step 6. Evaluation

The evaluation component contains three areas of concern: costs, activities, and outcomes. These more commonly are called fiscal, process, and outcome evaluation:

- Fiscal evaluation focuses on and determines cost accountability.
- Process evaluation determines program activity in terms of (1) the population receiving the benefits, by age, sex, race, or other demographic variables; (2) the program organization, staffing, and funding; and (3) the program location and timing. Process evaluation is a measure of program efforts or proposed activities rather than a program's effects or results.
- Outcome evaluation delineates program objectives in terms of effects to determine whether a change in health status has occurred as a result of the effort.

The following observations are relevant to program evaluation:

- Most management decisions are based on intuition rather than on facts.
- The purpose of evaluation is to answer the practical questions of administrators who want to know whether to continue a program, to extend it to other sites, to modify it, or to close it down.
- Evaluation is more productive when it is a continuous process, with a continuous feedback loop to the administrators, supervisors, and program managers who make the decisions. Routine evaluation reports should inform administrators about the efforts and results of policy and program decisions.

They should alert supervisors to service delivery trends and point to problems calling for corrective action.

Epidemiology directly contributes to health program evaluation in at least two ways.[55] First, the ideal design for evaluation remains the controlled clinical trial.[56, 57] Second, the measures of outcomes are almost necessarily epidemiological measures of the health status of the population.

In this regard, the contribution and use of epidemiology is essentially the same as that described in Step 1, to which the cyclical nature of the planning process now returns the operation.

SUMMARY

This chapter has examined the role of epidemiology in health services management, first by looking at the different uses of epidemiology, then by analyzing the nature of management. The conclusion is that the central feature of management is decision making. A global planning process whose aim is essentially to aid managerial decision making was described. It was noted that this planning process and the management process basically correspond. The planning process was used to examine epidemiology's contributions to health services management.

NOTES

1. J.P. Fox, C.E. Hall, and L.R. Elveback, *Epidemiology: Man and Disease* (Toronto: The Macmillan Company, 1970), 10.

2. J.N. Morris, *Uses of Epidemiology* (3rd. ed.) (Edinburgh: Churchill Livingstone, 1975), 121.

3. International Epidemiological Association, *Epidemiology—A Guide to Teaching Methods* (Edinburgh: Churchill Livingstone, 1973), 8.

4. D. Mowbray, "The Management Process," in *Epidemiology and Health,* ed. W.W. Holland and S. Gilderdale (London: Henry Kimpton Publishers, 1977), 155.

5. B.B. Lorgest, *Management Practices for the Health Professional* (2nd. ed.) (Reston, Va.: Reston Publishing Company, Inc. 1980), 39-49.

6. P.H. Levin, "On Decisions and Decision-Making," *Public Administration* 50, no. 19 (1972).

7. Mowbray, "Management Process," 157.

8. H. Mintzberg, "Organizational Power and Goals: A Skeletal Theory," in *Strategic Management: A New View of Business Policy and Planning,* ed. D.E. Schendel and C.W. Hofer (Boston: Little, Brown and Co., 1979), 64-80.

9. Mowbray, "Management Process," 155-156.

10. R.L. Ackoff, *A Concept of Corporate Planning* (New York: Wiley Interscience Publications, 1970), 1.

11. J. Friedmann, "A Conceptual Model for the Analysis of Planning Behavior," *Administrative Science Quarterly* 12 (1967): 225.

12. J. Roeber, "Objectives, Forecasts, and Plans," *The New York Times,* July 12, 1971.

13. R. Cyert and J.G. March, *A Behavioral Theory of the Firm* (Englewood Cliffs, N.J.: Prentice-Hall, Inc., 1963).

14. H.A. Simon, *Administrative Behavior* (New York: The Macmillan Company, 1957).

15. C.E. Lindblom, "The Science of Muddling Through," *Public Administration Review* 19 (1959): 79-99.

16. D. Braybrooke and C.E. Lindblom, *A Strategy of Decision* (Glencoe, Ill.: The Free Press, 1970), 268.

17. M.Q. Patton, *Utilization-Focused Evaluation* (Beverly Hills, Calif.: Sage Publications, Inc., 1978), 127-128.

18. G.E. Alan Dever, *Community Health Analysis* (Rockville, Md.: Aspen Systems Corporation, 1980), 409.

19. Henrik L. Blum, *Planning for Health* (New York: Human Sciences Press, Inc. 1981), 462.

20. H.G. Hicks, *The Management of Organizations: A Systems and Human Resources Approach* (New York: McGraw-Hill Book Company, 1976), 602.

21. Blum, *Planning,* 14.

22. R. Pineault, "La planification des services de santé: Une perspective épidémiologique," *Administration Hospitalière et Sociale,* Mars-Avril 1979, 6.

23. A. Donabedian, *Aspects of Medical Care Administration: Specifying Requirements for Health Care* (Cambridge, Mass.: Harvard University Press, 1973), 62.

24. E.G. Knox, ed., *Epidemiology in Health Care Planning* (Oxford, England: Oxford University Press, 1979), 47.

25. Donabedian, *Aspects of Medical Care,* 58-207.

26. Blum, *Planning,* 88-95.

27. Robin E. MacStravic, *Determining Health Needs* (Ann Arbor, Mich.: Health Administration Press, 1978), 268.

28. Carol Clemenhagen and Francois Champagne, "Program Planning in a Small Community Health Care Setting," *Health Care Management Review* 7, no. 1 (Winter 1982): 47-55.

29. R.A. Bell et al., "Service Utilization, Social Indicator, and Citizen Survey Approaches to Human Service Need Assessment," in *Evaluation of Human Service Programs,* ed. C.C. Attkisson et al. (New York: Academic Press, Inc., 1978), 256.

30. L.M. Siegel, C.C. Attkisson, and L.G. Carson, "Need Identification and Program Planning in the Community Context," in *Evaluation of Human Services Programs,* ed. C.C. Attkisson et al. (New York: Academic Press, Inc., 1978), 226-227.

31. Committee on Health Sciences, *Science for Health Services,* Science Council of Canada Report No. 22 (Ottawa: Science Council of Canada, 1974), 144.

32. Siegel, Attkisson, and Carson, "Need Identification," 227.

33. P.H. Rossi, H.E. Freeman, and S.R. Wright, *Evaluation: A Systematic Approach* (Beverly Hills, Calif.: Sage Publications, 1979), 108.

34. MacStravic, *Determining Health Needs,* 64-66.

35. L.W. Chambers, C.A. Woodward, and C. Dok, *Guide to Health Needs Assessment: A Critique of Available Sources of Health Care Information* (Ottawa: Canadian Public Health Association, 1980), 7.

36. Ibid, 9-10.

37. Siegel, Attkisson, and Carson, "Need Identification," 229.

38. Rossi, Freeman, and Wright, *Evaluation.*

39. A.L. Delbecq, A.H. Van de Ven, and D.H. Gustafson, *Group Techniques for Program Planning* (Glenview, Ill.: Scott Foresman and Company, 1977), 66.

40. Siegel, Attkisson, and Carson, "Need Identification," 247.

41. Delbecq, Van de Ven, and Gustafson, *Group Techniques,* 10.

42. Ibid, 11.

43. Siegel, Attkisson, and Carson, "Need Identification," 230.

44. MacStravic, *Determining Health Needs,* 58.

45. Henrik L. Blum, "Does Health Planning Work Anywhere, And If So, Why?" *American Journal of Health Planning* 3, no. 3 (July 1978): 43.

46. Ibid., 44.

47. Donabedian, *Aspects of Medical Care,* 164.

48. J.H.F. Brotherston, et al., "Planning of Health Services and the Health Team," in *The Theory and Practice of Public Health,* ed. W. Hobson (London: Oxford University Press, 1979), 634.

49. D.O. Anderson, "Priorities and Planning," in Holland and Gilderdale, *Epidemiology and Health,* 178.

50. Donabedian, *Aspects of Medical Care,* 165.

51. Ibid., 164-192. (See also Pineault, "La planification," 6.)

52. Donabedian, *Aspects of Medical Care,* 169.

53. Pineault, "La planification," 8.

54. Knox, *Epidemiology in Health Care,* 124.

55. Pineault, "La planification," 12.

56. D.P. Byar et al., "Randomized Clinical Trials: Perspectives on Some Recent Ideas," *The New England Journal of Medicine* 295 (1976): 74-80.

57. W. Spitzer, "What Is a Health Care Trial?" *Journal of the American Medical Association* 233 (1975): 161-163.

Epidemiological Measurement

RATES AND POPULATION AT RISK

An important aspect of any scientific endeavor, including epidemiology, is measurement. Measurement is an instrument to be used to answer research questions, not an end in itself. As seen in Chapter 3, health care managers can use epidemiology to answer questions relating to the type and amount of services they should offer to their catchment population as well as to the impact of these services. More precisely, this means using epidemiological principles, methods, and techniques to identify health problems, to determine priorities, and to evaluate services. This chapter examines the epidemiological measures appropriate to these tasks.

As noted in Chapter 2, epidemiology, public health, and health services management involve the consideration of both a numerator and a denominator. The numerator is the number of cases, deaths, services, and so forth and the denominator is the population from which the numerator is taken. The denominator generally is known as the population at risk of having something happen that would make such persons part of the numerator. A rate is simply the mathematical expression for the relation between the numerator and the denominator, together with some specification of time. For example:

$$\frac{\begin{array}{l}\textit{Number of events}\\ \textit{(cases, deaths, services)}\\ \textit{in a specified time period}\end{array}}{\begin{array}{l}\textit{Population at risk of}\\ \textit{experiencing the event}\end{array}} \times 10^{n}$$

The purpose of the multiplier (10^{n}) is simply to produce a rate that is manageable.[1] The number of events often is so small, in relation to the denominator, that it is easier to express the numbers per 1,000, 10,000, or other population.

Rates serve another important purpose. Epidemiological measurement, like all others, depends upon comparison.[2] Rates make possible a comparison of the number of events between populations and at different times. Numbers then are converted into rates to generate comparable indexes.

For example, if the number of deaths for two different groups of people or for a group at two different times are compared, the number may differ only because the size of the population at risk differs. By converting to a rate, such as deaths per 100,000 persons, the size effect is removed and the rates become comparable indexes.

GUIDELINES FOR USING RATES

Rates should be used and interpreted with caution. Some comments are warranted in this regard.

The Ecological Fallacy

This consists of generalizing the data collected in a particular area to all the individuals living in that area, associating an indicator with persons who were not included in its calculation, or making assertions about one unit of analysis based on the examination of another.

Babbie[3] gives several examples:

- Suppose data showed that counties whose voters were relatively young gave a female candidate a greater proportion of their votes than did counties with voters of older average age. It would be tempting to conclude that young voters were more likely to vote for the female candidate than were older voters, that age affected support for the woman. Such a conclusion would run the risk of committing the ecological fallacy, since it might have been the older voters in those "young" counties who voted for the woman.

- Similarly, if the data showed that crime rates were higher in cities having large black populations, they might not show whether the crimes actually were committed by blacks.

- If it were found that cerebrovascular disease rates were higher in a county with a large white population than one with a smaller white population, it still could not be known that whites actually had a higher cerebrovascular death rate than blacks.

Guidelines for avoiding such problems include: (1) deriving indicators from a denominator that encompasses the entire population group, or most of it, and

(2) applying indicators with subgroup denominators only to the persons in that subgroup.

Variations in Base

These may cause some problems in comparing rates. A proportion (say 5/100) is multiplied by 100 to become a percent (5 percent), by 1,000 to become an infant mortality rate (of 50), or perhaps by 10,000 to become a disease rate (of 500). A rate must be accompanied by an indication of its base to be meaningful. A statement that "the rate has doubled" should be answered with the question, "Rate per what?"

False Association

This comes about by forgetting that rates apply to aggregates and not to individuals. A neighborhood may have a high unemployment rate and a high alcoholism rate, and statistical tests would show an association between these factors. Yet the unemployed and the imbibers could be two entirely different groups of people.

Variance of Rates with Small Denominators

Rates based on very large populations may be interpreted as fixed numbers for purposes of comparison. But as the population base beomes smaller, statistical variation becomes more prominent as an explanation of differences.

The rate has implications of a probabilistic or predictive statement. The statement that two infants died out of 75 born, for example, is simply a statement of fact. To convert this to an infant mortality rate of 26—meaning 26 deaths per 1,000 live births—is by implication a statement of a long-run trend or prediction. Yet, if during the following year only one infant died out of 75 born (again a statement of fact), the infant mortality rate is only 13. This so-called large decrease is a result of statistical variation, and the magnitude of the drop is exaggerated because of the use of a base of 1,000.

Yearly infant mortality rates have been used in recent years as an indicator for hospitals as to their overall rating from a qualitative point of view. However, interpretations of the resulting data are questionable. Before conclusions are drawn, a time series for individual hospitals should be examined to avoid the risk of judgment based on small denominators. In addition it is very difficult to determine the total population at risk for any one hospital.

The problem of small denominator rates arises in any statistical analysis where numbers are converted to percentages (rates per hundred). It is common practice to stratify data by age, race, morbidity, or other factors and to compare percentages of some phenomena for the different strata. The resulting data may be meaningless. Most statisticians use guidelines to determine when percentages should or should not be computed. For example, percentages may not be given for any cell with fewer than ten observations.

Rate Advantages and Disadvantages

Last year the rate of disease X in the town was 10/1,000, but this year, because of an extensive effort, the community managed to reduce it to 5/1,000. What impression would that leave?

What if it were said that the rate was reduced from 100/10,000 to 50/10,000? or from 1000/100,000 to 500/100,000? Or 10,000/1,000,000 to 5000/1,000,000?

Sooner or later, it would be realized that they all were the same. And that would be correct. But how much more impressive it seems to cut 10,000 cases by half than to cut 10 cases by half.

EPIDEMIOLOGICAL IDENTIFICATION OF PROBLEMS

The epidemiologic assessment of health problems, as input to the determination of priorities and to subsequent program planning, may include three main categories of indicators: mortality, morbidity, and risk factors.

Mortality

Although mortality is far from being an ideal measure of the health of a population, it often is the most easily available and accessible—if not the only—indicator that can be used readily by health service managers (in addition to statistics on health service utilization and demographic data, discussed in Chapters 9 and 10).

Crude Rates

The simplest mortality measure is the crude death rate (CDR), stated as the number of deaths per unit of population (usually 1,000). All of these rates concern the number of deaths occurring during a specified time period, usually one year. Thus:

$$CDR = \frac{Total\ Deaths}{Population\ at\ Risk} \times 1,000$$

For example, the crude death rate for Georgia (1978) is derived as follows:

$$CDR = \frac{43,147 \text{ deaths}}{5,056,100 \text{ population}} \times 1,000 = 8.5 \text{ deaths}/1,000 \text{ population}$$

Specific Rates

A rate can be made specific for sex, age, race, cause of death, or a combination of these. These specific rates (SR) are illustrated in Table 4-1. Such specific rates usually are needed for understanding the epidemiologic aspects of disease and population dynamics.[4]

As the table shows, death rates vary greatly by race, sex, and age. Specific rates allow health care managers to target their programs to the appropriate population subgroups. Similarly, age/cause, sex/cause, and race/cause rates bring an even more revealing and useful picture of the mortality patterns.

As can be seen in the data for Georgia (1978), there are wide variations in the death rates for cancer and motor vehicle accidents by age groups. Without much further analysis, health service managers can have an indication that any program to reduce the impact of motor vehicle accidents should be directed toward the teen and young adult population.

Two other specific rates of a slightly different nature also are often used by epidemiologists: the case fatality rate (CFR) and the proportionate mortality rate (PMR):

$$CFR_{(\%)} = \frac{\text{Deaths by cause}}{\begin{array}{c}\text{Number of individuals with}\\ \text{the specified disease}\\ \text{(cause)}\end{array}} \times 100$$

This rate represents the risk of dying during a definite period of time for individuals who have the particular disease.[5] Case fatality rates also can be made specific for age, sex, race, or any other factors considered important.

The proportionate mortality rate (PMR) represents the proportion of all deaths resulting from a specific cause. It is useful because it permits estimation of the proportion of lives to be saved by reducing or eradicating a given cause of death. The PMR may be derived as follows:

$$PMR_{(\%)} = \frac{\text{Deaths by cause}}{\text{Total deaths}} \times 100$$

Although most authors refer to it as such, the PMR is not really a rate but a ratio, since the denominator is not the population at risk. A ratio usually compares the number of persons in a population with a specific characteristic to the number of persons in that same population without that characteristic.[6] Contrary to a rate, a ratio, therefore cannot be viewed as a probability statement. A hospital manager

Table 4-1 Specific Death Rates (SR)

Definition	Georgia, 1978
$SR_{race} = \dfrac{\text{Total deaths by race}}{\text{Population by race}} \times 1{,}000$	$SR_{white} = \dfrac{30{,}640}{3{,}797{,}500} \times 1{,}000 = 8.1$
	$SR_{black} = \dfrac{12{,}507}{1{,}258{,}600} \times 1{,}000 = 9.9$
$SR_{sex} = \dfrac{\text{Total deaths by sex}}{\text{Population by sex}} \times 1{,}000$	$SR_{male} = \dfrac{23{,}908}{2{,}445{,}100} \times = 9.8$
	$SR_{female} = \dfrac{19{,}239}{2{,}611{,}100} \times 1{,}000 = 7.4$
$SR_{age} = \dfrac{\text{Total deaths by age}}{\text{Population by age}} \times 1{,}000$	$SR_{10\text{-}14} = \dfrac{183}{448{,}800} \times 1{,}000 = 0.4$
	$SR_{40\text{-}44} = \dfrac{1{,}096}{269{,}700} \times 1{,}000 = 4.1$
$SR_{cause} = \dfrac{\text{Total deaths by cause}}{\text{Total population}} \times 100{,}000$	$SR_{cancer} = \dfrac{7{,}867}{5{,}056{,}100} \times 100{,}000 = 155.6$
	$SR_{mva^*} = \dfrac{1{,}523}{5{,}056{,}100} \times 100{,}000 = 3.1$
$SR_{age/ \atop cause} = \dfrac{\text{Total deaths by age and cause}}{\text{Population by age}} \times 100{,}000$	$SR_{15\text{-}24 \atop cancer} = \dfrac{68}{967{,}500} \times 100{,}000 = 7.0$
	$SR_{45\text{-}54 \atop cancer} = \dfrac{1{,}007}{502{,}100} \times 100{,}000 = 200.6$
	$SR_{15\text{-}24 \atop mva^*} = \dfrac{512}{967{,}500} \times 100{,}000 = 52.9$
	$SR_{45\text{-}54 \atop mva^*} = \dfrac{131}{502{,}100} \times 100{,}000 = 26.1$

*mva = motor vehicle accidents.

might calculate the proportion of deaths and/or operations for heart patients. This statistic compared with other such data would provide the manager with essential planning data.

Mortality measures traditionally used as health status indicators are shown in Table 4-2.

Adjusted or Standardized Rates

As stated previously, one of the purposes of epidemiologic measurement is the comparison between groups and time. Crude and specific death rates do not, however, lend themselves to such comparisons since they ignore the fact that different populations have different compositions, mostly in terms of age structure. Similarly, the age composition of a population varies in time, making the use of crude and specific rates more hazardous for comparison purposes.

The adjustment or standardization of rates is a statistical procedure that removes the effect of differences in composition.[7] Because of its marked effect on mortality (and morbidity), age is the variable for adjustment used most commonly. Sometimes other variables may need to be adjusted, instead of or in addition to age, such as sex and race, if the composition of the population to be compared is known or suspected to be dissimilar with regard to these variables.

Two basic methods of rate adjustment or standardization are the direct and the indirect. Although the following discussion deals with age adjustment, other variables can be adjusted by the same methods.

Direct Method: The direct method of age adjustment involves the application of the age-specific rates observed in each of the populations being compared to an arbitrarily chosen structure called the standard population. A standard population can be that of the United States, of a given state, or any other known population structure, including one or a combination of those being compared.

For example, a "U.S. Standard Million" sometimes is used, representing the composition of a hypothetical population of 1 million people having the same proportion in each age group as the United States has as a whole. Thus, in essence, the death rates in the populations to be compared are being recalculated by assuming that they have the same age distribution as the standard population's.

To illustrate, let it be said that the populations to be compared could have expected *x* and *y* numbers of deaths if they both had a "standard" age structure; that is, the same age distribution as the standard population selected. For instance, between 1971 and 1980, County A in Georgia had a death rate from acute myocardial infarction of 203 per 100,000 population. For the same period, the state rate was 152.7 per 100,000. This difference may result from a different age structure. To take away the effects of the age distribution, it is appropriate to age-adjust the county rate to the standard (state) age distribution. The direct method of age adjustment is shown in Table 4-3.

Table 4-2 Mortality Measures Most Used As Health Status Indicators

No.	Description of Indicator	Numerator	Denominator	Expressed per Number at Risk
1.	**Crude Death Rate** Crude; specific for age, race, sex, socioeconomic area, etc.	Number of deaths reported during a given time interval	Estimated midinterval population	1,000
2.	**Cause-Specific Death Rate** Crude by cause; specific for age, race, sex, socioeconomic area, etc.	Number of deaths assigned to a specific cause during a given time interval	Estimated midinterval population	100,000
3.	**Proportional Mortality Ratio** Crude by cause; specific for age, race, sex, socioeconomic area, etc.	Number of deaths assigned to a specific cause during a given time interval	Number of deaths from all causes reported during the same interval	100 (%)
4.	**Case Fatality Rate** Crude; specific for age, race, sex, socioeconomic area, etc.	Number of deaths assigned to a specific disease during a given time interval	Number of new cases of that disease reported during the same time interval	100 (%)
5.	(a). **Fetal Death Rate I** Crude; specific for age of mother, race, socioeconomic area, etc.	Number of fetal deaths of 28 weeks' or more gestation reported during a given time interval	Number of fetal deaths of 28 weeks' or more gestation reported during the same interval, plus number of live births during same interval	1,000
	(b). **Fetal Death Rate II** Crude; specific for age of mother, race, socioeconomic area, etc.	Number of fetal deaths of 20 weeks' or more gestation reported during a given time interval	Number of fetal deaths of 20 weeks' or more gestation reported during the same interval, plus number of live births during same interval	1,000

Table 4-2 continued

No.	Description of Indicator	Numerator	Denominator	Expressed per Number at Risk
6.	(a). **Fetal Death Ratio I** Crude; specific for age of mother, race, socioeconomic area, etc.	Number of fetal deaths of 28 weeks' or more gestation during a given time interval	Number of live births reported during the same time interval	1,000
	(b). **Fetal Death Ratio II** Crude; specific for age of mother, race, socioeconomic area, etc.	Number of fetal deaths of 20 weeks' or more gestation reported during a given time interval	Number of live births reported during the same time interval	1,000
7.	(a). **Perinatal Mortality Rate I** Crude; specific for age of mother, race, socioeconomic area, etc.	Number of fetal deaths of 28 weeks' or more gestation reported during a given time interval plus the reported number of infant deaths under 7 days of life during the same time interval	Number of fetal deaths of 28 weeks' or more gestation reported during the same time interval plus the number of live births occurring during the same time interval	1,000
	(b). **Perinatal Mortality Rate II** Crude; specific for age of mother, sex, socioeconomic area, etc.	Number of fetal deaths of 20 weeks' or more gestation reported during a given time interval plus the reported number of infant deaths under 28 days of life during the same time interval	Number of fetal deaths of 20 weeks' or more gestation reported during the same time interval plus the number of live births reported during the same time interval	1,000
8.	**Infant Mortality Rate** Crude; specific for race, sex, socioeconomic area, birth weight, cause of death, etc.	Number of deaths under one year of age reported during a given time interval	Number of live births reported during the same time interval	1,000

Table 4-2 continued

No.	Description of Indicator	Numerator	Denominator	Expressed per Number at Risk
9.	**Neonatal Mortality Rate** Crude; specific for race, sex, socioeconomic area, birth weight, cause of death, etc.	Number of deaths under 28 days of age reported during a given time interval	Number of live births reported during the same time interval	1,000
10.	**Postneonatal Mortality Rate** Crude; specific for race, sex, socioeconomic area, cause of death, etc.	Number of deaths from 28 days of age up to, but not including, one year, reported during a given time interval	Number of live births reported during the same time interval	1,000
11.	**Maternal Mortality Rate** Crude; specific for age of mother, race, socioeconomic area, etc.	Number of deaths assigned to causes related to pregnancy during a given time interval	Number of live births reported during the same time interval	10,000

Source: Reprinted from *Descriptive Statistics, Rates, Ratios, Proportions, and Indices,* U.S. Department of Health, Education, and Welfare, Public Health Service, Center for Disease Control, Atlanta, 1977, 3–8.

This means that the age-adjusted death rate from acute myocardial infarction is 182.24 per 100,000 in the county. This still is higher than the state rate but much less so than before age adjustment. Consequently, some of the difference between the state and county rates can be attributed to a different age distribution.

Indirect Method: The direct method of rate adjustment requires a knowledge of the age-specific death rates in all populations to be compared. If these age-specific rates are not known for the populations in which age adjustments are desired, or if the numbers are too small to produce stable rates, the indirect method of standardization (or adjustment) can be used.[8]

This indirect method is, in a sense, the reverse process: where the direct method applies the rates from the populations to be compared to a standard population structure, the indirect method applies the rates from the standard population (that is, a standard set of rates) to the distributions of the different populations to be compared.

Table 4-3 Direct Age Adjustment of Rates

Age Group	Age-Specific County Rate Per 100,000	State Population (1971–80)	Proportion of State Population	County Rates Times Proportion*
20–29	2.6	8,354,955	.1716	.45
30–44	45.1	9,015,340	.1851	8.35
45–59	312.0	7,080,165	.1454	45.36
60–74	832.5	4,715,510	.0968	80.61
>74	1,514.0	1,526,865	.0314	47.47
Total State Population		48,696,875		182.24 (Age-Adjusted Rate)

*The age-adjusted rate is the summation of this column.

In applying these standard rates to the populations of interest, it is possible to estimate the number of deaths (once again, the expected deaths) that would have occurred in these groups if the people who make them up had been dying at the same (age-specific) rate as those in the standard population. Addition of the age-specific expected deaths produces a total of expected deaths in each population that can be compared to the total observed deaths. This comparison usually is done by calculating the standardized mortality ratio (SMR), as follows:

$$SMR = \frac{Observed\ Deaths}{Expected\ Deaths} \times 100$$

If the SMR is greater than 100, it means that more deaths occurred in the population of interest than would be expected, based on the rates in the standard population. Similarly, a ratio less than 100 indicates fewer deaths than expected. For example, an SMR of 140 indicates 40 percent excess deaths as compared to the standard population, whereas an SMR of 85 indicates 15 percent fewer deaths.

Using the same example as before, the indirect age adjustment method of the rates in County A is as shown in Table 4-4.

The indirect age-adjusted rate in the county is 170.54 per 100,000. To calculate the SMR, it is necessary to use the actual number of deaths in the state (instead of the death rate). The product of those actual deaths times the ratio of the county population to the state population in each age group gives the expected number of deaths in the county in each age group, as in Table 4-5.

This means that if the county had the same age distribution as the state, 2,453 deaths from acute myocardial infarction could have been expected. The actual number of deaths was 2,912. Thus the age-adjusted SMR is derived as follows:

Table 4-4 Indirect Age Adjustment Method

Age Group	Age-Specific State Rate Per 100,000	County Population (1971–80)	Proportion of County Population	State Rates Times Proportion*
20–29	1.5	230,890	.1609	.24
30–44	27.2	246,305	.1716	4.67
45–59	217.4	230,460	.1606	34.91
60–74	680.9	156,880	.1093	74.44
>74	1,588.1	50,860	.0354	56.28
Total State Population		1,435,035		170.54 (Age-Adjusted Rate)

*The age-adjusted rate is the summation of this column.

$$SMR = \frac{2,912}{2,453} \times 100 = 118.7$$

The age-adjusted SMR indicates that, even in controlling for the age structure, there were proportionately 18.7 percent more deaths from acute myocardial infarction in the county than in the state.

The SMR has at least two distinct advantages over the direct method of rate adjustment.

First, knowledge of the age distribution of deaths in the population of interest is not required. Only the number of persons in each age group in this population and the age-specific death rate in the standard population are necessary. Since it often is much easier to obtain the data from the standard population (for example, the United States as a whole, or an individual state) than from a smaller population, this could be a major advantage.

Table 4-5 Application of SMR Calculations

Age Group	Deaths in State (D)	County Population (A)	State Population (B)	Expected Deaths (D × A/B)
20–29	125	230,890	8,354,955	3.45
30–44	2,451	246,305	9,015,340	66.96
45–59	15,390	230,460	7,080,165	500.95
60–74	32,110	156,880	4,715,510	1,068.27
>74	24,429	50,860	1,526,865	813.73
				2,453.36

Second, the SMR makes comparison among diseases much easier, since it is a ratio whose value is directly comparable across diseases. On the other hand, the results of direct standardization are adjusted rates with comparisons having direct meaning only for a given cause of death or disease.

Table 4-6 shows the advantages and disadvantages of crude, specific, and adjusted rates when used as health status indicators.

Morbidity and Risk Factors

Although mortality statistics are the most often used and most easily available health indicators, there can be no doubt they offer only an incomplete picture of the health problems of a population. For this reason, data on morbidity, showing the spread of disease, discomfort, and disability—both acute and chronic—also are necessary.

Incidence Rate

Morbidity data usually are presented through incidence and prevalence rates. An incidence rate (IR) indicates the rate at which people without a particular

Table 4-6 Advantages and Disadvantages of Using Crude, Specific, and Adjusted Rates for Health Status Indicators

Health Status Indicators	Advantages	Disadvantages
Crude rates	Easy to calculate. Summary rates. Widely used for international comparisons (despite limitations).	Because population groups vary in age, sex, race, etc., the differences in crude rates are not directly interpretable.
Specific rates	Applied to homogeneous subgroups. The detailed rates are useful for epidemiological and public health purposes.	Comparisons can be cumbersome if many subgroups are calculated for two or more populations.
Adjusted rates	Represent a summary rate. The differences in composition of groups are reviewed allowing unbiased comparison.	Not true rates (fictional). Magnitude of rates is dependent upon the standard million population chosen. Trends in subgroups can be masked.

Source: Adapted from *Epidemiology: An Introductory Text* by J.S. Mausner and A.K. Bahn with permission of W.B. Saunders Company, ©1974, 138.

disease develop it during a specified period of time; e.g., the number of new cases of a disease over a period of time, usually one year.[9] To illustrate:

$$IR = \frac{\textit{Number of new cases of a disease over a period of time}}{\textit{Population at risk (at midperiod)}} \times 1,000$$

Prevalence Rate

A prevalence rate (PR) measures the number of people in a population who have a particular disease. The point prevalence rate indicates the number of people who have the disease at a given point in time while the period prevalence rate (less commonly used) measures the number who had the disease over a period of time. These rates may be calculated as follows:

$$Point \; PR = \frac{\textit{Number of existing cases of a disease at a point in time}}{\textit{Total population}}$$

$$Period \; PR = \frac{\textit{Number of existing cases of a disease during a period}}{\textit{Total population}}$$

Period prevalence is constructed at a specific time plus new cases (incidence) and recurrences during a succeeding time period.[10] Both incidence and prevalence rates should be made specific for age, sex, race, or other important factors. They also can be adjusted by the same methods as for mortality rates. Incidence and prevalence rates obviously are closely related. Prevalence is a function of incidence and of duration of a disease (D). Thus:

$$PR = IR \times D$$

Similarly, mortality (crude death rate) is a function of the incidence and the case fatality rate:

$$CDR = IR \times CFR$$

Both incidence and prevalence rates are important and fundamental tools in assessing health problems of a population. The incidence rate is a direct indicator of risk: a high incidence rate indicates a high risk of disease. The prevalence rate can be used by health service managers as an indicator of workload or need for personnel and facilities. Contrary to the incidence rate, the prevalence rate does not necessarily reflect risk. A high prevalence may be the result of increased survival because of improved medical care or behavioral or environmental changes. Similarly, a low prevalence may reflect either a rapid fatal process or rapid and effective care.

Health service managers also need to look at risk factors, or phenomena, within each of the four dimensions of the health field: biology, life style, environment, and health care organization. (Chapters 8 and 9, on health service utilization and demography, respectively, deal more specifically with factors of biology and health care organization.) Life style and environmental factors can be described in a way similar to diseases—for example, an incidence rate for cigarette smoking or drug consumption, or the prevalence of rats or other pests presenting disease risks.

Data on morbidity and risk factors should be used as often as possible. The main problem, however, lies in obtaining the figures. Contrary to mortality data, specifics on morbidity often are not routinely reported and collected. Ways of obtaining information on morbidity and risk factors include using data collected by insurance plans, hospitals, employers, schools, or any other providers or third party organizations; using data from special surveys such as the United States National Health Survey, the Canadian Health Survey, the World Health Organization, those conducted by universities, health planning agencies, or others; and by conducting a special survey. That last alternative, of course, is complex and costly. Data concerning infectious diseases are available from the U.S. Public Health Service Centers for Disease Control as well as from state and county health departments.

Hospital Morbidity Data

Morbidity data that indicate various diagnostic categories are available in hospital records and should provide a particularly useful source of information for detecting changes in disease patterns. This source of information can be of major importance to the health service manager or administrator in a hospital or other health care facility.

The problem of time lag related to a discharge diagnosis is important to this aspect of morbidity data from hospital records. In certain situations, the admission diagnosis could be used by the health service manager for the investigation of the disease patterns. In both situations, however, the critical component is the lack of an appropriate denominator for determining population-at-risk. The numerator would be the number of cases categorized by diagnostic group. The difficulty comes when one tries to compute rates without really knowing the true population-at-risk. If the market area for a hospital is well defined, then it may be possible to utilize the population within that market area for the population-at-risk. At no time should a health care manager calculate at-risk rates using the denominator of the in-hospital population. A more likely statistic at that point in time would be a Proportionate Mortality Rate (PMR).

Various problems can be expected when estimating the incidence and prevalence of various diseases in the hospital setting. Basing estimates on hospital admissions will be less valid for chronic diseases than for those characterized as acute illness. Using in-hospital data will result in losing many cases of acute and minor illness that are diagnosed and treated in physicians' offices, outpatient departments, or ambulatory care settings. Thus, the concept of denominators is much more critical in the case of acute and minor illness than in the chronic case.

Because of these concerns, hospital records have been underutilized as a valuable source of information. To overcome some of these concerns, hospitals in a metropolitan or other common market area could join together in a common computer service. It would then be possible to have a systematic collection of admission and discharge diagnostic data. There are national systems and some state hospital associations that are currently utilizing this approach. The result of such endeavors is an *epidemiological surveillance system,* which provides many opportunities for the hospital to do effective health services planning and management.

Mortality and morbidity data may be referred to as health status indicators. A health status indicator is a single, unidimensional measure obtained from a single component (variable). Two or more variables also can be combined into a health status index: a composite measure summarizing data from two or more components (variables). Since an index allows the inclusion and weighting of the many dimensions of health (physical, mental, social), theoretically, it is preferable to single indicators. The construction of an index, however, requires elaborate statistical techniques and methodologies. Although this is an intense and burgeoning field of research, results that could be applied on a small scale by health service managers have yet to be described.[11, 12, 13]

THE SIGNIFICANCE OF RATES

The epidemiological approach to the determination of health problems rests on the comparison of mortality and morbidity rates in the population of concern to the health service manager with some other standard or target rate. The identification of a problem has meaning only in relation to some standard. A standard, then, refers to the value associated with a particular indicator (criterion) that is acceptable to the decision makers.

For example, an infant mortality rate of 20 per 1,000 has marginal meaning by itself. It is necessary to know something about the variability or stability of this rate. This rate then must be compared with an infant mortality rate in another geographical area or another time period or with some arbitrarily set standard or target value.

When comparing rates, the issue arises as to how much of a difference or deviation from the standard is significant. This involves three factors (discussed next): the variability of rates, the significance of the difference between two rates, and the significance of excess deaths.

The Variability of Rates

An observed mortality or morbidity rate cannot be taken as a true rate for an area. An observed rate is an estimate of the true rate and, as is the case with any estimate, is subject to chance variation. As Kleinman points out, the rationale is that the number of deaths in an area, for example, varies by chance depending upon the size of the population and the probability of death—the true mortality rate.[14] As the size of the population increases, the chance component becomes less important and the observed mortality rate becomes a better estimate of the true rate. For example, if an area has few deaths, the observed death rate may be very different from the true rate. Consequently, the variability of rates must be assessed. This can be done easily through basic statistical measures.

X = raw scores

$\overline{X}$ = the mean of a sample

$\sum$ = the sum of

Standard Deviation

This is the most important measure of dispersion about the mean value of a distribution and forms the basis for most statistical analysis. It consists of the square root of the sum of the squared deviations of each value from the mean, divided by the number of observations, or:

$$S = \sqrt{\left[\sum_{i=1}^{n} (X_i - \overline{X})^2\right] / n}$$

also: $S = \sqrt{\dfrac{\sum x^2}{n}}$

where: S = standard deviation

$(X_i - \overline{X})^2$ = subtract the mean value $\overline{X}$ from the value of X_i, then squared

n = number of observations

One unique property of the standard deviation in the normal distribution is that 68 percent of the observed values will fall within one standard deviation on either side of the mean, 95 percent within about two standard deviations, and 99 percent within three standard deviations. As is shown later, this property has important consequences for testing hypotheses and significance levels through statistical analysis.

$\overline{X} = \dfrac{\sum X}{n}$ $\sum x^2 = \sum X^2 - \dfrac{(\sum X)^2}{n}$

[sum of (squares) of deviation scores]

When measuring a population factor such as an infant mortality rate, it is helpful to estimate the true rate for the population. Since every value in the population cannot be measured, however, some smaller number of measurements is used and, from these, the true mean is estimated. Thus, when a population mean or some other population parameter is to be determined, a small sample of the total population is taken and the true population mean estimated from the sample. If all possible samples of a given size were taken from the same population, the result would be a distribution of sample means with the shape of a normal distribution.

Regardless of the shape of the population distribution, however, the distribution of the sample means will be about normal. This is expressed in the central limit theorem, which states that for almost all populations the sampling distribution of the means will be distributed about normally, given a sufficient sample size. Sufficient sample size generally is considered to be 30 or more elements. This theorem allows inferences to be drawn about population means and mortality rates from information extracted from samples in time or space.

Like a population distribution, a distribution of sample means also involves a variance. The variance of the sample mean is equal to the variance calculated from a sample, divided by the size of the sample used to calculate the variance:

$$S_{\bar{x}}^2 = S^2/n$$

STANDARD
ERROR
of
the MEAN

The square root of the variance of the sample mean is called the standard error of the mean, denoted:

$$S_{\bar{x}} = \sqrt{S^2/n} = S / \sqrt{(n)}$$

Where: $S_{\bar{x}}$ = standard error of the mean
S = standard deviation
$\sqrt{}$ = square root
n = number of observations

The standard error of the mean is the statistic that permits statements to be made regarding population estimates of the true mean with specified levels of confidence.

Similarly, the standard error of a rate is the standard deviation of the (theoretical) sampling distribution of the rate. The standard error is used to estimate the range within which the true population lies. This range is called the confidence interval, and the probability with which it is asserted that the true population rate is contained within that interval is called the degree of confidence.

The value most commonly used for the degree of confidence is .95, or 95 percent. This means users can be 95 percent confident that the true rate lies within the calculated confidence interval. To look at it another way, there is 95 percent probability that the confidence interval includes the true rate and 5 percent probability that it does not. When chance of error equals 5 percent and is not acceptable, then the 99 percent confidence interval is commonly used.

Confidence Intervals

The calculation of the confidence interval is based on the assumption that the distribution of the observed rates can be approximated by the standard normal curve. Elementary texts on statistics discuss the theoretical aspects of the construction of confidence intervals and of inferential statistics.[15, 16] This analysis is limited to three methods for the construction of confidence intervals.

Method 1: If a rate for a population at a given time has been computed, it can be considered a sample estimate of the true rate, or as a sample in time or space, thereby allowing confidence interval estimations to be used. An estimate of the true rate reflects the true rate plus random error. To construct a confidence interval for the rate, the following formula is used:[17]

> 95 percent confidence limits:
> $$\text{Upper limit} = 1,000/n[d + 1.96 \sqrt{(d)}]$$
> $$\text{Lower limit} = 1,000/n[d - 1.96 \sqrt{(d)}]$$

where: d = number of deaths upon which rate is based
$\quad\quad\quad n$ = denominator of rate (i.e., the target population)

Similarly, the 99 percent confidence limits are:

$$\frac{1,000}{n} [d \pm 2.58 \sqrt{(d)}]$$

The step-by-step procedure for calculating the 95 percent confidence interval is shown in Exhibit 4-1. For the 99 percent confidence interval, 1.96 is replaced with 2.58. If the death rate is greater than 100 per 1,000, $\sqrt{(d)}$ is replaced with $\sqrt{d[1-(d/n)]}$. If the rate is of some base other than 1,000 (10,000 or 100,000), this base is exchanged for 1,000 (above).

The procedure for calculating 95 percent confidence intervals using Method 1 is illustrated in Exhibit 4-2. The confidence interval calculated there shows that it is possible to be 95 percent confident that the true death rate lies between 6.46 and 8.88 deaths per 1,000.

Method 2: A 95 percent confidence interval for more than 30 observations also can be derived from the following formula:

$$CI = p \pm 1.96 \sqrt{[(p \times q)/n]}$$

where: CI = confidence interval
p = the rate
q = $(1-p)$
n = the population for the rate

To calculate the confidence interval:

1. Divide the rate (p) by 1,000 to put it on a per-person basis.
2. Multiply the rate (p) by 1 minus the rate (q): $p \times q$.
3. Divide the product of $p \times q$ by the population for the rate (n): $(p \times q)/n$.
4. Find the square root for the preceding quotient: $\sqrt{[(p \times q)/n]}$.
5. Multiply the preceding square root by 1.96. That is: $1.96 \times \sqrt{[(p \times q)/n]}$. (Multiply the product by the number used to get the rate to a per-person basis.)
6. To find the two specified confidence limits, add the preceding product to the rate for the high limit and subtract the product from the rate for the low limit. Thus, the confidence interval = rate $\pm 1.96 \sqrt{[(p \times q)/n]}$.

The procedure for calculating 95 percent confidence intervals using Method 2 is illustrated in Exhibit 4-3.

Method 3: The third and simplest method to calculate the confidence interval approximates the standard error of the rate. The standard error (SE) of a rate can be calculated easily:

$$SE = \frac{r}{\sqrt{d}}$$

where: r = the rate
d = observed number of deaths (upon which the rate is based)

The 95 percent confidence interval is constructed using the following formula:

$$CI_{(95\%)} = \text{rate} \pm (1.96 \times SE)$$

The 99 percent confidence interval would simply be:

$$CI_{(99\%)} = \text{rate} \pm (2.58 \times SE)$$

Exhibit 4-1 Calculating a Confidence Interval for a Population Rate

1.	Find the square root of d.	$\sqrt{d}$
2.	Multiply the square root of d by 1.96.	$1.96 \times \sqrt{d}$
3a.	For the upper limit, add d to $1.96\sqrt{d}$.	$d + 1.96\sqrt{d}$
b.	For the lower limit, subtract $1.96\sqrt{d}$ from d.	$d - 1.96\sqrt{d}$
4.	Divide 1,000 by n.	$1,000/n$
5a.	Multiply the quotient in # 4 $(1,000/n)$ by the sum in # 3a $(d + 1.96\sqrt{d})$ to get the upper limit.	
b.	Multiply the quotient in # 4 $(1,000/n)$ by the difference in # 3b to get the lower limit.	

Exhibit 4-2 Method 1 Procedure for Calculating 95 Percent Confidence
Interval for a Population Rate

In DeKalb County, Ga., in 1970, there were 155 deaths of white males aged 45 to 54 years. A total of 20,201 white males lived in the county. The death rate was 7.67 per 1,000:

$$(\frac{155}{20,201} \times 1,000)$$

The 95 percent confidence interval is:

$$CI = \frac{1,000}{n} [d \pm 1.96 \sqrt{d}]$$

1. $\sqrt{155} = 12.450$

2. $12.45 \times 1.96 = 24.402$

3a. $155 + 24.402 = 179.402$ (+ for high limit)

b. $155 - 24.402 = 130.598$ (− for low limit)

4. $1,000/20,201 = .0495$

5a. $.0495 \times 170.402 = 8.88$

b. $.0495 \times 130.598 = 6.46$

$$CI = 6.46 \text{ to } 8.88 \ (95\%)$$

Exhibit 4-3 Method 2 Procedure for Calculating a 95 Percent Confidence Interval for a Population Rate

---

Using the data for DeKalb County (Exhibit 4-2), the 95 percent confidence interval for the 1970 death rate among white males aged 45 to 54 is:

$$CI = p \pm 1.96 \sqrt{[(p \times q)/n]}$$

1. $7.67/1,000 = .00767$

2. $.00767 \times .99233 = .0076111$ (.99233 is obtained by subtracting .00767 from 1.00, as defined for q)

3. $.0076111/20,201 = .0000003$

4. $\sqrt{.0000003} = .0006138$

5. $1.96 \times .0006138 = .001203$ ($\times$ 1,000 = 1.20 (multiplying by 1,000 returns the rate to a per-1,000 population basis)

6. $7.67 + 1.20 = 8.87$ (high limit)
    $7.67 - 1.20 = 6.47$ (low limit)

$$CI = 6.47 \text{ to } 8.87$$

A step-by-step procedure to calculate the 95 percent confidence interval is as follows:

1. Find the square root of d: $\sqrt{d}$.
2. Calculate the standard error (SE): divide the rate (r) by the square root of d: ($\sqrt{d}$).
3. Multiply the SE by 1.96.
4. Add the preceding product to the rate for the high limit and subtract it for the low limit.

This procedure is illustrated in Exhibit 4-4.

The three methods described can be used to assess the variability of any rates, including the standardized mortality rate (SMR) and birth rates. Method 3 uses an approximation of the SE of a rate but it is the simplest and easiest to calculate and is more than adequate for use in health services management. Using Method 3, the SE of an SMR is:

$$SE = \frac{SMR}{\sqrt{d}}$$

where: d = number of observed deaths

and the SE of a birth rate (r) is:

$$SE = \frac{r}{\sqrt{b}}$$

where: b = number of births

Significance of Difference between Two Rates

When comparing a rate with an arbitrarily set standard, goal, or target value, the confidence interval for the observed rate (the rate to be compared with the standard) provides the significance of the difference: if the standard is included in the confidence interval of the observed rate, there is no significant difference at the level of confidence chosen.

The situation is somewhat more complex, however, when comparing rates of two different areas or of two different times for the same area. This requires a direct extension of the concept of a confidence interval. The objective is to determine whether a significant difference exists between the rates or whether the difference is caused solely by random effects. Different methods must be used depending upon whether or not the rates are independent.

Exhibit 4-4 Method 3 Procedure for Calculating a 95 Percent Confidence Interval for a Population Rate

Using the data from Exhibit 4-2:

1. $\sqrt{155}$ = 12.45

2. SE = 7.67/12.45 = .616

3. 1.96 × .616 = 1.21

4. 7.67 + 1.21 = 8.88 (high limit)

   7.67 − 1.21 = 6.46 (low limit)

   CI = 6.46 to 8.88

When Rates Are Independent

Two rates are said to be independent when they do not include any of the same observations or events (births, deaths, etc.) in their numerator. A death included in one death rate should not be included in a second rate. Thus, rates from overlapping time periods (e.g., from 1960 to 70 and 1965 to 75), or from geographical hierarchy (e.g., comparing a county rate to the one for the district or state it is in), are not independent. For example, independent rates are those from two different counties.

To determine whether there is a significant difference between two independent rates, the confidence interval for the ratio between the two rates, or the difference between the two independent rates is used.[18] The ratio between two rates is defined as:

$$R = r_1/r_2$$

where: R = ratio
r_1 = rate for Area 1 or Period 1
r_2 = rate for Area 2 or Period 2

The 95 percent confidence interval for the ratio (R) is defined as:

$$R \pm 1.96 \, R \, \sqrt{(1/d_1) + (1/d_2)}$$

where: d_1 = number of events (deaths, etc.) for Area 1 or Period 1 (i.e., the rate numerator)
d_2 = number of events for Area 2 or Period 2

To establish a significant difference, it must be determined whether the confidence interval contains one. If it does not, it can be stated that the two rates are significantly different. If the interval does contain one, it cannot be concluded that a significant difference exists. Kleinman gives the following example:[19]

Years	Number of Infant Deaths	Number of Live Births	Infant Mortality Rate per 1,000 Live Births
1961-65	200	5,000	40
1966-70	100	4,000	25
		$R = 40/25 = 1.6$	

The 95 percent confidence interval is:

$$1.96 \ R \ \sqrt{(1/d_1) + (1/d_2)} = 1.96 \ (1.6) \ \sqrt{(1/200) + (1/100)}$$

$$= 1.96 \ (1.6) \ (.1225) = .384$$

$$1.6 + .384 = 1.984 \ \text{(Upper limit)}$$

$$1.6 - .384 = 1.216 \ \text{(Lower limit)}$$

$$CI \ (95\%) = 1.216 \ \text{to} \ 1.984$$

Thus, the rate for 1961 to 1965 can be said, with 95 percent confidence, to be from 1.22 to 1.98 times the 1966 to 1970 rate. Since the interval does not contain one, there is a statistically significant difference in the area's infant mortality rate. On the other hand, if the interval did contain one, there would not be a statistically significant difference.

An alternate form of computing the 95 percent confidence interval for the ratio between two rates is to use the confidence intervals for each rate. If the confidence limit (CL) is defined as the value that is added to and subtracted from the rate to give the confidence interval, the formula is:

$$CL = 1.96 \times SE = 1.96 \times (r/\sqrt{d})$$

where: SE = standard error (see Method 3 for calculating a confidence interval)

The confidence interval for the ratio R, then, is:

$$CI = R \pm R \ \sqrt{\{[(CL_1/r_1)^2] + [(CL_2/r_2)^2]\}}$$

where: CL_1 = confidence level for rate 1
CL_2 = confidence level for rate 2
r_1, r_2 = rates for areas 1 and 2, respectively

In the previous example:

$$CL_1 = 1.96 \times (40/200) = 1.96 \times 2.828 = 5.54$$

$$CL_2 = 1.96 \times (25/100) = 1.96 \times 2.5 \ \ \ = 4.9$$

and:

$$CI = R \pm R \sqrt{(CL_1/r_1)^2 + (CL_2/r_2)^2}$$
$$= 1.6 \pm 1.6 \sqrt{(5.54/40)^2 + (4.9/100)^2}$$
$$= 1.6 \pm 1.6 \,(.147) = 1.6 \pm .235$$

$$\text{Upper limit} = 1.6 + .235 = 1.835$$
$$\text{Lower limit} = 1.6 - .235 = 1.365$$
$$CI = 1.365 \text{ to } 1.835$$

This confidence interval does not include one, which indicates that the two rates are significantly different at the 95 percent level. On the other hand, if the interval did contain one there would not be a statistically significant difference. The confidence interval (above) is slightly different from what would be obtained using the previous formula because in calculating the confidence limits through Method 3, an approximation of the standard error was used.

These two formulas for the construction of the confidence interval for the ratio between two independent rates are valid only when the rate in the denominator (r_2) is based on 100 or more events (deaths, etc.). An alternative way of testing the difference between two independent rates is to construct a confidence interval directly for the difference (and not for the ratio). The confidence interval for the difference between two independent rates $(D = r_1 - r_2)$ is given by:

$$D \pm \sqrt{CL_1^2 + CL_2^2}$$

where: D = difference between the two rates
CL_1, CL_2 = confidence limits for rates 1 and 2

The confidence limit (CL), then, is the value that is added to and subtracted from the rate to construct the confidence interval of the rate:

$$CL = 1.96 \times SE = 1.96 \times (r/\sqrt{d})$$

where d = number of deaths (for a death rate)

In this case, if the interval includes zero, it cannot be concluded that the difference between the two rates is significant. In the previous example:

$$D = r_1 - r_2 = 40 - 25 = 15$$

$$CL_1 = 5.54 \qquad CL_2 = 4.9$$

$$CI = D \pm CL_1{}^2 + CL_2{}^2$$

$$= 15 \pm 5.54^2 + 4.9^2$$

$$= 15 \pm 7.4$$

$$\text{Upper limit} = 15 + 7.4 = 22.4$$

$$\text{Lower limit} = 15 - 7.4 = 7.6$$

$$CL = 7.6 \text{ to } 22.4$$

The 95 percent confidence interval for the difference between the two rates ranges from 7.6 to 22.4. Since this interval does not include zero, there is 95 percent confidence that the difference between the two rates is significant.

Kleinman presents the following example:[20]

	Santa Cruz, California	DeKalb County, Georgia
Population (*n*), white males, 45-54	6,051	20,201
Number of deaths (*d*)	63	155
Death rate per 1,000	10.41	7.67

The confidence limits (95 percent) are as follows:

$$\text{Santa Cruz: } CL_1 = 1.96 \times (10.41/\sqrt{63}) = \pm 2.57$$

$$\text{DeKalb: } \quad CL_2 = 1.96 \times (7.67/\sqrt{155}) = \pm 1.21$$

The confidence interval for the difference between the two rates is:

$$\text{Difference: } D = 10.41 - 7.67 = 2.74$$

$$\text{Confidence interval} = D \pm \sqrt{(CL_1{}^2 + CL_2{}^2)}$$

$$= 2.74 \pm \sqrt{(2.57^2 + 1.21^2)}$$

$$= 2.74 \pm \sqrt{8.0690}$$

$$= 2.74 \pm 2.84$$

Thus, the 95 percent confidence interval would be ($-$ .10 to 5.58). Since the interval does include zero, it can be concluded that the rates for the two counties are not significantly different.

μ = the mean of a population

When Rates Are Not Independent

When comparing a rate to a standard rate (that is, when rates may not be independent), a slightly more complex formula is needed:[21]

$$\mu = (r - s) \sqrt{n/s - s^2}$$

where: r = the observed rate or rate to be compared
s = the standard rate (state, region, nation, etc.)
n = the denominator (population on which the rate is based)

The formula is calculated as follows:

1. Square (multiply by itself) the standard rate: s: $(s \times s = s^2)$. Change all rates to a per-person basis (divide by the rate's denominator).
2. Subtract the square of s from s: $s - s^2$.
3. Divide the denominator on which the rate is based, n, by the difference of $s - s^2$: $n/(s - s^2)$.
4. Find the square root of the quotient from the last step: $\sqrt{n/s - s^2}$.
5. Subtract the standard rate s from the observed rate, r: $r - s$.
6. Multiply the square root in the fourth step by the difference in the fifth step: $\mu = (r - s) \sqrt{n/s - s^2}$.

If μ exceeds 1.96, it can be concluded that the rate differs significantly at the 95 percent confidence level from the standard rate to which it is compared. If it exceeds 2.33, it is significantly different at the 98 percent level; and if it exceeds 2.58, it is significantly different at the 99 percent level. For example, a county has a population of 16,400 persons and a death rate of 20.9 per 1,000. The objective is to find out whether this is significantly different from the state rate of 16.8 per 1,000:

Observed rate, r = 20.9 per 1,000

Standard rate, s = 16.8 per 1,000

Population (denominator n on which the rate is based) = 16,400

1. $(.0168) = .0168 \times .0168 = .000282$
2. $.0618 - .000282 = .016518$
3. $16,400/.016518 = 992856.27$
4. $\sqrt{992856.27} = 996.42173$
5. $.0209 - .0168 = .0041$
6. $.0041 \times 996.42173 = 4.09$ (μ)

Since the value of 4.09 (μ) is greater than 2.58, it can be concluded that the difference between the rates is significant at the 99 percent confidence level—in other words, there is 99 percent confidence that the death rate in the county is higher than in the state.

When rates are based on a very few number of events (births, deaths, cases, etc.), the actual number of events is used instead of the rate:

$$\mu = (o - e)/\sqrt{e}$$

where: o = the observed number(s) to be compared
e = the standard number (state, region, nation, etc.)

To calculate this formula:

1. Find the square root of the standard number, e: $\sqrt{e}$.
2. Subtract the standard number, e, from the observed number, o: $o - e$.
3. Divide the difference between the observed and standard numbers (Step 2) by the square root of e: $(o - e)/\sqrt{e}$.

Thus, the significance of a higher infant mortality rate for a county as compared to the state may be determined by:

$$\mu = (o - e)/\sqrt{e}$$

Observed rate, o = 20.2 per 1,000 (65 deaths)

Standard rate, e = 17.5 per 1,000 (117 deaths)

1. $\sqrt{117} = 10.81$
2. $65 - 117 = -52$
3. $-52/10.81 = -4.81$

Since the value -4.81 in absolute terms (that is, without considering the sign) is greater than 2.58, it can be concluded that the two rates are significantly different at the 99 percent confidence level.

The Significance of 'Excess Deaths'

As noted, the epidemiological approach to the identification of health problems rests on comparisons. A problem is defined by an excess of morbidity or mortality. Although this discussion is limited to excess deaths, the same concepts and techniques can be applied to excess morbidity when the data are available.

The analysis of excess deaths requires two major steps. Initially, it must be determined whether or not there is a difference between the number of deaths expected and the number actually occurring. Once this difference is determined, the second step is to test it to ascertain whether it merely results from chance or actually is significant statistically. To conduct this analysis, the following data inputs are required:

1. Data on the population being investigated:

   - Population (demographic data, categorized by age, sex, race, occupation, or other specifics)
   - Mortality data by cause of death, either in actual number observed or in death rates

2. Data on the standard population

The standard population is the basis for comparing the group being investigated. The standard population can be the state's, the nation's, a county's, or some other geographical area larger than the group being analyzed. Data regarding the standard population must be identical, however, to those available for the group being studied.

If death rates are the desired area of investigation, then they must be available for the selected standard population. Similarly, if age breakdowns are used, they also must be available for the standard population. The standard, however, should resemble the population being investigated as closely as possible.

For example, if counties within a state are under scrutiny, the state should be used as the standard population. With these data, the expected number of deaths can be derived for the population being investigated. The next section provides two methodologies for testing the significance of differences between observed and expected deaths, using numbers and rates of deaths.

Determining the Number of Expected Deaths

Each of the methodologies in this section is statistically valid for health problem analysis and should produce the same results. The selection of one methodology over the other, therefore, depends solely upon the availability of data—and personal preference.

Utilizing the Actual Number of Deaths

The expected number of deaths can be calculated using the following formula:

$$E = P_1/P_2 \times D$$

where: E = expected deaths
P_1 = population being investigated
P_2 = standard population
D = actual deaths in standard population

The ratio, P_1/P_2, should be be age-sex-race specific: if the subject is deaths among white males 55 to 64, both P_1 and P_2 should refer to the number of white males of these ages; on the other hand, if deaths among the overall population are being looked at, P_1 and P_2 should refer to the total population.

For example, in Massachusetts between 1969 and 1973 there were 52 deaths from fires and flames among males aged 60 to 64. The state population for this group totaled 113,128 while the city being investigated had 4,055. Assuming that the risk of dying in a fire was the same in the city as the state as a whole, the expected number of deaths in the city was calculated as follows:

$$E = \frac{P_1}{P_2} \times D = \frac{4,055}{113,128} \times 52 = 1.9 \text{ deaths}$$

Thus, 1.9 (rounded to 2) is the expected number of deaths to males age 60 to 64 because of fires and flames. Comparing this expected number to the actual number of deaths (three in the city being investigated), a difference of one death is identified. To determine whether this death represents an excess, however, a test of significance must be performed.

Utilizing Death Rates

If death rates instead of actual number of deaths are available from the standard population, the expected number of deaths is given by:

$$E = P_1 \times M_2$$

where: P_1 = population being investigated
M_2 = specific death rate in the standard population

Since: $M_2 = \frac{D}{P_2}$, it can be seen this is algebraically equivalent to the previous method.

Testing the Significance of Results

In the previous example, Massachusetts had a death rate of 4.6/10,000 population among males aged 60 to 64 because of fires and flames:

$$E = 4,055 \times \frac{4.6}{10,000} = 1.9 \text{ (expected deaths)}$$

Once the difference between the expected and the observed (actual) deaths is determined, a statistical test must be applied to determine whether it has any significance. If the difference shows a statistical significance, then an elevated number of expected deaths is not likely to be a result of chance alone. Associated with significance level, however, there always is a certain possibility that X events in 100 could have occurred solely on the basis of chance.

Two approaches for testing this significance are presented in this section. In the first method, standard mortality ratios (SMRs) are developed and tested utilizing the standard error (SE) and confidence intervals (CI). The second method illustrates the chi-square "goodness-of-fit" test.

Although each of these methods is statistically sound for this purpose, the SMR can be used more easily by a wide range of health service managers with limited statistical backgrounds. It requires fewer restrictions than the chi-square test and is equally sound statistically. The SMR requires more subjective judgment in interpreting the results but the chi-square test is bound by more statistical parameters and thus is more rigorous. Although no subjective judgments are to be made, the chi-square test is more complex and may require some statistical expertise to perform.

Standardized Mortality Ratio (SMR)

The SMR has already been described in the indirect method of rate adjustment. It is calculated as follows:

$$SMR = \frac{Observed\ deaths}{Expected\ deaths} \times 100$$

An SMR of 100 indicates that the observed number of deaths equals the expected number of deaths. An SMR of 130 indicates 30 percent excess deaths, one of 90, 10 percent fewer deaths than expected.

The next step is to calculate the confidence interval of the SMR. Using Method 3 for the calculation of a 95 percent confidence interval (see Exhibit 4-4), the 95 percent confidence interval of an SMR is obtained by:

$$CI = SMR \pm (1.96 \times SE)$$

where: $SE = \dfrac{SMR}{\sqrt{d}}$

d = number of observed deaths

Data on observed and expected deaths in a county, as compared to a state, are presented in Table 4-7.

Table 4-7 Observed and Expected Deaths from Heart Disease for County A, by Age Group, 1970–74

Age Group	Observed Deaths	Expected Deaths
20–29	16	16
30–39	18	20
40–49	22	18
50–59	51	56
60–69	55	72
70–79	62	64
80–89	22	28
90 +	14	15
Totals	260	289

$$SMR = \frac{260}{289} \times 100 = 89.97$$

$$SE = \frac{SMR}{\sqrt{d}} = \frac{89.97}{\sqrt{260}} = 5.58$$

$$CI \ (95\%) = 89.97 \pm (1.96 \times 5.58)$$

$$\text{Upper limit} = 89.97 + 10.94 = 100.91$$

$$\text{Lower limit} = 89.97 - 10.94 = 79.03$$

$$CI = 79 \text{ to } 101$$

The interpretation of the confidence interval of an SMR is as follows:

1. If the lower and upper confidence limits are distributed above and below 100 (that is, if the lower limit is below 100 and the upper limit is above 100), then there is no significant difference between the observed and expected deaths.
2. If the lower confidence limit is above 100, then the observed deaths are significantly higher than expected (i.e., it is unlikely that the excess is merely a chance occurrence).
3. If the upper confidence limit is below 100, then the observed deaths are significantly fewer than expected.
4. If a confidence interval is quite wide, regardless of whether both limits are above or below 100, then more years of data are required, or the data should be grouped, before any conclusions can be reached. Although no clear-cut rules specify what constitutes a "wide" range, it is fair to say that a range of 50 or more would be excessive.

In the preceding example, the decision is difficult to make since the upper limit is barely above 100. It can only be concluded that the SMR seems moderately, although not significantly, low at the 95 percent confidence level (it would be significant, however, at the 90 percent level).

The Chi-Square (X^2) Test

The chi-square or "goodness-of-fit" test provides a way to compare an observed frequency with an expected frequency distribution. The formula for chi-square is:

$$X^2 = \Sigma \frac{(O - E)^2}{E}$$

where: X^2 = chi-square
Σ = sum across all groups
O = observed deaths
E = expected deaths

Table 4-8 presents the calculation of chi-square for the data presented in Table 4-7. The computed chi-square value of 6.97 is compared with a tabular value of X^2 with $(k - r)$ degrees of freedom, where k equals the number of categories that can be calculated $(O - E)^2/E$ (that is, the number of age groups in this example), and r equals the number of restrictions (quantities) that were determined from observed data and used in calculating the expected frequencies.[22]

In most cases, where the expected frequencies are determined by using one of the two methods just described, the only observed quantity involved in calculating the expected frequencies is the population (P_1). When this is the case, the degree of freedom is $(k - 1)$. In the example in Table 4-8, there are no restrictions since the expected frequencies were not calculated from observed data.

There are, then, eight degrees of freedom (eight age groups). The value of the X^2 for eight degrees of freedom at the 95 percent level is 15.507. If the calculated value (6.97) is less than the tabular value, as is the case here, then it can be said that there is no significant difference between the observed and the expected deaths. If it were greater than the tabular value, then the difference would be significant.

The results of both approaches (SMR and X^2) provide a statistically significant level allowing the health service manager to determine whether or not any excess deaths are indeed representative of a morbidity/mortality problem.

Evidence, Not Proof

Statistical significance provides evidence of differences, characteristics, or associations but does not provide proof. This is because statistical significance is based on several underlying assumptions, including those involving the properties

Table 4-8 Calculation of X^2 for Observed and Expected Deaths from Heart Disease for County A, 1970–74

Age Group	Observed Deaths	Expected Deaths	$\dfrac{(O - E)^2}{E}$
20–29	16	16	0.00
30–39	18	20	0.20
40–49	22	18	0.89
50–59	51	56	0.45
60–69	55	72	4.01
70–79	62	64	0.06
80–89	22	28	1.29
90 +	14	15	0.07
Totals	260	289	6.97

$x^2 = 0 + .20 + .89 + .45 + 4.01 + .06 + 1.29 + .07$
$x^2 = 6.97$

of the distribution and the sample results. In statistical significance testing, the concern is with the probability of making an error (or of being correct), given the results obtained.

Thus, if there is a 95 percent confidence level (or a 5 percent error level), what really is being said is that 95 times out of 100 the outcome would be a value that is within two standard errors of the true mean; 5 times out of 100 the resulting value would exceed two standard errors.

Further, if the value exceeds the established critical level and falls outside the range of likely values, two things are possible. Either the true mean is different from the one hypothesized (rejection of the false null hypothesis), or the true mean is not different from the one hypothesized; that is, the sample value selected falls in the 5 percent region only by chance (rejection of a true null hypothesis).

Of similar importance, statistical significance deals with probabilities based upon repeated sampling from a population. For any one sample, the true probability is either 0.0 or 1.0: either the sample statistic is a reliable estimate of the true population parameter, or it is not.

Although the confidence level (often referred to as α) indicates the probability of having a value exceeding the critical region by chance, it does not indicate the probability that the true statistic actually is different from the hypothesized one. The latter is the β probability or the power of the test, dealing with the ability to detect a false null hypothesis. Although the computation of the β probability is much more difficult than it is for α, it is important to realize that, once the desired α level and the sample size are set, the β level is fixed.

Since this β level value usually is not known and often is very small, it cannot be concluded that it is true, even when a null hypothesis is not rejected. Rather, it is said that the results are inconclusive or, more commonly, that the null hypothesis was not rejected. Thus, depending on the results from a test of significance, there is a greater likelihood of making an error—either rejecting a true null hypothesis or failing to reject a false null hypothesis. Any test for significance should consider these probabilities of error and the decision maker should weigh their consequences carefully.

Practical Significance and Decision Making

Where statistical significance is commonly reported in testing hypotheses or making inferences, based on the theory of sampling distributions and mathematics, serious concern also should be shown for its practical significance—the real impact or cost of a difference. Practical significance can be assessed only by someone familiar with the hypothesis being tested or with the program being evaluated.

It is possible that a difference may be statistically significant though so small as to be meaningless in terms of programmatic impact. This is especially true when dealing with large samples or rates based on large populations. Since statistical significance is a function of both sample size and population variation, it is quite possible that in a large sample any differences will be significant. Thus, consideration must be given to the real impact of a statistically significant difference on the program or population being tested.

A problem for the health care administrator, then, is the difference between statistical and practical significance. In health services, where data on large populations may be available, indexes such as means or rates may always be significantly different in a statistical sense. The health professional must decide whether the differences are of magnitude significant enough to justify action, such as revising a program.

A common problem in evaluation testing arises when a key index has increased significantly, according to a statistical expert, but the administrator senses that the size of the increase has no programmatic importance. Survey reports on populations often cite differences that are described as "significantly greater" and "significantly longer" but that, even to an untrained analyst, do not seem to matter much.

A final warning about repeated testing for significance: tests are designed so that the error probability in any one test is small. Yet, if several tests are made, it is quite likely that true null hypotheses based on chance occurrences may be rejected. Such repeated testing of a number of related factors often is done when searching for relationships rather than testing specific hypotheses. When statistical significance is found in such cases, the probability is quite high that chance occurrence has caused rejection.

SUMMARY

Health service managers can use many of the techniques and measurements presented here. The concept of a rate and population at risk are central to the analysis of problems related to the management of health services. This chapter has provided the tools and methods for epidemiological investigation into the effective delivery of health services.

The epidemiological measures of rates and their significance allow administrators to determine the magnitude of a problem and whether it warrants further analysis. A much more practical use for these statistical and epidemiological methods is to monitor current conditions and establish future needs. Finally, determining the significance of the results obtained may be more of a practical decision than a statistical one.

NOTES

1. P.E. Sortwell and J.M. Last, "Epidemiology," in *Maxcy-Rosenau Public Health and Preventive Medicine,* 11th ed., ed. J.M. Last (New York: Appleton-Century-Crofts, Inc., 1980), 14.

2. Ibid., 14.

3. E.R. Babbie, *The Practice of Social Research* (Belmont, Calif.: Wadsworth Publishing Co., 1979), 91.

4. Judith S. Mausner and Anita K. Bahn, *Epidemiology: An Introductory Text* (Philadelphia: W.B. Saunders Company, 1974), 136.

5. A.M. Lilienfeld, *Foundations of Epidemiology* (New York: Oxford University Press, 1976), 59.

6. A.A. Rimm et al., *Basis Biostatistics in Medicine and Epidemiology* (New York: Appleton-Century-Crofts, Inc. 1980), 287.

7. Mausner and Bahn, *Epidemiology: An Introductory Text,* 136.

8. Sortwell and Last, "Epidemiology," 25.

9. Mausner and Bahn, *Epidemiology: An Introductory Text,* 126.

10. Ibid., 127.

11. G.E. Alan Dever, *Community Health Analysis: A Holistic Approach* (Rockville, Md.: Aspen Systems Corporation, 1980), 80-85.

12. Jack Elinson and A.E. Siegmann, eds., *Socio-Medical Health Indicators* (Farmingdale, N.Y.: Baywood Publishing Company, Inc., 1979).

13. "1976 Health Status Indexes Conference—An Annotated Guide to the Papers," *Health Services Research* (Winter 1976), vol. 4, 335.

14. J.C. Kleinman, "Infant Mortality," *Statistical Notes for Health Planners,* vol. 2 (Washington, D.C.: National Center for Health Statistics, July 1976), 4.

15. Robert W. Broyles and Colin M. Lay, *Statistics in Health Administration,* vol. 1 (Rockville, Md.: Aspen Systems Corporation, 1979), 570.

16. Rimm et al., *Basic Biostatistics,* 37-42.

17. J.C. Kleinman, "Mortality," *Statistical Notes for Health Planners,* vol. 3 (Washington, D.C.: National Center for Health Statistics, February 1977), 6.

18. Kleinman, "Infant Mortality," 11.

19. Ibid., 11.

20. Kleinman, "Mortality," 7.

21. David E. Drew and E. Keeler, "Algorithms for Health Planners," *Hypertension,* vol. 6 (Publication No. R2215/6-HEW, The Rand Corporation, August 1977), 63.

22. Broyles and Lay, *Statistics,* 398.

Chapter 5

Identifying Problems, Determining Priorities

MANAGERS' USE OF MORTALITY INDICATORS

Several epidemiological measurements, techniques, and concepts have been described that are useful in identifying health problems. Based on some of those methods, this chapter presents a concrete, overall epidemiological approach that can be used easily by health service managers for identifying problems in their population. However, when appropriate, any of the alternatives discussed may be used.

This approach is centered on the standardized mortality ratio (SMR) as an initial screening device. The age-sex-race rates then are used within each diagnostic (cause-of-death) grouping. Table 5-1 presents the data for Georgia County A, Table 5-2 for the State of Georgia. Data for 10 years are used because, when dealing with small areas, there is too much variability to make annual rates significant. Similarly, cause-of-death diagnoses are grouped into larger diagnosis-related groups. Only actual number of deaths are used.

Calculations of the SMRs are shown in Table 5-3 and the construction of the 95 percent confidence intervals and the corresponding significance in Table 5-4.

Population data are not available for each year between 1971 and 1980. To construct the 10-year population, therefore, the 1970 and 1979 populations each were multiplied by five. The years selected are those available that best reflected the time period being analyzed.

Identifying the Problems

Table 5-4 shows definite problems in County A. Heart diseases in general and acute myocardial infarction in particular are significantly higher in the county than in the state. A substantially higher number of homicides also occur in the county as

110   EPIDEMIOLOGY IN HEALTH SERVICES MANAGEMENT

Table 5-1 Leading Causes of Death in County A, Georgia, 1971-1980
All Ages, Sexes, Races

Year	Heart Diseases*	Cerebro- vascular Disease	Lung Cancer	Motor Vehicle Accidents	All Other Accidents	Pneumonia	Homicide
1971	576 **(344)	247	45	49	55	44	34
1972	503 (305)	255	37	67	40	45	34
1973	568 (350)	248	40	54	35	40	46
1974	553 (308)	209	53	35	50	35	42
1975	588 (324)	168	61	48	37	36	35
1976	572 (309)	199	66	27	51	42	35
1977	536 (232)	206	51	47	48	56	27
1978	558 (262)	168	50	29	37	66	27
1979	554 (236)	144	73	46	34	22	26
1980	537 (243)	160	66	38	39	35	22
Totals	5,545 (2,913)	2,004	542	440	426	421	328

*Includes acute myocardial infarction, other ischemic heart disease, other heart disease, and diseases of the arteries.
**Numbers in parentheses indicate deaths from acute myocardial infarction.

Population: 1970 = 143,366, 1979 = 143,641.

compared to the state. Cancer of the lung, motor vehicle accidents, and other accidents are not higher (or significantly lower) than in the state. Pneumonia seems to be borderline—somewhat higher in the county but barely significant.

It should be noted that county and state mortality are being compared, so identification of problems is based on the state average. It might be desirable to apply another standard: for example, even though lung cancer is not higher in the county than in the state, it still could be considered a problem if the state incidence were regarded as too high. Furthermore, the analysis encompasses all ages, sexes, and races; although an SMR may not be significant for the overall population, it still might be important in a specific age, sex, or race group.

Table 5-2 Leading Causes of Death in Georgia, 1971-1980
All Ages, Sexes, Races

Year	Heart Diseases*	Cerebro- vascular Disease	Lung Cancer	Motor Vehicle Accidents	All Other Accidents	Pneumonia	Homicide
1971	14,594 **(7,639)	5,538	1,358	1,765	1,544	1,480	869
1972	15,070 (7,757)	5,910	1,420	1,885	1,512	1,428	953
1973	15,494 (7,705)	5,897	1,466	1,847	1,657	1,507	985
1974	15,529 (7,782)	5,647	1,528	1,570	1,526	1,196	1,024
1975	14,885 (7,217)	5,136	1,658	1,411	1,451	1,233	871
1976	15,198 (7,272)	5,253	1,790	1,302	1,400	1,248	793
1977	15,551 (7,226)	4,995	1,902	1,461	1,536	1,275	725
1978	15,835 (7,355)	4,882	2,090	1,523	1,403	1,348	749
1979	15,203 (7,142)	4,601	2,094	1,568	1,349	1,029	844
1980	15,508 (7,247)	4,513	2,269	1,504	1,561	1,151	808
Totals	152,867 (74,342)	52,372	17,575	15,836	14,939	12,895	8,621

*Includes acute myocardial infarction, other ischemic heart disease, other heart disease, and diseases of the arteries.
**Numbers in parentheses indicate deaths from acute myocardial infarction.

Population: 1970 = 4,587,930, 1979 = 5,151,445.

The next step, then, is to look at the specific rates. Although this analysis is limited to age-specific rates, it also is advisable to look at age-sex-race rates. Table 5-5 presents these age (life stage) rates. (A blank space does not represent zero deaths but unavailable data, since information was limited to the top 10 leading causes of death in each age group.)

Table 5-5 serves several purposes. It shows the age at which each cause of death is most prevalent. For example, motor vehicle accidents are the leading cause of death in adolescence and early adulthood while pneumonia is most prevalent in infants and in older adults. Health service managers can use these data to target a program specifically to the most appropriate group. It also is interesting to note that

Table 5-3 SMRs for Cause of Deaths in County A, Georgia, 1971-1980 All Ages, Sexes, Races

| Cause of Death | Calculation of Expected Deaths[1] | | | | Observed Deaths | SMR[2] |
| | A | B | C | D | E | F |
	Local Population[3] (P_1)	State Population[4] (P_2)	Actual Deaths in State (d)	Expected Deaths $\frac{Col\ A}{Col\ B} \times Col\ C$	Observed Deaths in Area	$\frac{Col\ E}{Col\ D} \times 100$
Heart disease	1,435,035	48,696,875	152,867	4,505	5,545	123
			*(74,342)	(2,191)	(2,913)	(133)
Cerebrovascular disease	1,435,035	48,696,875	52,372	1,543	2,004	130
Lung cancer	1,435,035	48,696,875	17,575	518	542	104.6
Motor vehicle accidents	1,435,035	48,696,875	15,836	467	440	94.2
All other accidents	1,435,035	48,696,875	14,939	440	426	96.8
Pneumonia	1,435,035	48,696,875	12,895	380	421	111
Homicide	1,435,035	48,696,875	8,621	254	328	129

1. Expected deaths = $\dfrac{P_1}{P_2} \times d$

   where: P_1 = local population
   P_2 = state population
   d = number of actual deaths in state (standard).

2. $SMR = \dfrac{Observed\ deaths}{Expected\ deaths} \times 100$.

3. 1971-80 local population = $(5 \times 143,366) + (5 \times 143,641)$. (Because we have 10 years of mortality data, we need 10 years of population data. One must match the numerator and denominator.)

4. 1971-80 state population = $(5 \times 4,587,930) + (5 \times 5,151,445)$.

*Numbers in parentheses indicate deaths from acute myocardial infarction.

Table 5-4 Confidence Interval and Significance, County A, Georgia, 1971-1980 All Ages, Sexes, Races

| | A | Standard Error[1] | | | Confidence Limits (Interval, 95%) | | | Significance |
| | | B | C | D | E | F | | |
Cause of Death	SMR (from Column F, Table 5-3)	Number of Observed Deaths	Square Root of Observed Deaths	$SE = \dfrac{Col\ A}{Col\ C}$	$SE \times 1.96$	Col A−Col E Lower Limit	Col A+Col E Upper Limit	+ if Lower Limit > 100 — if Upper Limit < 100 0 if UL >100, LL < 100
Heart diseases	123	5,545	74.46	1.65	3.2	119.8	126.2	+
	*(133)	(2,913)	(53.97)	(2.46)	(4.8)	(128.2)	(137.8)	+
Cerebrovascular disease	130	2,004	44.77	2.90	5.7	124.3	135.7	+
Lung cancer	104.6	542	23.28	4.49	8.8	95.8	113.4	0
Motor vehicle accidents	94.2	440	20.98	4.49	8.8	85.4	103.0	0
All other accidents	96.8	426	20.64	4.69	9.2	87.6	106.0	0
Pneumonia	111	421	20.52	5.41	10.6	100.4	121.6	(+)
Homicide	129	328	18.11	7.12	14.0	115.0	143.0	+

1. Standard error $(SE) = \dfrac{SMR}{\sqrt{d}}$

where: d = the number of observed deaths in area being investigated.

*Numbers in parentheses indicate deaths from acute myocardial infarction.

Table 5-5 Cause-Specific Mortality Rates by Life Stage, County A and
State of Gerogia, 1979-1980
Rates Are Expressed as Deaths Per 100,000 Population

					Cause of Death			
Life Stage	Area	Heart Diseases*	Cerebro-vascular Disease	Lung Cancer	Motor Vehicle Accidents	All Other Accidents	Pneumonia	Homicide
INFANCY	County	19.4	3.9	–	27.0	27.0	132.0	3.9
(under 1 year)		(–)						
	State	15.7	4.4	–	11.9	54.5	148.6	5.4
		(–)						
CHILDHOOD								
Early	County	3.1	–	–	12.5	19.7	9.4	3.1
(1 to 4 years)		(–)						
	State	2.1	.7	–	13.8	21.3	6.5	2.5
		(–)						
Later	County	1.9	1.1	–	12.9	10.3	.8	.8
(5 to 14 years)		(–)						
	State	.8	.4	–	13.6	11.6	1.3	1.2
		(–)						
ADOLESCENCE	County	1.5	1.5	–	56.3	31.1	–	14.1
(15 to 19 years)		(–)						
	State	2.2	1.1	.7	57.3	24.4	1.2	12.5
		(–)						
ADULTHOOD								
Early	County	8.2	3.5	–	45.9	19.9	3.5	47.2
(20 to 29 years)		(2.6)						
	State	4.6	2.6	–	49.6	24.0	2.6	31.2
		(1.5)						
Young	County	63.7	19.9	–	25.6	23.1	–	39.0
(30 to 44 years)		(45.1)						
	State	45.7	14.9	7.6	31.5	26.2	11.0	32.2
		(27.2)						
Middle	County	448.0	115.0	77.7	–	34.3	–	–
(45 to 59 years)		(312.0)						
	State	345.0	80.1	78.4	32.4	37.0	–	30.4
		(217.4)						
Late	County	1,409.0	450.7	160.6	–	–	77.8	–
(60 to 74 years)		(832.5)						
	State	1,257.0	367.5	184.4	–	–	67.0	–
		(680.9)						
Older	County	4,327.0	1,905.2	184.8	–	157.3	346.0	–
(over 74)		(1,514.0)						
	State	4,291.0	1,812.1	171.2	–	152.6	365.4	–
		(1,588.1)						

*Numbers in parentheses refer to deaths from acute myocardial infarction.

the data for heart diseases, including acute myocardial infarction, and cere-brovascular disease, are higher in the county than in the state from early to late adulthood but not in older adulthood.

The table also shows whether there is a problem in a specific age (or sex or race) group that does not show up in the overall SMR. In the example, this does not seem to be the case. If it were, however, the solution would be to calculate the specific SMR, to use the formula for testing the significance of the difference between two rates (not independent), or to calculate the confidence interval of the county rate if it is to be compared with an arbitrary standard (a goal or target).

Infant Mortality—An Example

Another important cause of death is infant mortality. Between 1976 and 1980, there were 11,830 births in County A, as compared to 427,973 in the state. In the county, 201 infant deaths occurred (rate = 17/1,000 births), while in the state there were 6,649 (15.5/1,000 births). The significance can be estimated using either the SMR or the direct comparison of the rates:

$$SMR = \frac{Observed\ deaths}{Expected\ deaths} \times 100$$

$$Expected\ deaths = \frac{P_1}{P_2} \times deaths\ in\ state = \frac{11,830}{427,973} \times 6,649 = 183.8$$

$$SMR = \frac{201}{183.8} = 109.4$$

The standard error (*SE*) is:

$$SE = \frac{SMR}{\sqrt{d}} = \frac{109.4}{\sqrt{201}} = 7.7$$

The confidence interval is:

$$CI = \pm\ 7.7 \times 1.96 = \pm\ 15.1$$

$$Upper\ limit = 109.4 + 15.1 = 124.5$$

$$Lower\ limit = 109.4 - 15.1 = 94.3$$

$$CI = 94.3\ to\ 124.5$$

Since the confidence interval includes 100, it can be concluded that there is no significant difference in infant mortality between county and state rates. The same conclusion can be reached using the following formula (see also Chapter 4):

$$\mu = (r - s)\sqrt{n/s - s^2}$$

where: r = county rate = 17.0/1,000 = .017

s = state rate = 15.5/1,000 = .0155

n = denominator of county rate = 11,830 births

$$= (.017 - .0155) \times \sqrt{\frac{11,830}{(.0155 - .00024)}} = 1.32$$

Since μ is smaller than 1.96, it can be concluded that the two rates are not significantly different at the 95 percent confidence level. It also is interesting to calculate the confidence interval of rates, allowing the comparison with an arbitrarily set standard or goal. For example, is the county rate significantly higher than a goal of 13 deaths per 1,000 births? The confidence interval is given by:

$$CI = rate + 1.96 \times SE$$

where:

$$SE = \frac{rate}{\sqrt{deaths}}$$

$$SE = \frac{17.0}{\sqrt{201}} = 1.2$$

$$CI = 17.0 \pm (1.96 \times 1.2) = 17.0 \pm 2.35$$

Upper limit = 17.0 + 2.35 = 19.35

Lower limit = 17.0 - 2.35 = 14.65

This means that, just by chance, the county rate may vary between 14.65 and 19.35, 95 percent of the time. It thus is significantly higher than a target value of 13.0.

In summary, health service managers can identify the specific health problems of their area by the following steps:

1. Calculate the SMRs across all ages, sexes, and races to determine the causes of death that are excessive as compared to a standard (state or other).
2. Look at the specific age-sex-race rates to determine further specific problems.
3. Calculate the significance of any difference found in Step 2.

DETERMINATION OF PRIORITIES

Once problems are identified, questions remain as to which should be addressed, which are the most important. Epidemiology can contribute to the determination of priorities.

Proportionate Mortality Ratio

The simplest and perhaps the preliminary epidemiological measure for determining priorities is the proportionate mortality ratio (PMR). As discussed earlier, the PMR represents the percentage of all deaths that result from a specific cause:

$$PMR = \frac{Deaths\ by\ cause}{Total\ deaths} \times 100$$

The PMR indicates the relative importance of causes of death and consequently provides an estimate of the number and population of lives saved by reducing or eradicating a specific cause. On the other hand, the PMR can be misleading since its magnitude depends on the number of deaths from causes other than the one under consideration. Mausner and Bahn give the following example:[1]

$\frac{31}{85} \times 100 = 36.5$

Age Group	Death Rate per 100,000 (All Causes)	(Accidents)	PMR for Accidents (%)
1- 4	85	31	36.5
65-74	3,739	89	2.4

Even though death rates from accidents are higher among the elderly, the proportion of deaths from that cause is greater for young children. This of course is because total deaths from all other causes are much higher in the elderly. Care must be exercised, therefore, when comparing PMRs across age groups.

In addition to the PMR, epidemiology provides two main sets of criteria for determining priorities: magnitude of the loss and amenability to prevention or reduction

Magnitude of Loss, Years of Life Lost

The development of priorities may be based on losses from death, from morbidity, or from both.[2] Losses may be expressed in terms of time, productive time, or income foregone. To each may be added losses because of the cost of care.

The years-of-life-lost (or YLL) indicator can be used to calculate the estimated number lost for each cause of death. The resulting ranking or prioritization of causes of death will be quite different from that obtained using the PMR, with only the crude number of deaths. This is because most deaths occur at an older age but many more life years are lost when death occurs at a younger age than expected. Since mortality in older age groups probably is least amenable to health services, the opposite might be true for morbidity or disability. The YLL thus might be a useful indicator in the prioritization of problems for purposes of health service management.[3] Figure 5-1 illustrates the ranking of causes of death in the United States, using both the crude number of deaths and the estimated years of life lost.

As shown in the left-hand bar, the four leading causes of death in 1977 were heart disease, malignant neoplasms (cancer), stroke, and accidents, poisonings, and violence. Together they accounted for four out of five deaths; of these heart disease caused about two in five, cancer one in five, and accidents one in ten. The respiratory diseases category also figures as numerically important.

The right-hand bar shows the impact of the six leading categories on years of life lost, based on life expectancy rates at each age. Heart disease and cancer again dominate; because they hit older age groups more frequently, however, they account for a smaller proportion of lost years than they do of deaths. Because children, teenagers, and young adults are the most frequent victims of accidents and violence, the proportion of potential years of life lost from those causes is almost twice as high as the proportion of deaths. Finally, deaths associated with congenital anomalies, including perinatal mortality, though relatively small in number, account for a sizable proportion of total years of potential life lost because they occur at the early end of the life span.

Basically, the YLL can be used in two ways: (1) to simply calculate the number of life years lost for each cause of death and compare the different causes or (2) to compare an area (county) with another standard (state), as was done with the SMR. The latter approach is referred to here as the YLL index, as opposed to the YLL indicator (described earlier).

Once again, the data for 1971-1980 from County A in Georgia are usable. It had been determined that heart diseases in general (particularly acute myocardial infarction), cerebrovascular disease, and homicide were definite problems. It now might be decided that the state rate for cancer of the lung was too high and that, even though the SMR for lung cancer was not significantly higher in the county than in the state, it still had to be considered a problem.

For purposes of this example, the priority analysis is limited to cerebrovascular disease, homicide, and lung cancer. Table 5-6 illustrates the calculation of the YLL indicator. Age 70 was chosen arbitrarily as the life expectancy, that is, the age to which the population normally could aspire. All deaths are assumed to occur at midpoint of the age groups so the expected number of years lost is calculated as 70 minus the midpoint of the age group. The table shows the cause of death costing the most years of life is homicide, followed by cerebrovascular disease, even though

Figure 5-1 Number and Percent Distribution of Selected Causes of
Death and Potential Years of Life Lost

(United States, 1977)

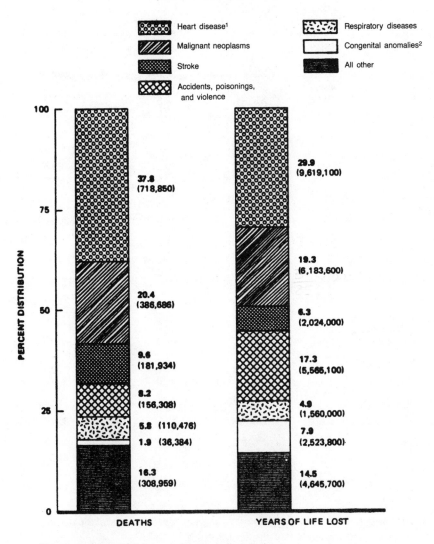

1. Diseases of the circulatory system excluding stroke.
2. Includes certain causes of perinatal mortality.

Source: Reprinted from *Health—United States, 1980,* by Department of Health and Human Services,
Public Health Service, National Center for Health Statistics, 1980, 270.

Table 5-6 Estimated YLL Indicators, County A, Georgia, 1971-1980

	Indicators	Age Group	Deaths		Average YLL		Estimated YLL
A.	Cerebro-	Under 1	1	x	69.5	=	69.5
	vascular	1-4	0	x	67.0	=	0
	disease	5-14	3	x	60.0	=	180.0
		15-19	2	x	52.5	=	105.0
		20-29	8	x	45.0	=	360.0
		30-44	49	x	32.5	=	1,592.5
		45-59	265	x	17.5	=	4,637.5
		60-74	707	x	2.5	=	1,767.5
		Over 74	969	x	0	=	0
		Totals	2,004				8,712.0
B.	Homicide	Under 1	1	x	69.5	=	69.5
		1-4	3	x	67.0	=	201.0
		5-14	2	x	60.0	=	120.0
		15-19	19	x	52.5	=	997.5
		20-29	109	x	45.0	=	4,905.0
		30-44	96	x	32.5	=	3,120.0
		45-59	70	x	17.5	=	1,225.0
		60-74	0	x	0	=	0
		Over 74	0	x	0	=	0
		Totals	300				10,638.0
C.	Cancer of	Under 1	0	x	69.5	=	0
	the Lung	1-4	0	x	67.0	=	0
		5-14	0	x	60.0	=	0
		15-19	1	x	52.5	=	52.5
		20-29	0	x	45.0	=	0
		30-44	0	x	32.5	=	0
		45-59	179	x	17.5	=	3,132.5
		60-74	252	x	2.5	=	630.0
		Over 74	94	x	0	=	0
		Totals	526				3,815.0

the latter accounts for almost seven times as many deaths as homicide does. Lung cancer is second in number of deaths but third in YLL.

To compare the county with the state in terms of YLL, using the YLL index, it is necessary to adjust for differing age distributions by calculating the expected number of deaths for each age group. The expected YLL then can be computed; the YLL index is the ratio of observed to expected YLL.

$$YLL \ index \ = \ \frac{Observed \ years \ of \ life \ lost}{Expected \ years \ of \ life \ lost} \ \times \ 100$$

Interpretation and calculation of the significance of the YLL index are identical to that of the SMR. Table 5-7 presents the calculation of the expected YLL.

Table 5-7 Expected YLL Index, County A, Georgia, 1971-1980

Indicators	Age Group	County Population (P₁)	State Population (P₂)	Deaths in State (D)	Expected Deaths (P₁/P₂ × D)	Average YLL	Expected YLL
A. Cerebro-	< 1	25,715	907,050	40	1.1	69.5	76.45
vascular	1-4	96,245	3,445,320	24	0.7	67.0	46.9
disease	5-14	262,680	9,128,030	37	1.1	60.0	66.0
	15-19	135,000	4,522,640	52	1.6	52.5	84.0
	20-29	230,890	8,354,955	214	5.9	45.0	265.5
	30-44	246,305	9,015,340	1,339	36.6	32.5	1,189.5
	45-59	230,460	7,080,165	5,669	184.5	17.5	3,228.75
	60-74	156,880	4,715,510	17,329	576.5	2.5	1,441.25
							6,398.0
B. Homicide	< 1	25,715	907,050	49	1.4	69.5	97.3
	1-4	96,245	3,446,320	85	2.4	67.0	160.8
	5-14	262,680	9,128,030	105	3.0	60.0	180.0
	15-19	135,000	4,522,640	565	16.9	52.5	887.25
	20-29	230,890	8,354,955	2,605	72.0	45.0	3,240.0
	30-44	246,305	9,015,340	2,899	79.2	32.5	2,574.0
	45-59	230,460	7,080,165	1,700	55.3	17.5	967.75
	60-74	156,880	4,715,510	0	0	2.5	0
							8,107.0
C. Cancer of	< 1	25,715	907,050	0	0	69.5	0
the lung	1-4	96,245	3,446,320	0	0	67.0	0
	5-14	262,680	9,128,030	0	0	60.0	0
	15-19	135,000	4,522,640	0	0	52.5	0
	20-29	230,890	8,354,955	0	0	45.0	0
	30-44	246,305	9,915,340	687	18.8	32.5	611.0
	45-59	230,460	7,080,165	5,549	180.6	17.5	3,160.5
	60-74	156,880	4,715,510	8,694	289.2	2.5	723.0
							4,495.0

$$Expected\ deaths = \frac{P_1}{P_2} \times D$$

where: P_1 = county population

P_2 = state population

D = deaths in the state

The YLL indexes (age adjusted) are as follows:

$$Cerebrovascular\ disease = \frac{8{,}712}{6{,}398} \times 100 = 136$$

$$Homicide = \frac{10{,}638}{8{,}107} \times 100 = 131$$

$$Cancer\ of\ the\ lung = \frac{3{,}815}{4{,}495} \times 100 = 85$$

The confidence interval for the YLL index is calculated as described previously:

$$95\%\ CI = YLL \pm 1.96 \times SE$$

where: $SE = \dfrac{YLL}{\sqrt{d}}$

Thus, for:

Cerebrovascular disease:

$$CI = 136 \pm 1.96 \times \frac{136}{\sqrt{2{,}004}} = 136 \pm 6$$

$$CI = 130\ to\ 142$$

Homicide:

$$CI = 131 \pm 1.96 \times \frac{131}{\sqrt{300}} = 131 \pm 15$$

$$CI = 116\ to\ 146$$

Cancer of the lung:

$$CI = 85 \pm 1.96 \times \frac{85}{\sqrt{526}} = 85 \pm 7$$

$$CI = 78 \text{ to } 92$$

This means it is possible to be 95 percent confident that from 30 to 42 percent more years of life are lost in the county than in the state because of cerebrovascular disease, from 16 to 46 percent more because of homicide, and significantly less—8 to 22 percent—from lung cancer.

It is interesting to note that the results of the YLL index are somewhat different from those of the SMR. The SMR for lung cancer indicates no important difference between the county and the state but the YLL index shows a significant deficit. This is because of two factors:

(1) the YLL index, unlike the SMR, emphasizes the differences in age-specific mortality in younger ages;
(2) the YLL index is age-adjusted, whereas the SMRs were not age-adjusted. This can be done in calculating the expected deaths for each age group, as for the YLL, instead of directly figuring the overall expected deaths across all ages. This age adjustment removes any variations in mortality that may occur because of a different age distribution in the county and in the state.

When data are available, the magnitude of loss for morbid conditions also can be calculated. Obviously, this is valuable information, since it is a direct indicator of the burden of diseases in the population. Such loss often is expressed in terms of disability days.

RISK FACTORS AND PRIORITIES

Another epidemiological strategy in the determination of priorities is to calculate losses because of risk factors. As should be clear by now, risk factors are the cornerstone of epidemiology. It has been shown earlier how the concept of causality is expanded in epidemiology by the concept of risk. It also has been shown how health can be conceived of as resulting from the interaction of multiple risk factors grouped in four health field dimensions. In that sense, risk factors are the key to an effective and efficient health strategy, mostly through preventive action.

In the planning and management of health programs, therefore, it is important to be able to estimate the impact of each risk factor on the population. This gives an estimate of the potential impact of a program directed toward some risk factors in reducing mortality and morbidity. Such estimates consequently help managers to determine the relative importance—prioritization—of each risk factor for which a program could be developed.

Absolute and Relative Risk

The incidence rate of a disease is a measure of risk. The incidence rate in a group of people exposed to a risk factor can be called the absolute risk of the disease. An even more meaningful action is to compare this risk with that of people who are not exposed to that factor. The ratio of the incidence rate in the exposed to the incidence rate in the nonexposed is called the relative risk (RR).

$$RR = \frac{Incidence\ rate\ among\ exposed}{Incidence\ rate\ among\ nonexposed}$$

Using the concept of relative risk, Doll and Hill studied death rates among British male physicians who smoked.[3a] Among heavy smokers, they found death rates of 1.66 per 1000 for lung cancer, 2.63 for other cancers, and 1.41 for other respiratory diseases. This compared with 0.07 (lung cancer), 2.01 (other cancers), and 0.81 (other respiratory diseases) among nonsmokers. Using the formula, the relative risk of lung cancer among heavy smokers in this survey is 23.7 (1.66 ÷ 0.07 = 23.7), for other cancers 1.3 (2.63 ÷ 2.01 = 1.3), and for other respiratory diseases, 1.7.

Doll and Hill also found death rates of 5.99 versus 4.22 (heavy smokers vs. nonsmokers) for coronary thrombosis (a RR of 1.4), and for other causes, rates of 7.19 vs. 6.11 (RR = 1.2). The rate for all causes of death in the survey is 18.84 for heavy smokers, contrasted with 13.25 for nonsmokers, giving a RR for all causes of 1.4.

In this particular example, relative risk is a measure that illustrates the association between nonsmokers and heavy smokers for certain causes of death in the physician population. In general, for all the causes, the risk of death is 1.4 times as great for heavy smokers as nonsmokers, and in particular for lung cancer, the risk of death for heavy smokers is almost 24 times as great as that of nonsmokers.[3b]

As described in Chapter 1, the three main types of epidemiological study are prospective, retrospective, and cross-sectional. Only prospective studies can provide an incidence rate by following a group of people (usually two groups, exposed and nonexposed) forward in time and observing the development of disease. With data from prospective studies, relative risk can be calculated with few problems. Cross-sectional studies provide a measure of the prevalence of disease at one point in time. An estimate of the relative risk can be calculated from such studies by obtaining the ratio of the prevalence rates between the exposed and the nonexposed.

Much more frequently, however, epidemiological data are derived from retrospective studies. In these, data are collected from two groups of people, one having a specific disease or condition and the other not having it, to determine whether they were or were not exposed to the same risk factors. For example, data can be collected from people who have lung cancer and from others, comparable in terms of age, sex, race, and other variables, who do not, to determine their smoking habits. From such studies, four categories are obtained:

	With the Disease (Cases)	Without the Disease (Controls)
Exposed	A	B
Nonexposed	C	D

It is known that a given number (A) of people with the disease have been exposed to the factor, a given number (B) without the disease also have been exposed, and so on. However, the population at risk is not known, so the incidence rates cannot be calculated. These four groups do not represent the total populations exposed and not exposed. However, the relative risk can be estimated by using the odds ratio, also known as the risk ratio or the cross ratio. The estimate of relative risk is obtained by:

$$RR = \frac{A \times D}{B \times C}$$

where: A, B, C, D are defined as above

For example, Doll and Hill did a retrospective study to determine the smoking habits of a group of lung cancer patients and of a matched group of patients with other diseases. They found the following (smokers were defined as those who had averaged at least one cigarette a day over the 10 years preceding the onset of the present illness):

	Patients with Lung Cancer	Patients with Other Conditions
Smokers	1,350	1,296
Nonsmokers	7	61

The relative risk can be estimated as:

$$RR = \frac{1,350 \times 61}{7 \times 1,296} = 9.08$$

This estimate represents a risk of lung cancer nine times greater among smokers than nonsmokers. It differs from the previous result because that was the relative risk among heavy smokers.

Attributable Risk

The number or proportion of cases of a disease, or a cause of death, attributable to a risk factor also can be calculated. The attributable risk can be defined as the difference between exposed and the nonexposed groups in the incidence rate of a disease or condition. The data show that the incidence of lung cancer attributable to heavy smoking is 1.59 per 1,000 (1.66 − .07). The rate of 1.59 per 1,000 is referred to as the excess risk.[4]

A proportion (ratio) is another way of expressing the attributable risk, known as the attributable risk percent (AR%). This represents the percentage of risk that can be attributed to the risk factor. The ratio can be calculated either for the exposed population (AR% in the exposed) or for the total population (AR% in the population).

$$AR \text{ in the exposed} = \frac{IR_e - IR_{ne}}{IR_e} \times 100$$

$$Population\ AR = \frac{IR_e - IR_{ne}}{IR_e + IR_{ne}} \times 100$$

where: IR_e = incidence rate among exposed

IR_{ne} = incidence rate among nonexposed

Using data from Doll and Hill's study of lung cancer produces this result:

$$AR \text{ in heavy smokers} = \frac{1.66 \times .07}{1.66} \times 100 = 95.8\%$$

Thus, 95.8 percent of deaths from lung cancer can be attributable to heavy smoking. The population AR% in this example cannot be calculated because the incidence rate of nonheavy smokers is lacking (only the incidence rate among nonsmokers is available). If the death rate from lung cancer among all smokers is .85/1,000 and among nonsmokers is .07/1,000 then:

$$AR\% \text{ in smokers} = \frac{.88 - .07}{.88} \times 100 = 92\%$$

$$Population\ AR\% = \frac{.88 - .07}{.88 + .07} \times 100 = 85\%$$

This means that 92 percent of deaths from lung cancer among smokers can be attributed to smoking and that 85 percent of lung cancer deaths among the total population also can be attributed to smoking. The latter figure (population attributable risk) represents the maximum proportion of lung cancer that can be assigned to cigarette smoking.

As for relative risk, the population AR% can be calculated even when incidence rates are not available (in retrospective studies):

$$Population\ AR\% = \frac{B\ (RR\ -\ 1)}{1\ +\ B\ (RR\ -\ 1)} \times 100$$

where: RR = relative ~~task~~ risk

B = proportion of those exposed in the population

For example, if the relative risk of lung cancer among smokers is 9.08, and it is known that 50 percent of the general population are smokers, then:

$$Population\ AR\% = \frac{.50\ (9.08\ -\ 1)}{1\ +\ .50\ (9.08\ -\ 1)} \times 100 = 80\%$$

Both attributable and relative risks can be helpful in determining priorities. Table 5-8 illustrates the relationship and complementary components of these epidemiological measures. In this example, smokers are at 12 times greater risk of dying from lung cancer than nonsmokers and at 1.4 times greater risk from

---

Table 5-8 Comparison of Relative and Attributable Risks

	Death Rates per 100,000	
	Lung Cancer	Cerebrovascular Disease
Smokers	85	599
Nonsmokers	7	422
Then,		
Relative risk =	$\frac{85}{7} = 12.1$	$\frac{599}{422} = 1.4$
Attributable risk = (excess risk)	$85 - 7 = 78/100{,}000$	$599 - 422 = 177/100{,}000$

Source: Adapted from *Epidemiology: An Introductory Text* by Judith S. Mausner and Anita K. Bahn with permission of W.B. Saunders Company, ©1974, 322.

cerebrovascular disease. It can be said that smoking influences the death rates from lung cancer much more than those from cerebrovascular disease. The attributable (excess) risks indicate, however, that 78 lung-cancer deaths and 177 cerebrovascular deaths per 100,000 are attributable to smoking. This means that smoking influences a greater number of deaths from cerebrovascular disease than from lung cancer.[5]

Relative risk thus is a better measure of the causal association between a risk factor and a disease (or cause of death) while the attributable risk gives an estimate of the possible reduction in morbidity and mortality from the elimination of the risk factor.

Amenability to Prevention or Reduction

The second set of epidemiological criteria that can be used in determining priorities is the amenability of the disease, problem, or risk factor to prevention or reduction or its sensitivity to a health program. Consequently, it is not of much use to consider a problem to be a priority if there is nothing that can be done about it.

Amenability can be conceived of as a relationship between inputs and outputs.[6] Inputs often are stated in terms of costs or expenditures, outputs in terms of the effects of the program on the problem or as the money value of such effects. This is known as a cost-benefit analysis.

Although cost-benefit analysis is popular, its regular use in health service management is far away. It is relatively easy to keep track of such costs but the measurement and valuation of benefits present several problems. However, health service managers still can consider the amenability of a health problem by relying on the judgment of experts or on the experience of others. For example, several estimates of the effectiveness of smoking cessation programs have been published. Similarly, the work of Rutstein and colleagues[7] and of the Canadian Task Force on the Periodic Health Examination[8] (both described in Chapter 2) can be used to determine the problems that are most amenable to prevention.

Magnitude of loss and amenability thus are two essentially independent properties jointly constituting guides for the determination of priorities.[9] Donabedian (Table 5-9) illustrates possible decision rules or bases for magnitude of loss and amenability to prevention or reduction.

PROBLEMS OF MEASUREMENT

This chapter and the previous one have presented several epidemiological measures to be used in health service management and analyzed their statistical and practical significance. A last issue remains: the quality of these measures.

For purposes here, distinctions are drawn among three components of the quality of a measure: its validity, its reliability, and its sensitivity.

Table 5-9 Deciding on Loss and Prevention

Magnitude of Loss	Amenability	Decision
High	High	High priority for delivery of service
High	Low	High priority for research
Low	High	Second priority for delivery of service
Low	Low	Second priority for research; lowest priority for delivery of service

Source: Reprinted from *Aspects of Medical Care Administration: Specifying Requirements for Health Care* by Avedias Donabedian with permission of the Harvard University Press, ©1973, 169.

Validity of a Measure

Validity refers to the extent a measure can measure what it purports to measure. Is it really measuring what was intended to be measured? The validity of epidemiological measures for identifying health problems is, of course, a big issue: Are they really measuring "health problems?" The answer is even more difficult since it is not really known what "health" is.

The validity of a measure has four dimensions: face, and the three Cs, content, criterion, and construct.

Face validity refers to apparent, common-sense validity: does the measuring appear to be doing what it is supposed to be doing? For example, if the number of parking tickets is used as an indicator of the health of a community, that poses a big problem with face validity even though it really may be right (by some as yet unexplainable phenomenon). Face validity is important mostly in terms of the acceptability of results to outsiders.

Content validity refers to the extent of measuring all aspects, dimensions, or components of what is intended to be measured. This is, of course, the major drawback to health indicators or single measures of health. For example, an infant mortality rate unquestionably is not a content valid measure of health, even though infant mortality often is used as the single indicator. There is no way to assess the content validity of a measure mathematically. The only guideline is to break down what is to be measured into as many components as possible. For example, if the subjects are physiological, psychological, and social health, indicators can be found for each. These indicators can be used either separately or combined into a health index.

Criterion validity refers to the extent to which it is possible to explain or predict what is wanted to be measured (a distinction can be made between predictive and concurrent criterion validity). This can be assessed by looking at the correlation of the measure with some other criteria, either retrospectively or futuristically (when those criteria become available). For example, the predictive criterion validity of smoking can be assessed as a health problem indicator by looking at the association between smoking and death. In this case, the relative and attributable risks associated with smoking demonstrate that smoking is a good predictor of health problems.

Finally, construct validity refers to the general definition of validity: that is, the extent to which managers are really measuring what they say they are. Several methods have been proposed to assess construct validity. These all are complex, however, and are well described in other excellent sources.[10, 11, 12] In general, all of these methods aim to correlate the measure to be construct-validated with other measures that are known to be construct-valid.

An oversimplified example would be if an attempt were made to devise a new aptitude scale, perhaps a shorter version. It is known that several such scales have been construct-validated. If the new scale correlated highly with the others, then there could be relative confidence in its construct-validity.

Reliability of a Measure

Reliability refers to the reproducibility or constancy of the measure. If a measure is used several times, how close will be the different results? This is not directly related to validity, however. A classic example is a weight scale: suppose a person is weighed five times in quick succession and the measurement always is the same. It could be said that the scale was reliable. However, it might be maladjusted and add 20 pounds to the real weight—five times in quick succession. Even though reliable in its consistency the scale would not give a valid measure. Assessment of the reliability of a single indicator is quite straightforward: repeated applications of the indicator must correlate together closely. For multidimensional indexes, some statistical techniques are available. [13, 14, 15]

Sensitivity of a Measure

The sensitivity of a measure refers to its ability to include a great proportion of what it is measuring. This is the opposite of its specificity, or its ability to exclude as much false information as possible. Infant mortality rates, for example, are sensitive indicators since they include most of the routinely reported infant deaths and omit many "false" deaths, i.e. deaths that could not be allocated to another group.

Sensitivity and specificity most often relate to screening measures. A screening measure (or test) can be either sensitive or specific. A sensitive screening measure should be wide enough to include as many real cases of the disease as possible; in doing so, however, it also will include a high number of false cases (it will not be specific).

SUMMARY

Two of the major problems facing all decision makers, including health service managers, is the identification of a problem and the resulting difficulty of determining priorities. This chapter shows how the SMR—the standardized mortality rate—a simple but reliable method, can be used to identify various problems from an epidemiological perspective. The determination of priorities may be accomplished by several methods, of which the PMR, years of life lost, risk factors, and amenability to prevention are discussed.

Each is useful and valid for priority setting in health management. Certainly all techniques and methods are subject to variability and errors, so for this reason the concepts of validity, reliability, and sensitivity are discussed. It is contended here that health service managers using these epidemiological measures will be more sophisticated in the analysis of health care utilization.

NOTES

1. Judith S. Mausner and Anita K. Bahn, *Epidemiology: An Introductory Text* (Philadelphia: W.B. Saunders Company, 1974), 188.

2. Avedias Donabedian, *Aspects of Medical Care Administration: Specifying Requirements for Health Care* (Cambridge, Mass.: Harvard University Press, 1973), 165.

3. J.C. Kleinman, "Infant Mortality," *Statistical Notes for Health Planners*, vol. 2 (Washington, D.C.: National Center for Health Statistics, July 1976), 12.

3a. Richard Doll and A.B. Hill, "A Study of the Aetiology of Carcinoma of the Lung," *British Medical Journal*, 1952, 1271-1286.

3b. Richard Doll and A.B. Hill, "Lung Cancer and Other Causes of Death in Relation to Smoking. A Second Report on the Mortality of British Doctors," *British Medical Journal*, 1956, 1071.

4. D.F. Austin and S.B. Werner, *Epidemiology for the Health Sciences* (Springfield, Ill.: Charles C Thomas, Publisher, 1974), 53.

5. Doll and Hill, *Carcinoma of the Lung*.

6. Donabedian, *Aspects of Medical Care*, 170.

7. D.D. Rutstein et al., "Measuring the Quality of Medical Care—A Clinical Method," *The New England Journal of Medicine* 294 (March 11, 1976), 582-588.

8. Minister of Supply and Services, Health and Welfare Canada, *The Periodic Health Examination Monograph—Report of a Task Force to the Conference of Deputy Ministers of Health* (Ottawa: 1980), 194.

9. Donabedian, *Aspects of Medical Care*, 169.

10. June C. Nunnally and Robert L. Durham, "Validity, Reliability, and Special Problems of Measurement in Evaluation Research" in *Handbook of Evaluation Research*, ed. Elmer L. Struemling and Maria Guttentag (Beverly Hills, Calif.: Sage Publications Inc., 1975), 289-305.

11. Ibid., 305-311.

12. E.G. Carmines and R.A. Zeller, *Reliability and Validity Assessment* (Beverly Hills, Calif.: Sage Publications, Inc. 1979), 76.

13. Ibid.

14. G.W. Bohrnstedt, "A Quick Method for Determining the Reliability and Validity of Multiple-Item Scales," *American Sociological Review, 34* (August 1969), 39.

15. L.S. Cronbach, "Coefficient Alpha and the Internal Structure of Tests," *Psychometrika* 16 (1951), 297.

Chapter 6

Descriptive Epidemiology: Person

THE PATTERNS OF DISEASE AND HEALTH

Descriptive epidemiology is concerned with the observation and description of the occurrence, distribution, size, and progression of health and causes of disease and death in populations. Chapter 5 showed how health service managers can use epidemiological measures to determine the occurrence and size of health problems in a population of interest. The basic premise of epidemiology, however, is that disease and health do not occur randomly but in patterns reflecting the operation of the underlying causes.[1]

These patterns of occurrence can be described in answering three broad questions: Who is affected? Where does the problem occur? When does the problem occur? The answers give managers a more detailed understanding of health problems in their communities and serve in the development of programs (program planning) to meet these needs.

Knowledge of the distribution and progression of health and disease in the population increases the effectiveness of programs by allowing, among other things, the identification of specific target groups.

This chapter examines the distribution of disease by person (who); Chapter 7 deals with place (where) and time (when) of occurrence. The use of the term disease is broadened here to encompass such other problems as motor vehicle and all other accidents, homicide, and suicide, all of which are included in epidemiological statistics as causal factors in deaths and other conditions that impact on health.

The distribution of health and disease in a population is a function of many attributes and characteristics of its members. These factors can be grouped into three sets of variables: demographic, social, and life style.

DEMOGRAPHIC VARIABLES

Age, sex, and racial or ethnic origin are the three main demographic variables that characterize the distribution of health and disease in a population.

The Role of Age

Age is the personal attribute most strongly related to disease occurrence. In fact, age association is so strong that it almost always is necessary to control (eliminate) the effect of differences in age distribution when comparing disease occurrences in two populations, or at two points in time, through age adjustment of rates—unless, of course, there is confidence that the age distributions are quite similar. Some diseases may occur almost exclusively in a particular age group, others over a wider age span but tending to be more prevalent at certain levels than at others.

The relationship between age and disease occurrence may be examined in several ways. Age-specific rates can (1) measure the risk of disease in each group, (2) examine the leading diseases in each group, and (3) trace the age progression of a particular disease.

Life Stage Disease Patterns

Table 6-1 lists the leading age-specific (life stage pattern) health problems in the state of Georgia (1975-77), whereas Tables 6-2, 6-3, 6-4, and 6-5 rank the life stage (age) specific mortality rates for males and females, white and black and others for the United States (1975-77). Definite patterns are peculiar to each age group (the influence of race and sex is discussed in the next sections). The problems of infancy are primarily congenital and are related to immaturity. During childhood, accidents (motor vehicle and other), infectious diseases, and homicide and other forms of violence and abuse are the most prevalent problems. The major killers of adolescence are motor vehicle accidents, other accidents, suicide, and homicide. Alcohol and drug abuse, as well as unwanted pregnancies, also are characteristic problems. As individuals grow older, accidents, homicide, and suicide slowly are replaced as major killers by chronic diseases, mostly heart, stroke, and cancer.

Age-Specific Rates

Age-specific rates also can be used to trace the progression of a particular disease through the life stages. Figure 6-1 shows death rates per 1,000 for white and nonwhite males and females, by age. It demonstrates that death rates in all four groups are high at infancy but decline rapidly, then increase gradually after age 10 and exponentially after age 40. Chronic diseases often show a dramatic relationship to age, as in Figure 6-2 (lung cancer) and Figure 6-3 (hypertension).

Table 6-1 Leading Age-Specific Health Problems

Georgia, 1975-77

Life Stage and Age	Health Problems	Life Stage and Age	Health Problems
Infancy *(birth through first year)*	Anoxia and hypoxia Low birth weight Congenital anomalies Pneumonia Accidents Infant sudden death syndrome Down's syndrome Hyaline membrane disease Phenylketonuria (PKU)	**Early Adulthood** (20-29 years)	Homicide Suicide Anxiety Depression Mental illness Motor vehicle/other accidents Cancers Ischemic heart disease Complications of pregnancy Cirrhosis of the liver Nervous conditions Back, limb, and hip injuries Gallbladder disease
Early Childhood *(1-4 years)*	Accidents Infectious diseases Child abuse Lead poisoning Development attrition		
Childhood *(5-12 years)*	Accidents Cancers Influenza and pneumonia Homicide Leukemia Morbidity (infection of ear, nose, throat, other) Malnutrition Dental disease	**Young Adulthood** *(30-44 years)*	Ischemic heart disease Motor vehicle accidents Cancers Stroke Heart attack Homicide Suicide Mental illness Depression
Adolescence *(13-19 years)*	Adolescent pregnancy Alcohol Drug abuse Motor vehicle accidents All other accidents Suicide Homicide Venereal diseases Dental disease Mental/emotional problems Sports injuries	**Middle Adulthood** *(45-59 years)*	Ischemic heart disease Heart attack Cancers Stroke Cirrhosis of the liver Diabetes Motor vehicle accidents Suicide Respiratory conditions Hypertension

Table 6-1 continued

Georgia, 1975-77

Life Stage and Age	Health Problems	Life Stage and Age	Health Problems

Late Adulthood *(60-74 years)*	Ulcer
	Frequent constipation
	Hypertension
	Hernia
	Upper gastrointestinal
	  disorders
	Gallbladder conditions
	Respiratory conditions
	Ischemic heart disease
	Stroke
	Heart attack
	Diabetes
	Cancers
	Influenza and pneumonia
	Chronic obstructive
	  pulmonary disease
	  (COPD)
		Older Adulthood *(75+ years)*	Hernia
			Dependency
			Frequent constipation
			Gallbladder conditions
			Senility
			Arthritis
			Rheumatism
			Heart conditions

Source: G.E. Alan Dever, "Passages: Predictability of Mortality through the Life Stages," Georgia Department of Human Resources, Division of Public Health, 1980, 399.

Disease Pyramids

The disease pyramid is an alternate method of examining diseases by age as well as by sex and race. Constructed in the same manner as a population pyramid, the disease pyramid shows which age groups are affected by diseases. It provides an immediate visual analysis of disease mortality by age, sex, and race. It can illustrate the dominance of a specific age, sex, or race for the selected disease (Figure 6-4). Specific target groups may be identified, depending upon the specificity of the age groups involved.

For example, an inverted pyramid indicates a disease that is concentrated in the older ages while one that bulges to the left of the central axis at midpoint indicates that a disease such as cirrhosis of the liver occurs predominantly in males of middle age. The pyramid, however, does not give the absolute risk of dying by age, sex, and race because its values are not weighted according to distribution of the population for each of those groupings.

Table 6-2 Causes of Death by Life Stages, U.S., 1975-1977

White Males

	Infancy (First Year)			Early Childhood (Ages 1-4)			Childhood (Ages 5-12)	
Rank	Cause of Death	Rate¹	Rank	Cause of Death	Rate¹	Rank	Cause of Death	Rate¹
1	Conditions of birthing	439.3	1	Accidents (other than motor vehicle)	19.3	1	Accidents (other than motor vehicle)	10.1
2	Congenital anomalies	286.7	2	Motor vehicle accidents	10.8	2	Motor vehicle accidents	9.9
3	Infective and parasitic diseases²	61.6	3	Congenital anomalies	8.5	3	Leukemia	3.3
4	Influenza and pneumonia	52.6	4	Cancer (except leukemia)	3.8	4	Cancer (except leukemia)	3.1
5	Accidents (other than motor vehicle)	30.3	5	Influenza and pneumonia	3.1	5	Congenital anomalies	2.3
6	Diseases of the circulatory system	27.6	6	Infective and parasitic diseases²	3.0	6	Infective and parasitic diseases²	1.0
7	Heart disease	21.9	7	Leukemia	2.3	7	Influenza and pneumonia	0.9
8	Meningitis	15.7	8	Meningitis	2.0	8	Heart disease	0.7
9	Motor vehicle accidents	7.8	9	Homicide	1.8	9	Homicide	0.7
10	Homicide	4.3	10	Heart disease	1.7	10	Stroke	0.5
	All causes	1,511.9		All causes	70.9		All causes	38.7

Table 6-2 continued

	Adolescence (Ages 13-19)			Early Adulthood (Ages 20-29)			Young Adulthood (Ages 30-44)	
Rank	Cause of Death	Rate[1]	Rank	Cause of Death	Rate[1]	Rank	Cause of Death	Rate[1]
1	Motor vehicle accidents	38.1	1	Motor vehicle accidents	56.9	1	Heart disease	54.7
2	Accidents (other than motor vehicle)	20.6	2	Accidents (other than motor vehicle)	33.3	2	Ischemic heart disease	46.5
3	Suicide	7.4	3	Suicide	27.0	3	Heart attack	32.8
4	Homicide	4.5	4	Homicide	14.7	4	Motor vehicle accidents	28.7
5	Cancer (except leukemia)	4.0	5	Heart disease	4.6	5	Accidents (other than motor vehicle)	27.3
6	Leukemia	2.2	6	Leukemia	2.0	6	Suicide	24.0
7	Congenital anomalies	1.7	7	Stroke	1.7	7	Homicide	14.0
8	Heart disease[3]	1.5	8	Ischemic heart disease	1.6	8	Cirrhosis of the liver	13.3
9	Influenza and pneumonia	1.1	9	Influenza and pneumonia	1.6	9	Lung cancer	9.4
10	Infective and parasitic diseases[2]	0.7	10	Congenital anomalies	1.6	10	Cancer of digestive system	6.9
	All causes	92.8		All causes	176.3		All causes	246.8

Middle Adulthood (Ages 45-59)			Late Adulthood (Ages 60-74)			Older Adulthood (Ages 75+)		
Rank	Cause of Death	Rate[1]	Rank	Cause of Death	Rate[1]	Rank	Cause of Death	Rate[1]
1	Heart disease	418.4	1	Heart disease	1,628.6	1	Heart disease	5,789.5
2	Ischemic heart disease	377.8	2	Ischemic heart disease	1,487.6	2	Ischemic heart disease	5,296.2
3	Heart attack	258.6	3	Heart attack	909.0	3	Heart attack	2,159.3
4	Lung cancer	102.3	4	Lung cancer	354.7	4	Stroke	1,670.0
5	Cancer of digestive system	57.4	5	Stroke	262.4	5	Influenza and pneumonia	643.4
6	Cirrhosis of the liver	48.5	6	Cancer of digestive system	241.3	6	Cancer of digestive system	567.7
7	Stroke	37.9	7	COPD[4]	94.4	7	Lung cancer	421.4
8	Accidents (other than motor vehicle)	33.8	8	Influenza and pneumonia	78.9	8	Cancer of genitalia	383.6
9	Suicide	29.1	9	Cancer of genitalia	77.9	9	Diseases of arteries and capillaries	377.4
10	Motor vehicle accidents	24.4	10	Cirrhosis of the liver	66.7	10	COPD[4]	221.2
	All causes	1,007.3		All causes	3,755.1		All causes	12,763.9

1. Life stage specific rates are per 100,000 population.
2. Includes bacillary dysentery and amebiasis; tuberculosis, all forms; whooping cough; meningococcal infections; septicemia; measles; syphilis and sequelae; enteritis and other diarrheal diseases; other.
3. Heart disease categories are mutually inclusive; i.e., "heart disease" includes ischemic heart disease and heart attack, and "ischemic heart disease" includes heart attack.
4. COPD = chronic obstructive pulmonary disease.

Source: U.S. Department of Health, Education, and Welfare, National Center for Health Statistics, *Vital Statistics of the United States*, Vol. II, 1975-1977, Hyattsville, Md.

Table 6-3 Causes of Death by Life Stages, U.S., 1975-1977

Black and Other Males

	Infancy (First Year)			Early Childhood (Ages 1-4)			Childhood (Ages 5-12)	
Rank	Cause of Death	Rate[1]	Rank	Cause of Death	Rate[1]	Rank	Cause of Death	Rate[1]
1	Conditions of birthing	811.3	1	Accidents (other than motor vehicle)	28.5	1	Accidents (other than motor vehicle)	17.0
2	Congenital anomalies	304.4	2	Motor vehicle accidents	15.1	2	Motor vehicle accidents	15.0
3	Infective and parasitic diseases[2]	157.6	3	Congenital anomalies	9.5	3	Cancer (except leukemia)	3.2
4	Influenza and pneumonia	152.0	4	Influenza and pneumonia	7.1	4	Congenital anomalies	2.3
5	Accidents (other than motor vehicle)	66.5	5	Homicide	7.1	5	Leukemia	1.8
6	Diseases of the circulatory system	48.2	6	Infective and parasitic diseases[2]	4.4	6	Homicide	1.8
7	Heart disease	39.7	7	Heart disease	3.3	7	Infective and parasitic diseases[2]	1.2
8	Meningitis	36.1	8	Cancer (except leukemia)	2.8	8	Influenza and pneumonia	1.1
9	Homicide	14.3	9	Meningitis	2.6	9	Heart disease	1.0
10	Motor vehicle accidents	8.4	10	Leukemia	1.7	10	Stroke	0.4
	All causes	2,931.3		All causes	108.1		All causes	54.1

	Adolescence (Ages 13-19)			Early Adulthood (Ages 20-29)			Young Adulthood (Ages 30-44)	
Rank	Cause of Death	Rate[1]	Rank	Cause of Death	Rate[1]	Rank	Cause of Death	Rate[1]
1	Accidents (other than motor vehicle)	25.9	1	Homicide	122.1	1	Homicide	106.7
2	Homicide	23.8	2	Motor vehicle accidents	53.4	2	Heart disease	99.5
3	Motor vehicle accidents	20.5	3	Accidents (other than motor vehicle)	49.2	3	Ischemic heart disease	69.4
4	Suicide	4.1	4	Suicide	25.2	4	Accidents (other than motor vehicle)	57.0
5	Cancer (except leukemia)	3.6	5	Heart disease	13.7	5	Cirrhosis of the liver	48.0
6	Heart disease[3]	3.2	6	Cirrhosis of the liver	6.9	6	Motor vehicle accidents	42.7
7	Congenital anomalies	1.8	7	Influenza and pneumonia	4.5	7	Heart attack	35.8
8	Influenza and pneumonia	1.6	8	Stroke	4.3	8	Stroke	25.5
9	Leukemia	1.5	9	Ischemic heart disease	4.0	9	Suicide	18.5
10	Infective and parasitic diseases[2]	1.3	10	Congenital anomalies	1.8	10	Lung cancer	18.0
	All causes	103.3		All causes	354.1		All causes	616.6

Table 6-3 continued

	Middle Adulthood (Ages 45-59)			Late Adulthood (Ages 60-74)			Older Adulthood (Ages 75+)	
Rank	Cause of Death	Rate[1]	Rank	Cause of Death	Rate[1]	Rank	Cause of Death	Rate[1]
1	Heart disease	520.3	1	Heart disease	1,636.4	1	Heart disease	3,836.0
2	Ischemic heart disease	428.7	2	Ischemic heart disease	1,389.6	2	Ischemic heart disease	3,301.7
3	Heart attack	206.6	3	Heart attack	616.8	3	Stroke	1,332.4
4	Lung cancer	171.5	4	Stroke	478.2	4	Heart attack	1,156.3
5	Stroke	114.3	5	Lung cancer	383.6	5	Cancer of genitalia	494.5
6	Cancer of digestive system	113.2	6	Cancer of digestive system	336.9	6	Cancer of digestive system	493.3
7	Cirrhosis of the liver	87.5	7	Cancer of genitalia	176.9	7	Influenza and pneumonia	453.3
8	Homicide	70.6	8	Influenza and pneumonia	124.4	8	Lung cancer	320.9
9	Accidents (other than motor vehicle)	69.0	9	Diabetes	94.3	9	Diseases of the arteries and capillaries	229.3
10	Influenza and pneumonia	46.5	10	Accidents (other than motor vehicle)	86.2	10	Diabetes	157.9
	All causes	1,717.7		All causes	4,548.0		All causes	9,666.1

1. Life stage specific rates are per 100,000 population.
2. Includes bacillary dysentery and amebiasis; tuberculosis, all forms; whooping cough; meningococcal infections; septicemia; measles; syphilis and sequelae; enteritis and other diarrheal diseases; other.
3. Heart disease categories are mutually inclusive; i.e., "heart disease" includes ischemic heart disease and heart attack, and "ischemic heart disease" includes heart attack.

Source: U.S. Department of Health, Education, and Welfare, National Center for Health Statistics, *Vital Statistics of the United States,* Vol. II, 1975-1977, Hyattsville, Md.

Table 6-4 Causes of Death by Life Stages, U.S., 1975-1977

White Females

Infancy (First Year)			Early Childhood (Ages 1-4)			Childhood (Ages 5-12)		
Rank	Cause of Death	Rate[1]	Rank	Cause of Death	Rate[1]	Rank	Cause of Death	Rate[1]
1	Conditions of birthing	315.0	1	Accidents (other than motor vehicle)	12.3	1	Motor vehicle accidents	6.5
2	Congenital anomalies	251.6	2	Congenital anomalies	8.9	2	Accidents (other than motor vehicle)	4.6
3	Infective and parasitic diseases[2]	50.5	3	Motor vehicle accidents	8.5	3	Leukemia	2.3
4	Influenza and pneumonia	42.8	4	Cancer (except leukemia)	3.0	4	Congenital anomalies	2.3
5	Accidents (other than motor vehicle)	22.7	5	Influenza and pneumonia	3.0	5	Cancer (except leukemia)	2.1
6	Diseases of the circulatory system	20.5	6	Infective and parasitic diseases[2]	2.7	6	Influenza and pneumonia	0.8
7	Heart disease[3]	15.9	7	Leukemia	1.9	7	Homicide	0.7
8	Meningitis	12.1	8	Heart disease[3]	1.4	8	Infective and parasitic diseases[2]	0.7
9	Motor vehicle accidents	8.2	9	Homicide	1.4	9	Heart disease[3]	0.6
10	Homicide	3.8	10	Meningitis	1.2	10	Stroke	0.4
	All causes	1,169.7		All causes	56.0		All causes	26.6

Table 6-4 continued

	Adolescence (Ages 13-19)		Early Adulthood (Ages 20-29)		Young Adulthood (Ages 30-44)	
Rank	Cause of Death	Rate[1]	Cause of Death	Rate[1]	Cause of Death	Rate[1]
1	Motor vehicle accidents	14.7	Motor vehicle accidents	14.6	Heart disease	14.3
2	Accidents (other than motor vehicle)	4.7	Suicide	7.5	Breast cancer	13.4
3	Cancer (except leukemia)	2.7	Accidents (other than motor vehicle)	5.7	Suicide	11.0
4	Homicide	1.9	Homicide	4.2	Motor vehicle accidents	9.2
5	Suicide	1.8	Heart disease[3]	2.3	Ischemic heart disease	8.7
6	Leukemia	1.5	Stroke	1.5	Stroke	7.1
7	Congenital anomalies	1.4	Leukemia	1.4	Cancer of genitalia	6.9
8	Influenza and pneumonia	1.0	Influenza and pneumonia	1.3	Accidents (other than motor vehicle)	6.7
9	Heart disease[3]	0.9	Congenital anomalies	1.1	Cirrhosis of the liver	5.9
10	Infective and parasitic diseases[2]	0.6	Cirrhosis of the liver	0.5	Heart attack	5.7
	All causes	38.9	All causes	60.5	All causes	132.7

Middle Adulthood (Ages 45-59)			Late Adulthood (Ages 60-74)			Older Adulthood (Ages 75+)		
Rank	Cause of Death	Rate[1]	Rank	Cause of Death	Rate[1]	Rank	Cause of Death	Rate[1]
1	Heart disease	112.7	1	Heart disease	692.3	1	Heart disease	4,263.3
2	Ischemic heart disease	90.3	2	Ischemic heart disease	610.8	2	Ischemic heart disease	3,877.1
3	Breast cancer	59.3	3	Heart attack	343.2	3	Stroke	1,577.5
4	Heart attack	57.6	4	Stroke	179.7	4	Heart attack	1,329.3
5	Cancer of digestive system	38.5	5	Cancer of digestive system	149.0	5	Cancer of digestive system	390.0
6	Lung cancer	37.3	6	Breast cancer	97.5	6	Influenza and pneumonia	388.4
7	Cancer of genitalia	32.8	7	Lung cancer	74.1	7	Diseases of arteries and capillaries	342.7
8	Stroke	30.8	8	Cancer of genitalia	69.8	8	Diabetes	178.4
9	Cirrhosis of the liver	22.9	9	Diabetes	53.3	9	Accidents (other than motor vehicle)	151.2
10	Suicide	13.3	10	Influenza and pneumonia	35.1	10	Breast cancer	147.1
	All causes	518.0		All causes	1,839.2		All causes	8,951.0

1. Life stage specific rates are per 100,000 population.
2. Includes bacillary dysentery and amebiasis; tuberculosis, all forms; whooping cough; meningococcal infections; septicemia: measles; syphilis and sequelae; enteritis and other diarrheal diseases; other.
3. Heart disease categories are mutually inclusive; i.e., "heart disease" includes ischemic heart disease and heart attack, and "ischemic heart disease" includes heart attack.

Source: U.S. Department of Health, Education, and Welfare, National Center for Health Statistics, *Vital Statistics of the United States,* Vol. II, 1975-1977, Hyattsville, Md.

Table 6-5 Causes of Death by Life Stages, U.S., 1975-1977

Black and Other Females

	Infancy (First Year)		Early Childhood (Ages 1-4)		Childhood (Ages 5-12)	
Rank	Cause of Death	Rate[1]	Cause of Death	Rate[1]	Cause of Death	Rate[1]
1	Conditions of birthing	647.3	Accidents (other than motor vehicle)	21.0	Accidents (other than motor vehicle)	7.9
2	Congenital anomalies	281.4	Motor vehicle accidents	10.9	Motor vehicle accidents	7.9
3	Infective and parasitic diseases[2]	135.2	Congenital anomalies	10.2	Congenital anomalies	2.6
4	Influenza and pneumonia	124.2	Homicide	6.5	Cancer (except leukemia)	2.3
5	Accidents (other than motor vehicle)	56.7	Influenza and pneumonia	6.1	Homicide	1.7
6	Diseases of the circulatory system	47.3	Infective and parasitic diseases[2]	4.2	Leukemia	1.5
7	Heart disease[3]	36.3	Cancer (except leukemia)	3.1	Influenza and pneumonia	1.4
8	Meningitis	35.7	Heart disease[3]	2.7	Infective and parasitic diseases[2]	1.2
9	Homicide	12.2	Meningitis	1.5	Heart disease[3]	1.1
10	Motor vehicle accidents	8.4	Leukemia	1.4	Stroke	0.5
	All causes	2,456.5	All causes	88.7	All causes	35.5

	Adolescence (Ages 13-19)			Early Adulthood (Ages 20-29)			Young Adulthood (Ages 30-44)	
Rank	Cause of Death	Rate[1]	Rank	Cause of Death	Rate[1]	Rank	Cause f Death	Rate[1]
1	Homicide	7.2	1	Homicide	24.1	1	Heart disease	45.4
2	Motor vehicle accidents	6.9	2	Motor vehicle accidents	11.7	2	Ischemic heart disease	27.1
3	Accidents (other than motor vehicle)	6.1	3	Accidents (other than motor vehicle)	11.3	3	Cirrhosis of the liver	24.3
4	Cancer (except leukemia)	3.1	4	Heart disease	7.3	4	Stroke	20.8
5	Heart disease[3]	2.3	5	Suicide	6.3	5	Homicide	19.5
6	Influenza and pneumonia	1.5	6	Stroke	3.8	6	Breast cancer	15.5
7	Suicide	1.4	7	Cirrhosis of the liver	3.8	7	Heart attack	12.9
8	Congenital anomalies	1.3	8	Influenza and pneumonia	2.8	8	Accidents (other than motor vehicle)	12.3
9	Leukemia	1.2	9	Leukemia	1.4	9	Cancer of genitalia	12.2
10	Infective and parasitic diseases[2]	1.0	10	Ischemic heart disease	1.4	10	Motor vehicle accidents	10.1
	All causes	45.6		All causes	121.6		All causes	289.0

Table 6-5 continued

	Middle Adulthood (Ages 45-59)		Late Adulthood (Ages 60-74)		Older Adulthood (Ages 75+)	
Rank	Cause of Death	Rate[1]	Cause of Death	Rate[1]	Cause of Death	Rate[1]
1	Heart disease	269.1	Heart disease	1,101.4	Heart disease	3,123.9
2	Ischemic heart disease	210.0	Ischemic heart disease	924.1	Ischemic heart disease	2,701.2
3	Heart attack	94.9	Stroke	404.1	Stroke	1,274.7
4	Stroke	90.8	Heart attack	378.5	Heart attack	856.3
5	Cancer of the digestive system	62.4	Cancer of the digestive system	190.4	Cancer of the digestive system	322.8
6	Breast cancer	57.9	Diabetes	144.0	Influenza and pneumonia	236.2
7	Cancer of genitalia	46.4	Cancer of genitalia	98.1	Diabetes	230.3
8	Cirrhosis of the liver	41.1	Breast cancer	85.3	Diseases of the arteries and capillaries	196.6
9	Lung cancer	40.2	Lung cancer	67.2	Cancer of genitalia	117.6
10	Diabetes	38.9	Influenza and pneumonia	54.4	Breast cancer	104.9
	All causes	958.6	All causes	2,878.3	All causes	7,135.6

1. Life stage specific rates are per 100,000 population.
2. Includes bacillary dysentery and amebiasis; tuberculosis, all forms; whooping cough; meningococcal infections; septicemia; measles; syphilis and sequelae; enteritis and other diarrheal diseases; other.
3. Heart disease categories are mutually inclusive; i.e., "heart disease" includes ischemic heart disease and heart attack, and "ischemic heart disease" includes heart attack.

Source: U.S. Department of Health, Education, and Welfare, National Center for Health Statistics, *Vital Statistics of the United States*, Vol. II, 1975-1977, Hyattsville, Md.

Figure 6-1 Death Rates Per 1,000 by Age, Race, and Sex, U.S., 1968
(Semilogarithmic Scale)

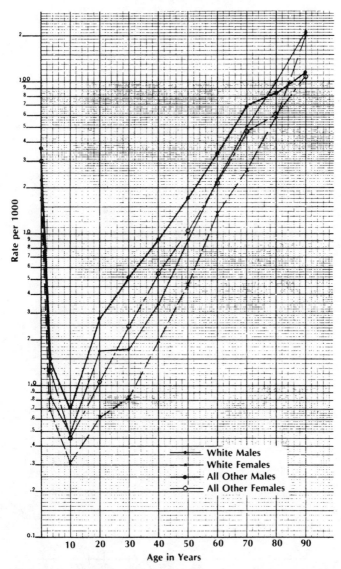

Source: Reprinted from *Epidemiology: An Introductory Text* by Judith S. Mausner and Anita K. Bahn with permission from W.B. Saunders Company, © 1974, p. 44. Based on *Vital Statistics of the United States, 1968,* vol. IIA. National Center for Health Statistics, U.S. Government Printing Office, 1972.

Figure 6-2 Age Specific Rates for Lung Cancer, U.S., 1950-1969
Whites, Per 100,000

Age	Males	Females
0- 4	0.08	0.06
5- 9	0.03	0.02
10-14	0.04	0.03
15-19	0.08	0.06
20-24	0.22	0.11
25-29	0.51	0.23
30-34	1.95	0.74
35-39	5.67	2.06
40-44	15.04	4.72
45-49	33.43	8.39
50-54	66.66	12.50
55-59	113.21	16.84
60-64	167.49	21.08
65-69	206.52	25.71
70-74	219.25	31.87
75-84	191.28	38.62
85+	120.82	38.74

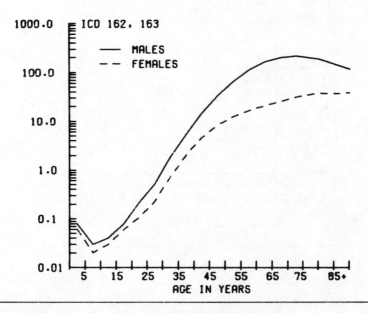

Source: Reprinted from *Atlas of Cancer Mortality for U.S. Counties, 1950-69*, by T.J. Mason, F.W. McCay et al., U.S. Department of Health, Education, and Welfare, National Institutes of Health (DHEW Publication No. [NIH] 75-780, 1975), 81.

Figure 6-3 Percent of Hypertensive Persons by Age, Race, and Sex, U.S., 1974

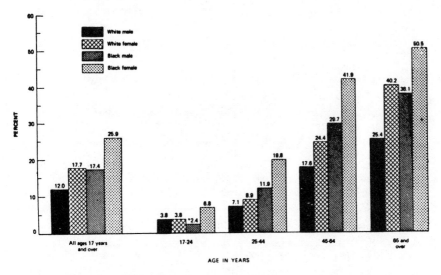

Source: Reprinted from *Advance Data—Hypertension: U.S. 1974*, U.S. Department of Health, Education, and Welfare, November 8, 1976, 2.

Cohort Analysis

Both age-specific rates and disease pyramids thus trace the progression of a particular disease through the age groups by showing the relationship between age and disease rates, as they occur simultaneously in time.[2] This process is known as current or cross-sectional analysis. Different people thus are involved in each age group.

By contrast, cohort analysis, although showing disease progression through the different age groups, follows a specific bloc of people (a cohort) through time. Several cohorts usually are identified and followed as they pass through different ages during part, or all, of their life span. Both current and cohort analysis should produce same results except when the frequency of the disease under consideration has been changing over time.[3] Then a cohort analysis will show a truer picture of the relationship of age, or aging, on the progression of disease.

The now-classic example of this is Frost's study of tuberculosis in Massachusetts for the years 1880 to 1930.[4] Figure 6-5 shows the results of three cross-sectional analyses of the mortality rates of tuberculosis in 1880, 1910, and 1930. As for the relationship between age and tuberculosis, the three curves produce quite different

Figure 6-4 Disease Pyramids, Georgia, 1970-1974

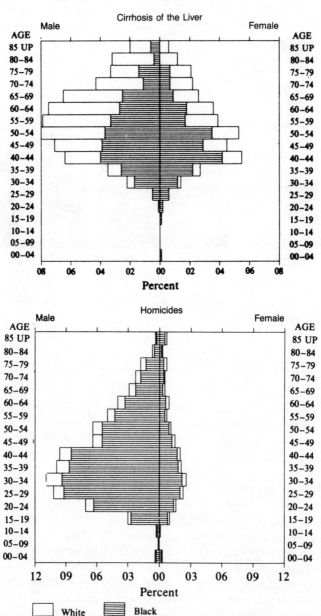

Source: Reprinted from "Disease Patterns of the 70's," *Health Services Research and Statistics,* Georgia Department of Human Resources, Division of Physical Health, August 1976. 116, 121, 137.

Figure 6-5 Cross-Sectional Analysis of Tuberculosis Death Rates
Massachusetts

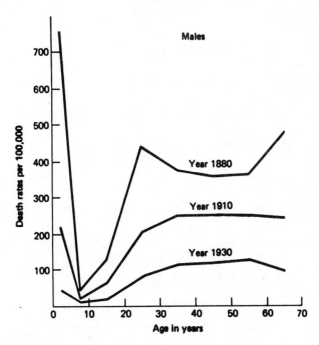

Source: Reprinted from "The Age Selection of Mortality from Tuberculosis in Successive Decades" by W.H. Frost with permission of the *American Journal of Hygiene,* © 1939, vol. 30, 91-96.

results. Although all three show a high incidence in childhood, the current (cross-sectional) analysis of 1880 death rates shows a peak between ages 20 and 30 and another after about age 55. In contrast, the 1910 analysis shows a quite steady incidence in adulthood while the 1930 curve shows a small but steady increase through adulthood, peaking between 50 and 60. How can these seemingly contradictory relationships between age and death rates from tuberculosis be explained?

A cohort analysis provides the answer. In Figure 6-6, each curve represents the death rates from tuberculosis experienced by the cohort of persons born between 1861-1870 (" cohort 1870"); 1871-1880 ("1880"); 1881-1890 ("1890"); 1891-1900 ("1900"); and 1901-1910 ("1910"). All curves show the same basic relationship between age and tuberculosis: in addition to a high incidence in early childhood, all cohorts experienced their highest death rates between ages 20 and 30, with a steady decrease thereafter. No increase is evident in older adulthood, nor is there a steady rate through adulthood.

Figure 6-6 Cohort Analysis of Tuberculosis Death Rates

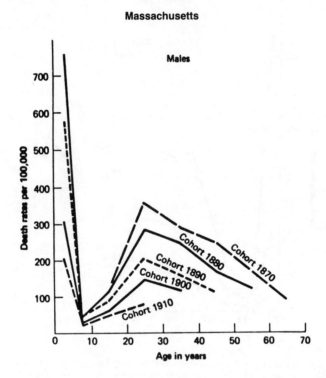

Massachusetts

Source: Reprinted from "The Age Selection of Mortality from Tuberculosis in Successive Decades" by W.H. Frost with permission of the *American Journal of Hygiene,* © 1939, vol. 30, 91-96.

Frost concludes that adults and older adults have a higher rate in the cross-sectional analysis than they should have had, as shown from the results of the cohort analysis, because they belong to an older cohort with overall (through all ages) higher death rates. For example, persons in the 50 to 60 age group in the 1930 analysis (Figure 6-5) belong to the 1880 cohort (that is, born between 1871 and 1880), which had a greater exposure to tuberculosis than any other succeeding groups.

This study supports the hypothesis that mortality from tuberculosis in adult life is predominantly endogenous (that is, resulting from activation of latent foci) and determined largely by the degree of infection received in early life.[5]

The Role of Sex

Males and females have different mortality and morbidity patterns. The simplest way to examine these different patterns is to use the sex ratio: the ratio of male to female cases. Table 6-6 illustrates the sex ratios for selected causes of death.

Figure 6-7 illustrates the importance of classifying male/female ratios. These ratios of more than 3, 2-2.99, 1-1.99, and less than 1 aid in the identification of a problem by sex. Today, as in 1959-61 (Figure 6-7), death rates almost always are higher among males than females, except for diabetes, hypertension, and a few types of cancers (Table 6-7). In utero and neonatal death rates also are higher for males. These rates are true for both whites and blacks. Life expectancy also is quite a bit greater in females and the difference is widening. A female born in 1979 could

---

Table 6-6 Male, Female Mortality Rates, U.S., 1971

Selected Causes

Cause	Mortality Rate†			Ratio of Male to Female Rate
	Total	Male	Female	
Emphysema and bronchitis	10.2	18.6	3.7	5.0
Respiratory cancer	29.4	51.8	11.0	4.7
Homicide	10.0	16.3	4.0	4.1
Buccal cavity and pharyngeal cancer	3.1	4.9	1.6	3.1
Tuberculosis	1.8	2.9	1.0	2.9
Motor vehicle accidents	26.6	39.5	14.4	2.8
Other accidents	25.3	37.6	13.8	2.7
Urinary cancer	5.6	8.5	3.2	2.7
Peptic ulcer	3.0	4.6	1.8	2.6
Suicide	11.9	17.2	7.1	2.4
Cirrhosis of the liver	14.7	20.4	9.8	2.1
Ischemic heart disease	226.8	314.8	153.9	2.0
Influenza and pneumonia	19.3	24.9	14.8	1.7
Leukemia	5.7	7.1	4.5	1.6
Digestive cancer	34.8	42.8	28.4	1.5
Nephritis and nephrosis	3.3	3.4	2.8	1.4
Cerebrovascular diseases	65.7	72.5	60.2	1.2
Diabetes mellitus	13.8	13.2	14.2	0.9

°From Division of Vital Statistics, National Center for Health Statistics, unpublished data, 1971.

†Annual rates per 100,000 population, age-standardized.

Source: Reprinted from *Epidemiology: An Introductory Text* by Judith S. Mausner and Anita K. Bahn with permission of W. B. Saunders Company, ©1974, 47. (Based on unpublished 1971 data of the U.S. Department of Health, Education, and Welfare, National Center for Health Statistics, Division of Vital Statistics.)

Table 6-7 Ratio of Male to Female Age-Adjusted Cancer Death Rates, U.S., 1959-1961

By Primary Site for Whites

Primary Site (ICD Code)	Male/Female Ratios
	Ratios 3 or More
Larynx (161)	10.50
Bronchus and lung specified as primary and unspecified (162.1, 163)	6.79
Esophagus (150)	4.13
Tongue (141)	4.00*
Buccal cavity and pharynx (140–148)	4.00
Nasopharynx (146)	3.00
Parotid gland (142.0)	3.00
	Ratios 2–2.99
Bladder and other urinary organs (181)	2.89
Mediastinum (164)	2.84
Other malignant neoplasm of skin (191)	2.20
Lymphatic leukemia (204.0)	2.11
Bone (196)	2.00
	Ratios 1–1.99
Stomach (151)	1.97
Kidney (180)	1.94
Liver, primary (155.0)	1.83
Hodgkin's disease (201)	1.77
Pancreas (157)	1.68
Other and unspecified leukemia (204.4)	1.60
Rectum (154)	1.56
Lymphosarcoma and reticulosarcoma (200)	1.54
Leukemia and aleukemia (204)	1.54
Other endocrine glands (195)	1.50
Liver (primary, secondary, and unspecified) (155.0, 156)	1.50
Nose, nasal cavities, middle ear, and accessory sinuses (160)	1.50
Brain and other parts of nervous system (193)	1.50
Other forms of lymphoma and mycosis fungoides (202, 205)	1.50
Multiple myeloma (203)	1.45
Acute leukemia (204.3)	1.45
Myeloid leukemia (240.1)	1.44
Small intestine including duodenum (152)	1.33
Melanoma of skin (190)	1.27
Monocytic leukemia (204.2)	1.20
	Ratios Less Than 1
Large intestine, except rectum (153)	0.98
Thyroid gland (194)	0.67
Gall bladder and extrahepatic gall ducts including ampulla of Vater (155.1)	0.56
Breast (170)	0.01

*Based on crude death rates.

Reprinted from A. M. Lilienfeld, *Foundations of Epidemiology,* with permission of Oxford University Press, ©1976, 96.

expect to live 7.7 years longer than a male born in the same year, although a female born in 1930 enjoyed only a 3.5-year advantage.[6]

The sex ratio assumes that the population is divided equally by sex. This of course is not the case. Although more males are born alive than females (106 males to 100 females), from age 20 on females exceed males in each age group and the relative difference increases with advancing age.[7] Consequently, age-specific and sex-specific rates are more useful than sex ratios in comparing health problems of males and females.

An interesting aspect of the influence of sex on disease is that, although mortality rates are higher in males, morbidity rates usually are higher in females. For females, both reported morbidity and physician visits are higher in all age groups. These sex differences may be caused by many factors. Some diseases, such as hemophilia, are genetically sex linked. Hormonal and reproductive factors also can play a role in either predisposing a given sex toward a particular disease or providing protection against it.

For example, the greater occurrence of coronary heart disease in young men than in young women may be linked to some hormonal factors, perhaps protection of the women by estrogens before menopause.[8] Men and women also have different life styles, which may explain some differences. For instance, the greater incidence of lung cancer in males can be related to the fact that men smoke more cigarettes than women. However, these statistics are changing rapidly. The sex ratio of lung cancer should decrease as more women begin to feel the effects of long-term smoking. Similarly, the higher incidence of cirrhosis of the liver may be explained by the fact that men consume more alcohol than do women.

Finally, the higher morbidity and lower mortality in women may result in part from their lower case fatality rate; that is, some diseases have a less lethal effect on women than men. Since women consume more health services than men, however, it also may stem from the fact that women seek medical care at an earlier stage of a disease.[9, 10] As Mausner and Bahn point out, depression provides a good example of contradictory sex differences in morbidity and mortality rates;[11] rates for many forms of depression are higher in women than in men, as is the rate of attempted suicide.[12]

Racial or Ethnic Origin

The examination of specific health statistics may be controversial, especially when related to ethnic or minority groups. Nevertheless, Haynes states that:

> We should insist that adequate statistics be maintained so that health planners do not lose sight of special problems of minority groups. Only by such special focus will minority problems receive due attention. Representing a relatively small percentage of the total population, it is

easy for minority problems to be ignored. This must not happen. We must oppose those within minority groups who wish to conceal special problems, and we must oppose those of the majority group who want to ignore these problems.[13]

Adequate health care for all is the goal of any health agency. To reach this goal, the agency must know the disease patterns that reflect the health status of the population it serves. Definite differences exist in mortality and morbidity among races. In some cases, such as sickle-cell anemia, disease is determined genetically. In most instances, however, differences are related to socioeconomic status. Regrettably, socioeconomic data often are difficult to gather and are available only every ten years (census period). Even so, racial or ethnic origin can be useful as an indicator of groups with particular deficiencies in health care.

As shown in Figure 6-1, blacks have a higher death rate than whites at every age group except that of 75 and over. Cause-specific death rates (Tables 6-2 to 6-5) for hypertensive heart diseases, cerebrovascular accidents, tuberculosis, syphilis, homicide, and accidental deaths all are higher among blacks. Infant mortality rates are twice as high for black infants as they are for whites. Black infants are about two and a half times as likely as whites to have very low birth weight (1,500 grams or fewer). Whites have higher death rates for arteriosclerotic heart disease, suicide, and leukemia. Whites and blacks also have different rates for several forms of cancer; for example, black females have a higher incidence of cervical cancer, white females of breast cancer.

SOCIAL VARIABLES

In addition to personal attributes, a group of factors referred to as social variables also influences a population's health. These social variables include socioeconomic status, occupational exposures, other environmental health hazards, marital status, and other family-related characteristics.

Socioeconomic Status

Socioeconomic status, or social class, is a multidimensional construct that has long been used, often with quite a bit of controversy, to rank or stratify a population in terms of wealth (poverty and affluence), prestige, and power. There is extensive literature both on how to conceptualize and measure socioeconomic status and on its relationship to mortality and morbidity. It is generally believed that socioeconomic status is best measured by some mixture of income, education, and occupational data. In many instances it is appropriate to combine these variables into a socioeconomic status index while at other times it is necessary to use them as single indicators. Since all these variables seem to be consistently related to health in the same manner, they are not distinguished here.

One review of the relationship between social class and health starts: "Social class gradients of mortality and life expectancy have been observed for centuries, and a vast body of evidence has shown consistently that those in the lower classes have higher mortality, morbidity, and disability rates."[14] As is demonstrated, however, there are some specific exceptions to this general statement.

There is little doubt that socioeconomic status is negatively associated with overall mortality rates. Table 6-8 shows the standardized mortality ratios for males and females, white and nonwhite, as a function of educational level.[15] For all of these groups, a lower educational level is associated with higher mortality. For example, white males with little education have a death rate 15 percent higher than the average and 64 percent more than their counterparts with higher education. The difference is even more striking for white females with low education: 60 percent more than average, 105 percent more than the group with higher education.

Table 6-9 shows the relationship between social class and selected causes of death (again using standardized mortality ratios) in England and Wales. In this study, social class was measured on a scale of five occupational levels. The standardized mortality ratios were age-adjusted to remove any effects of differing age distribution. The table demonstrates clearly that for all selected causes of death except coronary heart disease, the mortality ratios are progressively higher as the social class level decreases. For bronchitis, the mortality ratios in the lower class are seven times higher than in the higher class. Although not included in Table 6-9, mortality ratios from infectious and parasitic diseases and infant mortality rates also are higher in the lower socioeconomic groups.

The same relationship holds true for morbidity. Higher rates of morbidity from a vast array of conditions have been observed in lower socioeconomic groups. Table 6-10 shows the relationship between prevalence of hypertension and social class. Using either income or educational level, this example shows lower socioeconomic groups have higher prevalence rates of hypertension.

It can be hazardous to try to explain the relationship between socioeconomic status and health. Syme and Berkman comment:

> There can be little doubt that the highest morbidity and mortality rates observed in the lower social classes are in part due to inadequate medical care services as well as to the impact of a toxic and hazardous physical environment. There can be little doubt also that these factors do not entirely explain the discrepancy in rates between the classes. . . . That so many different kinds of diseases are more frequent in lower class groupings directs attention to generalized susceptibility to disease and to generalized compromises of disease defense systems.[16]

Life changes, life stresses, and particularly the way people cope with such stress, probably are an important part of this negative social and psychological environment.

Coping, in this sense, refers not to specific types of psychological responses but to the more generalized ways in which people deal with problems in their everyday life. It is evident that such coping styles are likely to be products of environmental situations and not independent of such factors. Several coping responses that have a wide range of disease outcomes have been described. Cigarette smoking is one such coping response that has been associated with virtually all causes of morbidity and mortality; obesity may be another coping style associated with a higher rate of many diseases and conditions; Pattern A behavior is an example of a third coping response that has been shown to have relatively broad disease consequences.[17]

Data on the socioeconomic level of their surrounding population thus can be helpful to health service managers. Even though the reasons might be poorly understood, lower socioeconomic groups do in fact have higher mortality and morbidity rates for the great majority of diseases. Dividing the population according to such levels would be helpful in identifying target groups, in planning the

Table 6-8 Standardized Mortality Ratios by Educational Level, U.S., 1960 Whites and Nonwhites, 25 to 64 Years of Age

| Sex and Race | Educational Level | | |
	Lowest	Highest[1]	Differential[2]
Male			
White	115	70	64%
Nonwhite	114	87	31%
Female			
White	160	78	105%
Nonwhite	126	74	70%

1. For whites, the highest educational level was defined as "4 or more years of college," for nonwhites, "high school or college."

2. The differential (for white males, above) may be calculated as follows:

$$\frac{115 - 70}{70} = 64\%$$

Source: Reprinted from "Social Class, Susceptibility, and Sickness" by S.L. Syme and L.F. Berkman with permission from the American Journal of Epidemiology, © July 1976, vol. 104, no. 1, 1.

Table 6-9 Standardized Mortality Ratios by Social Class

Selected Causes of Death, Males 15-64 Years of Age, England and Wales, 1961

Causes of Death	Social Class				
	I Profes- sionals	*II* Inter- mediate	*III* Skilled Labor	*IV* Semi- Skilled	*V* Unskilled Labor
Tuberculosis	40	54	96	108	185
Stomach cancer	49	63	101	114	163
Lung cancer	53	72	107	104	148
Coronary heart disease	98	95	106	96	112
Bronchitis	28	50	97	116	194
Accidents (excluding motor vehicle)	43	56	87	128	193
All other causes	76	81	100	103	143

Source: Reprinted from *Prevention Health, Everybody's Business,* with permission of The Department of Health and Social Security, London, 1976, 52.

location of satellite or new facilities, and in tracing the general patterns of health and disease in a population. Data by census tract can be obtained from Federal publications. Occupation, income, or education can be used as indicators, although education has been shown to be the best predictor.[18, 19, 20]

Occupational and Environmental Hazards

In addition to being an indicator of socioeconomic status, occupation is linked to health in other ways. Both the occupational environment and the everyday life

Table 6-10 Prevalence Rates of Hypertension, U.S., 1971-1975

By Income and Educational Levels, Persons 25-74 Years of Age

Income	Prevalence Rate per 100	Education	Prevalence Rate per 100
Under $3,000	32.1	Under 5 years	36.6
Under $5,000	29.6	5-8 years	27.0
$5,000-$9,999	18.1	9-12 years	15.9
$10,000 or more	13.8	13 years or more	13.7

Source: Reprinted from *Hypertension in Adults, U.S., 1971-1975,* U.S. Department of Health and Human Services, Vital Health Statistics Data from the National Health Survey, Series 11, Number 221, 1981 (Public Health Service Document No. 81-1671), 16.

environment can influence health through specific risks associated with noxious agents and general working or living conditions. (Environmental and occupational epidemiology is the topic of Chapter 12.) It is important to stress at this point that the identification of occupational exposures and other environmental health hazards is an integral part of describing the "person" characteristics of health and disease in a population.

Marital Status, Family-Related Variables

Family-related variables have been the subject of many epidemiological studies.[21] Among such variables, marital status often is linked to mortality and morbidity. The overall mortality rate in both men and women is higher (in decreasing order) among the divorced, the widowed, and the single; it is lowest among married persons.[22] This trend is also true for admission rates to psychiatric hospitals for males while the widowed female shows the highest rate for admission.

As Table 6-11 shows, most diseases are more frequent in single than married males and females. This is true for most cancers, cardiovascular diseases, tuberculosis, suicides, and venereal diseases. The best known exception to this is cancer of the cervix, which is more than twice as common among married than single women.[23]

MacMahon, Pugh, and Ipsen suggest three explanations of the relationship between marital status and mortality rates.[24]

1. Persons in poor health, or in the presymptomatic stages of ill health, tend to remain single.
2. Persons who "live dangerously" and are consequently exposed to a wide variety of disease-producing agents and situations tend to remain single.
3. Differences in the ways of life of single and married persons result from the presence or absence of the married state and are causally related to certain diseases. For example, there is more interpersonal contact and life is more routine in a family (married state). One's spouse, and other family members, may provide psychological and physical support, perhaps contributing to better health.

For women, marital status also may be related to health through differences in sexual exposure, pregnancy, childbearing, and lactation.[25] This explains why cancer of the cervix is more common in married than single women. Early sexual experience and frequency of intercourse appear to be decisive factors in the emergence of cervical cancer. By contrast, breast cancer is more frequent in single than married women: in married women, hormonal balance, ensured by early age at first pregnancy and artificial menopause before the age of 40, seems to lower the risk of breast cancer.

Table 6-11 Mortality Rates in Single and Married Whites, U.S., 1949-1951*

Selected Causes of Death	Males		Females	
	Single	Married	Single	Married
Respiratory tuberculois	96.7	22.7	25.0	11.4
Tuberculosis, other forms	3.4	1.3	1.8	0.8
Syphilis	14.8	6.6	2.0	2.2
Malignant neoplasms, total	260.0	207.1	470.4	182.5
Buccal and pharynx	13.7	7.0	1.6	1.8
Digestive organs	115.7	87.6	73.0	65.5
Respiratory system	44.5	33.5	7.8	7.2
Breast	0.7	0.4	54.0	33.2
Genital organs	23.7	25.0	40.0	38.2
Urinary system	15.5	13.3	6.6	5.8
Leukemia	8.0	8.8	5.6	5.8
Diabetes mellitus	21.9	18.3	16.5	29.0
Vascular lesions of central nervous system	182.1	138.9	136.6	124.7
Rheumatic heart disease	28.7	18.6	23.8	17.4
Arteriosclerotic heart disease	525.6	409.9	212.0	179.1
Chronic nephritis	33.0	23.1	20.2	18.4
Influenza and pneumonia	73.5	27.0	34.1	18.3
Peptic ulcer	21.5	11.8	3.8	2.4
Motor vehicle accidents	61.9	33.7	11.0	10.8
Other accidents	99.2	46.1	36.4	21.1
Suicide	43.7	20.5	7.7	6.2

*Average annual rates per 100,000 population.

Source: Reprinted from *Epidemiologic Methods* by B. MacMahon, T.F. Pugh, and J. Ipsen with permission of Little, Brown, & Co., © 1960, 135. (Data are from the National Center for Health Statistics, Division of Vital Statistics, 1956.)

Although the relationship between marital status and health is well documented it should weaken somewhat since most characteristics of married life—possibly responsible for the positive impact on health—seem to be spreading out to other life styles (such as unmarried individuals living together) and becoming less specific to the wedded role. Early sexual experience and frequency of intercourse (as well as lack of multiple partners) no longer are characteristic of married life. Similarly, with the emergence of the extended family, as opposed to the nuclear family (as predicted by Toffler[26]), psychological and physical support should not be characteristics specifically restricted to married life.

Family Size, Birth Order, and Maternal Age

Other variables associated with health status are family size, birth order, and maternal age. These variables refer to the "family of origin," or the family into which a person is born or spends the formative years, as opposed to the "family of procreation," in the case of marital status.[27]

Family size is associated first with health through the impact of multiple pregnancies on women's condition. Family size also is linked to contagious diseases since the concentration of persons and subsequent multiple contacts facilitate their propagation. Finally, family size is highly correlated with socioeconomic status, large families being more common among the poor. This also may work in the opposite direction: large family size can influence the socioeconomic status and, consequently, the health status, nutrition of all members, and children's growth and development.

Maternal age is strongly involved with infants' health. Very young mothers (under 20 years of age) have a greater incidence of producing infants who have low birth weight and/or are immature (Table 6-12). This high incidence may be explained by both biological and socioeconomic factors.[28] In general, very young teenage mothers are both physiologically immature and of low socioeconomic status. Older mothers (over 40) with no previous pregnancies, or very few, also are more likely to have babies of low birth weight.

Table 6-12 Births and Percent of Infants Weighing 2,500 Grams or Less, U.S., 1978

According to Race and Age

Age (Years)	White		Black	
	Births	% 2,500 Grams or Less	Births	% 2,500 Grams or Less
Less than 15	4,512	10.9	6,068	16.9
15-19	380,060	8.1	151,001	14.6
15	15,756	9.8	12,525	15.1
16	40,776	9.1	22,754	15.0
17	74,425	8.5	32,038	14.7
18	108,074	8.0	39,933	14.5
19	141,029	7.4	43,571	14.2
20-24	914,772	5.9	196,731	12.7
25-29	860,209	5.2	121,613	11.4
Total	2,155,041	6.0	469,345	12.9

Source: Reprinted from *Health, United States, 1980,* U.S. Department of Health and Human Services, Public Health Service, National Center for Health Statistics, Division of Vital Statistics, 20.

The greatest problem associated with older mothers, however, is congenital malformation. Many congenital malformations, including anencephalus, hydrocephalus, and clubfoot are more frequent in both younger and older mothers. Some other malformations, such as those of the circulatory system and Down's syndrome, are more frequent in older mothers. Further, the relationship between maternal age and Down's syndrome is indeed striking. It is a direct relationship.

Birth order is a variable that is thought to influence infants' health. Although almost everything, including intelligence,[29] is related to birth order, studies of the subject seem to have many biases.[30, 31, 32] Figure 6-7 shows the relationship between stillbirth rates, birth order, and age of mother. In this case, both variables are shown to be associated with stillbirth rates.

Family-related variables, mostly marital status and maternal age, thus are significant personal characteristics to be investigated in describing the health problems of a population.

LIFE STYLE VARIABLES

Life style is an important determinant of health and should be an integral part of the epidemiological framework. Life style variables can be used in the same way as demographic and social variables to describe the personal aspects of the distribution of health in a population. These also can be a focus for intervention: some life style variables are so closely associated with mortality and morbidity that they represent a very real potential for effective and efficient health services action.

Life style refers to the individual and societal behavior patterns that are at least partly under individual control and that demonstrably influence personal health.[33] Somers writes that the rationale for linking health and life style can be summarized in three statements:[34]

1. The major causes of death, serious illness, and disability in the developed nations today [1980] are chronic disease and violence.
2. Behind most chronic disease, disability, and premature death are many environmental and behavioral factors, potentially amenable to prevention. [This is illustrated in Tables 6-1 and 6-13, which list the risk factors for the major causes of death and disease by life stage.]
3. A few individual and societal life style patterns constitute the major behavioral risk factors involved in chronic disease and severe disability.

Contrary to popular belief, the number of serious behavioral risk factors is limited. Those of major importance include cigarette smoking, alcohol and drug abuse, inadequate nutrition, lack of adequate physical activity, irresponsible use of motor vehicles, and irresponsible use of guns and other manifestations of violence.

Figure 6-7 Stillbirth Rates by Birth Order and Age of Mother

Missouri 1972-74

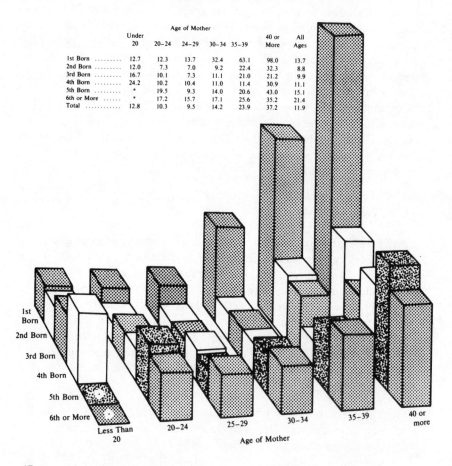

	Age of Mother						
	Under 20	20–24	24–29	30–34	35–39	40 or More	All Ages
1st Born	12.7	12.3	13.7	32.4	63.1	98.0	13.7
2nd Born	12.0	7.3	7.0	9.2	22.4	32.3	8.8
3rd Born	16.7	10.1	7.3	11.1	21.0	21.2	9.9
4th Born	24.2	10.2	10.4	11.0	11.4	30.9	11.1
5th Born	*	19.5	9.3	14.0	20.6	43.0	15.1
6th or More	*	17.2	15.7	17.1	25.6	35.2	21.4
Total	12.8	10.3	9.5	14.2	23.9	37.2	11.9

*Rate not shown because of extremely small numbers in cell.

Source: Reprinted from Missouri Monthly Vital Statistics, Department of Social Services, Missouri Center for Health Studies, 1975, 3.

Cigarette Smoking

No single measure would lengthen the life or improve the health of Americans more than eliminating cigarette smoking.[35] This was clearly demonstrated in the

Table 6-13 Major Causes of Death, Risk Factors, U.S., 1977

Major Causes of Death, 1977		
Cause	*Percent of All Deaths*	*Risk Factor*
Heart disease	37.8	Smoking,[1] hypertension,[1] elevated serum cholesterol[1] (diet), lack of exercise, diabetes, stress, family history
Malignant neoplasms	20.4	Smoking,[1] worksite carcinogens,[1] environmental carcinogens, alcohol, diet
Stroke	9.6	Hypertension,[1] smoking,[1] elevated serum cholesterol,[1] stress
Accidents other than motor vehicle	2.8	Alcohol,[1] drug abuse, smoking (fires), product design, handgun availability
Influenza and pneumonia	2.7	Smoking, vaccination status[1]
Motor vehicle accidents	2.6	Alcohol[1], no seat belts,[1] speed,[1] roadway design, vehicle engineering
Diabetes	1.7	Obesity[1]
Cirrhosis of the liver	1.6	Alcohol abuse[1]
Arteriosclerosis	1.5	Elevated serum cholesterol[1]
Suicide	1.5	Stress,[1] alcohol and drug abuse, gun availability

1. Major risk factors.

Source: Reprinted from *Health, United States, 1980*, U.S. Department of Health and Human Services, Public Health Service, data from *Office of Disease Prevention and Health Promotion*, 274.

previous chapter (see relative and attributable risks). Nearly 18 percent of all U.S. mortality now is related to smoking.[36] Tobacco's contribution to cancer deaths is estimated at 30 percent. Cigarette smokers' cancer death rates are more than double those of nonsmokers. Heavy smokers (more than one pack a day) have three to four times greater excess risk of cancer mortality. Table 6-14 shows the projected distribution of smoking-related deaths for several causes of death.

Contrary to what the cigarette industry might contend, the relationship between smoking and health has been documented ad nauseam. Scientific proof does not

Table 6-14 Projected Distribution of Smoking-Related Deaths, U.S. Population

Cause	Mortality Distribution 1977 Population	Tobacco-Related Mortality	
		Number	% of Total
Diseases of the heart	82,080,000	24,624,000	30
Brochitis/emphysema	2,160,000	1,836,000	85
Arteriosclerosis	3,672,000	1,212,000	33
Cancer of the oral cavity	670,000	469,000	70
Cancer of the esophagus	734,000	220,000	30
Cancer of the pancreas	2,160,000	756,000	35
Cancer of the larynx	368,000	184,000	50
Cancer of the lung	9,051,000	7,874,000	87
Cancer of the kidney	793,000	159,000	20
Cancer of the bladder	1,050,000	494,000	47
Other diseases	113,262,000	—	—
Total	216,000,000	37,828,000	18

From Gori GB: Unpublished Data, National Cancer Institute, 1977.

Source: Anne R. Somers, "Life-Style and Health" in Public Health and Preventive Medicine, 11th ed., ed. John M. Last, N.Y.: Appleton-Century-Crofts, 1980), 1049.

come from a perfect experiment but from a gradually evolving body of facts and knowledge. The cut-off point when something can be considered as proved is arbitrary.[37] In the case of the relationship between smoking and health, this point has long since been reached.

Possible intervention strategies against cigarette smoking are discussed in Chapter 9, on marketing. It is important to stress at this point that smoking is one of the most important personal characteristics influencing health and that every health care provider, manager, and organization should make every effort to produce an impact on this habit.

A 1982 report of the U.S. Department of Health and Human Services[38] says smokers of lower tar cigarettes have statistically lower death rates from lung cancer than do those who use higher tar brands, although they still are significantly higher than rates for nonsmokers. Even after many years of cigarette smoking, stopping reduces cancer risk substantially compared with that of continuing users. The more years individuals can refrain from smoking after stopping, the greater the reduction in excess cancer risk. Fifteen years after stopping, lung cancer risk is reduced to nearly the level of nonsmokers. The same reduction in risk is observed for other cancer sites associated with smoking.

Alcohol and Drug Abuse

An estimated 10 percent of the adult population has drinking problems, and 16 percent of all adults report that they, or someone in their family, drink more than they should.[39] Furthermore, the effects of alcohol abuse on health are severe. Somers reports that alcoholism is "the most devastating sociomedical problem faced by human society short of war and malnutrition."[40] Alcohol is a major factor in liver disease, peptic ulcer, and other gastrointestinal disorders, nervous system damage, heart disease, nutritional disorders, motor vehicle accidents, homicides, and suicides.[41, 42] It also is a factor in child abuse, battered spouse, and in the outcome of pregnancy (low birth weight, fetal alcohol syndrome).

Drug abuse involves legal and illegal drugs, prescribed and nonprescribed. Although medical problems, including mortality, related to heroin and barbiturates, have been declining, the use of cannabinoids (marijuana, hashish) has been increasing, with unclear health consequences. The use of central nervous system stimulants, including amphetamines and cocaine, as well as caffeine in cola beverages, coffee, tea, and cocoa, may represent even a great health hazard. Stimulants of the central nervous system have an effect on the cardiovascular system and on the metabolic rate. Caffeine also has been shown to interfere with normal hormonal secretions, to be associated with bladder cancer, and is thought to be associated with pancreatic cancer, although the latter has yet to be demonstrated conclusively.[43]

Drugs prescribed by physicians, such as hypnotics, tranquilizers, stimulants, and sleeping pills also are often abused, leading to psychological and physical dependence. Many over-the-counter drugs such as aspirin, cold remedies, and even laxatives, largely among the older adult population, tend to be abused, with potentially damaging health consequences.

Nutritional Inadequacies

There is increasing evidence that nutritional habits are strongly related to health and disease, most notably coronary heart disease and cancer. Obesity might be the most prevalent form of malnutrition in the industralized countries and is associated with many health problems, including heart disease. It is estimated that about 80 million American adults are obese. Furthermore, juvenile-onset obesity, which is particularly serious, is increasingly prevalent.[44]

The most common health problem in the world may be the high consumption of sugar, long associated with dental disease.[45] The heavy use of salt is associated with hypertension, and of fat, particularly saturated, and cholesterol with atherosclerosis and coronary heart disease.

Less well known is the significant relationship between nutrition and many forms of cancer. A recent study estimates that diet is associated with 70 percent of all cancers.[46] It is thought that diet is not a primary causative factor but enhances tumor growth and alters the body's reponse to carcinogens.

Fat intake (usually estimated as exceeding 45 percent of total calories) is associated with cancers of the colon, prostate, breast, and large bowel. High protein intake is linked to an increased risk of breast, endometrium, ovary, prostate, large bowel, pancreas, and kidney cancer. In addition, low-protein diets have been shown in animal studies to inhibit tumor development. Low fiber consumption is thought to be associated with colon-rectal cancer.

There is, finally, some concern that chemical carcinogens may be present in food additives and in industrial food preparation (such as chemical decaffeination). Nitrosamines, aflatoxins, and polycyclic hydrocarbons, among others, are potentially carcinogenic. Some studies suggest that Vitamin A (more specifically, caratonene) and Vitamin C are potentially protective against chemical carcinogens.[47]

Inadequate Physical Activity

Lack of adequate physical activity may be related to health and disease in several ways. Epidemiological evidence, although as yet inconclusive, suggests a protective effect against coronary death from regular, current, and vigorous physical activity.[48] Conversely, lack of physical exercise would seem to aggravate coronary problems. In any case, there is little doubt that inactivity leads to obesity and its associated health problems.

Physical activity may play an even greater role in morbidity. Data from a 1981 Canadian health survey show that "sedentary" persons are much more likely than "very active" ones to exhibit behavior related to ill health; that is, consultations with health professionals, use of medication, activity limitation, and disability days.[49] The association between physical activity and behavior related to morbidity seems strongly slanted toward age. In general, the level of physical activity is not strongly related to behavior denoting ill health for persons under 45. However, those 45 and over who are very active are significantly less likely to display behavior linked to ill health.[50] This seems to point to some long-term preventive potentials of physical activity.

Another study on the benefits of regular exercise in the elderly shows an improvement in social and cultural life, fewer physician visits, and fewer medications for those who undertake regular exercise.[51] As Berg writes, "Few interventions offer as much in the prevention of disability as the use of regular, properly planned physical exercise for the elderly."[52]

Irresponsible Use of Motor Vehicles

Motor vehicle accidents are an important public health problem since they are the leading cause of death in adolescence and early adulthood and a consistently important one throughout all ages. Most of this mortality, as well as correspondingly high morbidity, can be related to irresponsible use.

The single most important human factor identified with fatal motor accidents is the use of alcohol,[53, 54] which may be the cause of about half of those deaths. Although no data are available to substantiate this, it is reasonable to expect that drugs (other than alcohol) also may be involved in many motor vehicle accidents.

Another aspect of irresponsible usage is that only 20 percent of the drivers in the United States use seat belts although all new models of cars are equipped with them.[55] It has been shown conclusively that the use of seat belts reduces significantly the injury rates from car accidents.[56] The same may be said concerning motorcycle helmets.[57, 58] Even more striking, a 1974 survey found proper child-safety restraints in use for only 7 percent of the almost 9,000 automobile passengers under 10 years of age in the study.[59]

A final aspect of irresponsible use may be driving speed. For two years following the 1973 Arab oil embargo and the national imposition of the 55-mile-per-hour speed limit, the motor vehicle accidental death rate fell.[60]

Irresponsible Use of Guns and Other Manifestations of Violence

Deaths related to violence account for a large proportion of total deaths in the nation. A 1980 Federal publication reports "that homicide constitutes a major cause of death for American children is shocking, especially because it serves as merely one measurable indicator of child abuse and neglect."[61] The United States has one of the highest homicide rates in the industrial world—five times the rate for most European countries and Japan.[62] Since the mid-60s, there has been a direct relationship between increased handgun availability and increased gun-related crimes in the United States.[63] As Somers writes:

> It is often said that "violence as a way of life" or "violence as a way of problem solving" are normal aspects of American life. It is difficult to distinguish between deliberate violence and irresponsibility. In any case, the results are frequently disability, psychological suffering, and premature death.[64]

SUMMARY

This concludes the discussion of some of the major life style factors associated with health and disease. Even though it might be difficult at times to see the importance of some of these factors to health service management, their impact on a population's disease pattern is sufficient to warrant the attention and concern of all involved in health care delivery. These life style factors should be considered initially in describing the health problems of a community.

This chapter has reviewed demographic, social, and life style variables that describe those affected by the diseases prevalent in a population. The information can help health service managers gain a better understanding of the problems faced by their populations of interest and develop comprehensive programs to solve them. The life style variables are the major areas where institutions can become actively involved in setting up prevention programs.

The health field concept treats life style as a major determinant of health that must undergo change if improvements in physical and mental status are to occur. Descriptive epidemiology (Person) is the cornerstone of analysis for health service managers. The multiple variables considered are most important to the subsequent utilization of services but more important are the ones that must be used for market analysis in view of health promotion and disease prevention.

NOTES

1. J.P. Fox, C.E. Hall, and L.R. Elveback, *Epidemiology: Man and Disease* (London: The MacMillan Company, 1970), 185.

2. G.D. Friedman, *Primer of Epidemiology* (New York: McGraw-Hill Book Company, 1974), 54.

3. B. MacMahon, T.F. Pugh, and J. Ipsen, *Epidemiologic Methods* (Boston: Little, Brown, & Co., 1960), 88.

4. W.H. Frost, "The Age Selection of Mortality from Tuberculosis in Successive Decades," *American Journal of Hygiene* 30 (1939): 91–96.

5. MacMahon et al., *Epidemiologic Methods*, 90.

6. Bureau of the Census, *Social Indicators III*, U.S. Department of Commerce (Washington, D.C.: U.S. Government Printing Office, December 1980), 59.

7. Fox et al., *Epidemiology: Man and Disease*, 195.

8. Friedman, *Primer*, 58.

9. Judith S. Mausner and Anita K. Bahn, *Epidemiology: An Introductory Text* (Philadelphia: W.B. Saunders Company, 1974), 48.

10. Fox et al., *Epidemiology: Man and Disease*, 196.

11. Mausner and Bahn, *Epidemiology: An Introductory Text*, 49.

12. C. Silverman, *Epidemiology of Depression* (Baltimore: The Johns Hopkins University Press, 1968), 142.

13. A.M. Haynes, *Urban Health*, Minorities and Health Statistics, Atlanta, Georgia (June 1975), 14.

14. S.L. Syme and L.F. Berkman, "Social Class, Susceptibility, and Sickness," *American Journal of Epidemiology* 104, no. 1 (July 1976): 1.

15. E.M. Kitagawa and P.M. Hauser, *Differential Mortality in the United States* (Cambridge, Mass.: Harvard University Press, 1973), 84.

16. Syme and Berkman, "Social Class," 4-5.

17. Ibid., 5.

18. Henrik L. Blum, *Planning for Health* (New York: Human Sciences Press, Inc., 1981), 23.

19. M.H. Naji and E.H. Stockwell, "Socioeconomic Differentials in Mortality by Cause of Health," *Health Services Reports* 88, no. 5 (1973): 449-456.

20. Victor R. Fuchs, "The Economics of Health in a Postindustrial Society," *The Public Interest* 56 (Summer 1979): 3-20.

21. J.P. Fox, "Family-Based Epidemiological Studies," *American Journal of Epidemiology* 99 (1974): 165-179.

22. "Death Rates in Canada Lowest Among Married Persons," *Statistical Bulletin of the Metropolitan Life Insurance Company* 54 (August 1973): 4-6.

23. C.E. Martin, "Marital and Coital Factors in Cervical Cancer," *American Journal of Public Health* 57 (1967): 803.

24. MacMahon et al., *Epidemiologic Methods*, 135.

25. Mausner and Bahn, *Epidemiology: An Introductory Text*, 56.

26. Alvin Toffler, *The Third Wave*.

27. Mausner and Bahn, *Epidemiology: An Introductory Text*, 57.

28. J.C. Kleinman, "Trends and Variations in Birth Weight," *Health, United States, 1981*, 19.

29. L. Belmont and F.A. Marola, "Birth Order, Family Size, and Intelligence," *Science* 182 (1973): 1096-1101.

30. Mausner and Bahn, *Epidemiology: An Introductory Text*, 58.

31. C. Schooler, "Birth Order Defects: Not Here, Not Now," *Psychological Bulletin* 78 (1972): 161.

32. J.R. Huguenard and G.E. Sharples, "Incidence of Congenital Pyloric Stenosis in Birth Series," *Journal of Chronic Diseases* 35 (1972): 727.

33. Anne R. Somers, "Life Style and Health," *Maxcy-Roseneau Public Health and Preventive Medicine*, 11th ed., ed. John M. Last (New York: Appleton-Century-Crofts, Inc. 1980), 1047.

34. Ibid., 1047.

35. Julius R. Richmond, "Health for the Future." Speech presented to Women's National Democratic Club, Washington, D.C., February 19, 1980, quoted in *Health, United States, 1980*, U.S. Department of Health and Human Services, Public Health Service (Washington, D.C.: U.S. Government Printing Office, December 1980), 294.

36. G.B. Gori, unpublished data, National Cancer Institute, 1977, quoted in Somers, "Life Style and Health," 1049.

37. K. Popper, *The Logic of Scientific Discovery*, 3rd. ed. (London: Hutchinson, 1972).

38. Office on Smoking and Health, *The Health Consequences of Smoking: Cancer*, A report of the Surgeon General, U.S. Dept. of Health and Human Services, Public Health Service (Washington, D.C.: U.S. Government Printing Office, 1982).

39. Health-United States, December 1980, U.S. DHHS, PHS (81-1232), 296.

40. Somers, "Life Style and Health," 1049.

41. P. Cole, "Coffee-Drinking and Cancer of the Lower Urinary Tract," *The Lancet* (1971): 1335-1337.

42. "A Population-Based Study of Bladder Cancer," in *Host Environment Interactions in the Etiology of Cancer in Man*, ed. R. Doll and I. Vodopija (Lyon, France: International Agency for Research on Cancer, 1973), 83-87.

43. Somers, "Life Style and Health," 1050.

44. G.S. Leske, L.W. Ripa, and M.C. Leske, "Dental Public Health," in Last, *Maxcy-Roseneau*, 1423.

45. T.H. Maugh, "Vitamin A: Potential Protection from Carcinogens," *Science* 186 (1974): 1198.

46. Cancer Research Supplement. Workshop Conference on Nutrition in Cancer Causation and Prevention—Sponsored by the American Cancer Society, Fort Lauderdale, Florida, October 18-20, 1982, Joseph P. Lowenthal, ed., Vol. 43, No. 5 (May 1983), 2390s.

47. S.S. Minvish et al., "Ascorbate-Nitrite Reaction: Possible Means of Blocking the Formation of Carcinogenic N-Nitroso Compounds," *Science* 177 (1972): 65.

48. H. Blackburn and R.F. Gillum, "Heart Disease," in Last, *Maxcy-Roseneau*, 1180.

49. Health and Welfare Canada and Statistics Canada, *The Health of Canadians—Report of the Canada Health Survey* (Ottawa: Minister of Supplies and Services, 1981), 72.

50. Ibid.

51. W. Lederer, *"Get Physically Fit," Parks and Recreation* (October 1978).

52. R.L. Berg, "Prevention of Disability in the Aged," in Last, *Maxcy-Roseneau*, 1295.

53. Secretary of Transportation, *Alcohol and Highway Safety—A Report to the Congress* (Washington, D.C.: U.S. Government Printing Office, August 5, 1968).

54. J.A. Waller, "Injury as a Public Health Problem," in Last, *Maxcy-Roseneau*, 1556.

55. Richmond, "Health for the Future," 295.

56. R.S. Roberts, L.W. Gerson, and T. Delmore, "The Effect of the Province of Ontario's Compulsory Seatbelt Legislation in an Urban Area," *Canadian Journal of Public Health* 70 (January-February 1979), 28-33.

57. C.S. Watson, P.L. Zador, and A. Wilks, "The Repeal of Helmet Use in the U.S., 1975-1978," *American Journal of Public Health* 70, no. 6 (June 1980): 579-585.

58. A. Muller, "Evaluation of the Costs and Benefits of Motorcycle Helmet Laws," *American Journal of Public Health* 70, no. 6 (June 1980): 586-592.

59. A.F. Williams and P.L. Zador, "Injuries to Children in Automobiles in Relation to Seating Location and Restraint Use," *Accident Analysis and Prevention* 9 (1977): 69-76.

60. Somers, "Life Style and Health," 1051.

61. Health-United States, December 1980, U.S. DHHS, PHS (81-1232), 276.

62. Somers, "Life Style and Health," 1052.

63. U.S. General Accounting Office, *Handgun Control: Effectiveness and Costs* (Washington, D.C.: U.S. Government Printing Office, 1978).

64. Somers, "Life Style and Health," 1052.

Chapter 7

Descriptive Epidemiology: Place and Time

PLACE: WHERE DISEASE OCCURS

The preceding chapter dealt with the individual characteristics that may affect disease patterns—the person. Disease occurrence also may be characterized in terms of where it occurs (place) and when (time).

Therefore, the second major issue in descriptive epidemiological studies of a community is: Where does disease occur? As in person-related characteristics, the quest again is for a pattern of disease occurrence, this time in relation to geography.

The method of analysis involves mapping disease patterns and making comparisons between geographic areas in tables, graphs, and charts. Relationships between location and disease have long been used as a basis for hypotheses of the etiology of diseases. Another objective is to assist health services managers in identifying problem areas.

Differences in occurrence of a disease between places may be caused by many factors such as the physical and biological environment inherent in the areas compared or in the characteristics of the inhabitants.[1] Epidemiologists concerned with the biology of disease are, or at least traditionally have been, mostly concerned with the physical and biological environment causative factors.

Those that depend upon specific environmental factors and conditions are called place diseases.[2] Obvious examples are parasitic and infectious diseases; less-well-known ones[3] include endemic goiter in iodine-deficient inland regions, histoplasmosis in inland river valleys where humidity is high, and mottled dental enamel, a condition related to the fluoride content of water and whose geographical pattern of occurrence led to the identification of the role of fluoride in preventing dental caries.

Multiple sclerosis also shows a distinctive geographical distribution pattern, with rare incidence between the equator and 30 to 35 degrees latitude, increasing with distance from the equator in both northern and southern hemispheres. The prevalence rate of multiple sclerosis is six times higher in Winnipeg, Man., than in New Orleans, and 2.4 times higher in Halifax, N.S., than in Charleston, S.C.[4]

Relationships between place and disease also may result from the personal characteristics of the inhabitants. There are numerous examples of this. The lower cardiovascular death rate in Japan as compared to the United States has been related to diet (intake of cholesterol). The overall lower mortality rate in Utah, mostly from heart disease and cancer, has been associated with the particular life style of the large Mormon population. A somewhat more "exotic" example is the geographical pattern of kuru, a rapidly fatal neurologic disease. This is limited to one area of New Guinea among one tribal group and results from cannibalistic practices. As the area has come under control of the Australian government and as cannibalism has been discouraged, kuru has been disappearing.[5]

The importance of location of disease for administrative, as opposed to biologic, purposes stems from the fact that, as Donabedian writes, "certain features of social organization conspire to concentrate particularly vulnerable populations in certain areas, notably the urban ghetto and some rural sections of the country. The association is often so close that mere residence in certain areas may constitute presumptive evidence of unmet need."[6]

In other words, there tend to be clusters of person factors (as described in Chapter 6) in certain places. In this sense, the location or place of disease is particularly relevant to health services managers since they can use it as an aggregate indicator of multiple risk factors in a particular population subgroup.

Mortality differences between places also can be caused by differences in survivorship, that is, in case fatality rates resulting from differences in medical services and facilities.[7] Mortality and morbidity differences may be artifactual (nonreal), stemming from differences or errors in reporting and diagnosis (errors in the numerators) or in the population census (errors in the denominators).

Analysis of disease patterns by place may be done using either natural or political boundaries. Natural boundaries are likely to be more useful when investigating environmental causative factors such as climate, water, soil, etc.[8] However, it often is more convenient to use political boundaries, either on an international, national, state, or local level. This is most essential if the expected results are to be used for the allocation of resources and money.

International Comparisons

International comparison of disease serves several purposes. It allows the monitoring of each country's health status. It is used in etiological studies to look at associations between disease and environmental conditions as well as person factors. It also provides some estimate of potential improvement in the countries that do not have the lower rates.

Interpretation of differences among countries may be hazardous, however, since major variances in reporting and diagnosis are likely. Small differences in specific causes of death probably are insignificant but it is hard to discuss very large differences such as can be observed for several diseases.

Tables 7-1 and 7-2 show the overall mortality rates among men and women in selected countries. Since all of these countries have reasonably good vital statistics systems, the differences are interesting. These death rates have been age-adjusted to control for the effect of varying age composition.

During 1976-1977, mortality rates among men and women were lowest in the Scandinavian countries and the Netherlands, followed in order by Canada, the United States, and the Northwestern European countries. The order varies somewhat for specific age groups. At ages under 25, the lowest rates again were in the Scandinavian countries and the Netherlands, followed by the Northwestern European countries, then Canada and the United States. At ages 65 and over, the lowest mortality among men, the leader was Canada, followed by the United States, the Scandinavian countries and the Netherlands, and the Northwestern European countries. Among women, 65 and older, the United States had the lowest rate.

The international differences are sometimes very wide for specific diseases and causes of death. The incidence of infectious and parasitic diseases of course varies strikingly between tropical and temperate areas. There are many less easily explainable differences in chronic, noninfectious diseases.

Table 7-3 shows the ranking of various countries in terms of several cancer sites. The top rates range from 6.8 to 267.9 times higher than the lowest. Some countries—Scotland, Ireland, and Denmark—have high cancer rates for many different sites. Others such as Spain and Hong Kong have low rates for almost all sites, with Thailand at the bottom (best) in every category listed here. Still others have a low rate for certain causes of death and a very high one for others. For example, Japan has low rates for male colon and female breast cancer, as well as for male leukemia, but it has the highest rates for male stomach cancer.

Rates for the United States and Canada are exactly the opposite of Japan: among the higher ones for male colon and female breast cancer and among the lowest for male stomach cancer. Some countries such as Canada and Australia, geographically far apart but sharing a common heritage as well as comparable industrialization and life styles, have almost identical rates for all causes of death listed in Table 7-3.

As noted earlier, international comparisons often are used to study the etiology of diseases. For example, international comparisons show that the incidence of colon, rectum, stomach, and breast cancer is high where there is a low level of selenium in the soil.[9,10] A useful etiological tool when life style or environmental factors are suspected is the study of migrants. Studies of Japanese migrants to Hawaii and California show that they soon are likely to have the high breast cancer rates of women in the United States.[11,12,13] Studies of immigrants also have been used to implicate dietary practices in many forms of cancer.[14,15]

Table 7-1 Mortality among Men in Selected Countries, 1966-1967 and 1976-1977

Average Annual Death Rate per 1,000 Population

Country	1966-67					1976-77				
	All Ages	Ages Under 25	Ages 25-44	Ages 45-64	Ages 65 and Over	All Ages	Ages Under 25	Ages 25-44	Ages 45-64	Ages 65 and Over
United States										
White	9.1	1.8	2.5	14.4	69.0	7.9	1.5	2.2	12.1	61.4
Nonwhite	12.6	3.0	6.4	22.3	72.6	10.6	2.3	5.3	19.5	60.3
Total	9.5	2.0	2.9	15.2	69.2	8.2	1.6	2.5	12.9	61.3
Canada	8.3	1.9	2.2	12.3	64.2	7.7	1.5	2.0	11.5	61.2
Denmark	7.8	1.4	1.6	10.7	66.6	7.4	1.0	1.7	10.7	62.6
Norway	7.1	1.3	1.7	9.6	60.7	7.0	1.1	1.5	9.7	60.3
Sweden	7.0	1.2	1.8	8.9	61.0	6.8	.9	1.8	9.3	59.4
Netherlands	7.3	1.4	1.5	10.4	61.3	7.2	1.0	1.3	10.0	63.7
Weighted Average	7.3	1.3	1.6	9.9	62.0	7.1	1.0	1.5	9.9	61.6
United Kingdom										
England and Wales	8.9	1.5	1.6	12.7	77.0	8.3	1.2	1.4	11.9	73.5
Northern Ireland	9.1	1.7	1.8	13.2	76.8	9.8	1.7	2.2	13.9	82.1
Scotland	10.0	1.6	2.2	15.2	81.9	9.5	1.3	2.0	14.6	80.2
Belgium	9.2	1.8	2.1	13.7	74.8	8.9	1.4	1.9	12.6	76.1
France	8.6	1.5	2.5	13.2	67.2	8.1	1.3	2.4	12.4	63.2
Germany, Federal Republic	9.2	1.9	2.2	12.9	75.3	8.7	1.6	2.2	11.8	72.7
Switzerland	8.0	1.6	1.9	10.8	66.2	7.0	1.2	1.6	9.5	59.8
Weighted Average	8.9	1.7	2.1	13.0	73.3	8.4	1.4	2.0	12.1	70.2

1. Adjusted on basis of age distribution of the United States total population, 1940.
2. Belgium and France—1977 data not available; 1976 figures used.

Source: Reprinted from *Statistical Bulletin* with permission of the Metropolitan Life Insurance Company, 62, no. 4, October-December 1981, ©1981, 11, based on data from U.S. Department of Health, Education and Welfare, Public Health Service, National Center for Health Statistics, and *World Health Statistics Annual.*

Table 7-2 Mortality among Women in Selected Countries, 1966-1967 and 1976-1977

Average Annual Death Rate per 1,000 Population

Country	1966-67					1976-77				
	All Ages	Ages Under 25	Ages 25-44	Ages 45-64	Ages 65 and Over	All Ages	Ages Under 25	Ages 25-44	Ages 45-64	Ages 65 and Over
United States										
White	5.3	1.1	1.3	6.8	45.3	4.3	0.8	1.1	6.2	35.5
Nonwhite	8.5	2.0	3.7	14.6	52.1	6.3	1.5	2.4	10.9	40.5
Total	5.7	1.2	1.6	7.6	45.8	4.6	.9	1.3	6.7	36.0
Canada	5.1	1.2	1.2	6.4	43.3	4.3	.8	1.0	5.6	37.5
Denmark	5.4	.9	1.2	6.4	49.4	4.6	.6	1.1	6.3	40.2
Norway	4.7	.8	.8	4.9	45.3	4.1	.6	.7	4.6	38.9
Sweden	4.8	.7	1.0	5.1	45.5	4.1	.6	.9	4.8	38.6
Netherlands	4.8	.8	1.0	5.3	44.7	4.1	.6	.8	4.8	38.4
Weighted Average	4.9	.8	1.0	5.4	45.8	4.2	.6	.9	5.0	38.8
United Kingdom										
England and Wales	5.4	1.0	1.1	6.7	49.0	5.1	.8	1.0	6.5	46.3
Northern Ireland	6.0	1.2	1.3	7.1	54.1	6.0	1.0	1.2	7.7	52.9
Scotland	6.3	1.1	1.4	8.1	55.0	5.8	.8	1.2	8.2	49.9
Belgium	5.8	1.2	1.2	6.8	52.2	5.3	.9	1.1	6.1	48.7
France	5.0	1.0	1.3	6.0	43.6	4.4	.8	1.1	5.1	39.3
Germany, Federal Republic	5.8	1.2	1.3	6.8	62.2	5.1	.9	1.1	6.0	46.4
Switzerland	5.1	1.0	1.0	5.6	47.2	4.0	.7	.8	4.5	37.7
Weighted Average	5.5	1.1	1.2	6.5	48.8	4.9	.8	1.1	5.9	44.4

1. Adjusted on basis of age distribution of the United States total population, 1940.
2. Belgium and France—1977 data not available; 1976 figures used.

Source: Reprinted from *Statistical Bulletin* with permission of the Metropolitan Life Insurance Company, 62, no. 4, October-December 1981, ©1981, 12, based on data from U.S. Department of Health, Education and Welfare, Public Health Services, National Center for Health Statistics, and *World Health Statistics Annual.*

Variations within Countries

As opposed to international comparisons, which are useful mainly for etiological purposes, variations within countries are most appropriate for administrative purposes, although, as is noted later, they can and have often been used in analyzing the etiology of diseases. Variations within a country, on a national, state, or local level, can be used advantageously in the management and planning of health services.

Variations between U.S. States

There are many geographical differences in mortality patterns within the United States.[16] In general, mortality rates are higher in the East, particularly the Southeast. For blacks and for white males, the highest rate areas for all natural causes are largely in the Southeast. For white females, they more often are in the Middle Atlantic states and in the Chicago area. The Southeast has a particularly high incidence of cardiovascular diseases (Figure 7-1) and ischemic heart disease.

Table 7-3 Death Rates of Selected Countries, from Highest to Lowest

Age-Adjusted Death Rates Per 100,000 Population in Parentheses (Rounded)

	Cancer—1976-1977	
All sites, Males	*All sites, Females*	*Colon & Rectum, Males*
Scotland (270)	Denmark (171)	Ireland (36)
Belgium (267)	Scotland (166)	New Zealand (33)
France (256)	Ireland (161)	Scotland (33)
England & Wales (252)	England & Wales (156)	Denmark (32)
Switzerland (237)	New Zealand (151)	England & Wales (30)
Denmark (232)	Belgium (148)	Belgium (29)
Hong Kong (230)	Israel (141)	Canada (29)
Ireland (225)	Sweden (141)	Australia (28)
New Zealand (221)	Argentina (137)	France (28)
U.S.A. (214)	U.S.A. (136)	Switzerland (27)
Poland (213)	Canada (135)	U.S.A. (26)
Argentina (212)	Switzerland (134)	Sweden (25)
West Germany (212)	West Germany (134)	Norway (23)
Canada (211)	Norway (131)	West Germany (23)
Australia (210)	Australia (129)	Israel (21)
Sweden (198)	Poland (126)	Argentina (20)
Spain (192)	Hong Kong (125)	Hong Kong (17)
Norway (188)	France (125)	Japan (15)
Japan (187)	Spain (110)	Poland (15)
Israel (171)	Japan (109)	Spain (7)
Thailand (37)	Thailand (25)	Thailand (4)

Table 7-3 continued

Breast, Females	Cancer—1976-1977 Stomach, Males	Leukemia, Males
Denmark (34)	Japan (70)	Denmark (8.9)
England & Wales (34)	Poland (45)	Canada (8.8)
Ireland (32)	West Germany (34)	France (8.7)
Scotland (31)	Ireland (25)	Israel (8.7)
New Zealand (30)	Scotland (25)	New Zealand (8.5)
Israel (29)	England & Wales (25)	Switzerland (8.1)
Switzerland (29)	Argentina (24)	Belgium (8.0)
Canada (28)	Norway (24)	Australia (8.0)
Belgium (28)	Belgium (23)	Sweden (7.9)
U.S.A. (27)	Sweden (21)	West Germany (7.3)
Australia (25)	France (20)	Scotland (6.9)
Argentina (24)	New Zealand (19)	Poland (6.8)
Sweden (24)	Denmark (19)	Argentina (6.7)
France (23)	Israel (18)	England & Wales (6.6)
Norway (23)	Spain (16)	Norway (6.6)
West Germany (19)	Canada (16)	Ireland (6.2)
Poland (16)	Australia (16)	U.S.A. (5.6)
Spain (16)	Switzerland (12)	Japan (4.8)
Hong Kong (11)	U.S.A. (9)	Hong Kong (3.8)
Japan (6)	Hong Kong (6)	Spain (2.8)
Thailand (1)	Thailand (2)	Thailand (0.6)

Source: CA-A Cancer Journal for Clinicians, "*Cancer around the World* 1976-1977." Reprinted with permission. Vol. 32, no. 1, January-February 1982, 26-27.

Several factors may explain these geographical differences within the United States. Many counties classified as mining areas and/or having a history of mining have high rates for all causes of death and all natural causes. However, since these rates are high for both males and females, they cannot be attributed solely to the occupational risks of mining.

Various hypotheses have been proposed[17] to explain this association between mining and mortality rates. They illustrate the use of the geographical description of disease patterns in etiological reasoning. One hypothesis is that the presence of large coal or metal ore deposits, and particularly the mining of them, in some way disturbs the environment sufficiently to increase the risk of dying in middle age. The causal factor could be the exposure to the coal or metal itself or, possibly more likely, to byproducts or waste substances (such as sulfur) including trace substances (possibly arsenic) in the ores. The mode of transmission might be through water, especially drinking water, or air pollution. In some areas, mine waste has

Figure 7-1 Death Rates for Cerebrovascular Disease, U.S., 1968-1972*

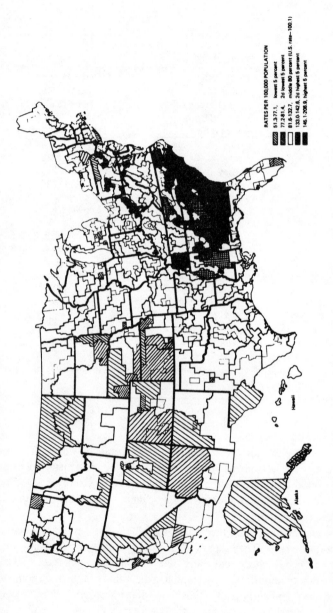

RATES PER 100,000 POPULATION

51.3-77.1,	lowest 5 percent
77.2-81.4,	2d lowest 5 percent
81.5-132.7,	middle 80 percent (U.S. rate—100.1)
133.0-142.6,	2d highest 5 percent
145.1-208.9,	highest 5 percent

*Among white males age 35-74 (age-adjusted) in the 50 lowest and 50 highest mortality rate state economic areas (ICDA 430-438).

Source: Reprinted from *Geographic Patterns in the Risks of Dying and Associated Factors—Ages 35-74 Years—U.S. 1968-1972*, U.S. Department of Health and Human Services, Public Health Service, National Center for Health, Statistics, Vital and Health Statistics Analytical Series 3, no. 18, September 1980.

been used to surface country roads, thereby increasing the potential for air pollution in contrast to places where the waste is simply dumped in huge piles.

Cultural or socioeconomic factors also may be considered. Individuals who move into mining counties are not necessarily at the same risk as individuals who pursue other occupations or work in other industries. Further, mining tends to be a boom-or-bust type of economy, which may have stressful effects on humans.

An alternate hypothesis may be proposed for some "history of mining" counties, particularly those with substantial outmigration over the years: That the able-bodied, more aggressive individuals would tend to move away in search of employment and that the remaining persons aged 35-74 would include a higher than usual proportion of those with chronic diseases or vague ill health that detracted from their willingness to look elsewhere for jobs. Thus, in some instances it may be appropriate to consider the hypothesis that the high rates in counties with a history of mining result largely from selective outmigration.

Another factor that seems related to the geographical distribution of diseases is altitude. Elevation above sea level is associated to a moderate but statistically significant extent with death rates for various diseases, but especially for cancer. The lowest rate areas to a large extent are in high plains areas.

Hypotheses proposed to explain the high rate area of the Southeast ("the enigma of the Southeast") [18] involve cultural characteristics, the availability of patient care resources, the content of the drinking water, atmospheric variables, and geochemistry and geobotany.

Another factor related to the geographical distribution of disease is the degree of urbanization. (Urban-rural differences are examined next.)

As an example of the use of this type of analysis, it should be noted that this information could have been included in the example in Chapter 4 on the identification of health problems in a Georgia county. That example calculated the standardized mortality ratios for the leading causes of death in county A using the state of Georgia as the "standard." The Southeastern states, including Georgia, have high rates of cerebrovascular and ischemic heart diseases. Consequently, since Georgia rates are problematic, it would be interesting to use another standard, such as the United States rate, for the identification of a cerebrovascular disease or ischemic heart disease problem in a particular county.

In other words, a standardized mortality ratio of 100 in a Georgia county for cerebrovascular disease or ischemic heart disease, when using that state as standard, still indicates a problem. Similarly, the problem identified in county A (SMR for cerebrovascular disease = 130) is even more important than previously thought.

Variations within States

There are wide variations in disease patterns within many of the states. However, contrary to variations between states, those within a state probably are more associated with differences in clustering of "person" factors, with degree of urbanization, and with availability of health care resources than with physical and biological environmental conditions. As an example of within-state variations, Figure 7-2 shows the distribution of neonatal mortality in Georgia.

An important component of variations in disease patterns is the difference between urban and rural areas. Urbanization has long been associated with higher

Figure 7-2 Neonatal Mortality in Georgia, by Health District, 1970-1974

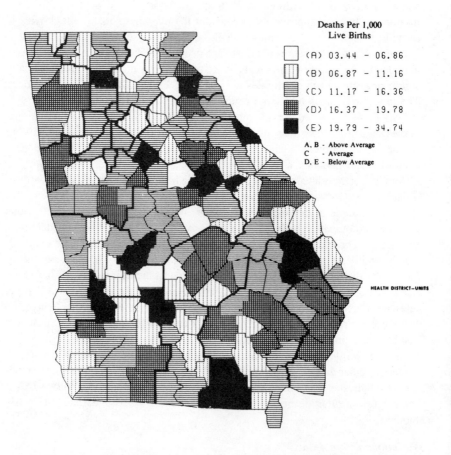

Deaths Per 1,000
Live Births

☐ (A) 03.44 - 06.86
▦ (B) 06.87 - 11.16
▦ (C) 11.17 - 16.36
▦ (D) 16.37 - 19.78
■ (E) 19.79 - 34.74

A, B - Above Average
C   - Average
D, E - Below Average

HEALTH DISTRICT—UNITS

Source: Reprinted from "Disease Patterns of the 70s," *Health Services Research and Statistics,* with permission of Georgia Department of Human Resources, Division of Physical Health, August 1976, 31.

mortality rates. This characterization of cities as notoriously unhealthy places[19] came about in the early days of modern public health practice when the high population density in urban areas made their inhabitants particularly vulnerable to epidemic diseases.

With the shift in disease patterns from infections to chronic diseases, urban-rural differences seem to have become less pronounced and more specific. A recent analysis of urban and rural mortality from all causes in Georgia showed rural counties were 29 percent higher than urban counties.[20] This difference was even greater in younger age groups, diminishing with age. In the over-64 population, the urban mortality rate was significantly higher than the rural rate.

Although much of the rural/urban difference in overall mortality is attributed to the larger proportion of older rural residents, the age-race adjusted rural rate still is significantly higher than the urban rate. Furthermore, age-specific and race-specific differences in rural health problems (Table 7-4) include congenital anomalies and perinatal-related deaths, motor vehicle and other accidents, and heart and cerebrovascular diseases. Specific urban health problems include homicides and cancer.

Other studies have shown higher infant and maternal mortality rates in rural areas.[21,22] Higher cancer rates in urban areas have been documented in several studies[23,24,25] and often have been related to exposure to industrial pollutants.[26,27] The evidence concerning heart disease, however, is more contradictory. Some studies have shown higher urban disease rates[28,29] involving the "stress of urban living" as a causative factor while other studies have reported higher rural disease rates.[30,31]

Local Variations

Health services managers, as noted, need data on local patterns of disease occurrence. Local variations in noninfectious disease incidence primarily reflect differences in person-related factors, notably socioeconomic status. Place of disease patterns in small areas is best analyzed using census divisions, since denominator data are available and rates can be computed; socioeconomic information also is available. Mapping by census tracts can help health services managers target specific populations and areas in need and allocate resources and provide facilities accordingly.

Analysis by place on a local level also is most appropriate when dealing with outbreaks of infectious diseases. A classic example of an epidemiological analysis by place is John Snow's study of cholera in London in 1848-54. Snow mapped the exact location of cholera deaths occurring during a 10-day period in 1848 (Figure 7-3). Through visual analysis of the distribution of cases, Snow noted the clustering of deaths around the Broad Street pump, from which residents received their water supply. After removal of the pump handle, no new cholera cases were reported. This fact, coupled with Snow's earlier work, suggested that cholera was transmitted by contaminated water.

By determining the relationship between location and disease, many place-related studies attempt to accomplish the same thing Snow did: discover the etiological factors of a disease.

A more recent example is the outbreak of Legionnaires' disease in Philadelphia in July 1976, when 182 persons attending an American Legion convention were affected by pneumonia caused by a previously unrecognized bacterium. It is

Table 7-4 Significant Problems[1] by Age and Race Groups (Georgia, 1979)

Age Group	Race	Rural (non-SMSA)[2]	Urban (SMSA)[2]
0-14	White	Perinatal-related Motor vehicle accidents	
	Nonwhite		
15-44	White	Motor vehicle accidents, other accidents, congenital anomalies	Homicide
	Nonwhite		
		Other accidents	
45-65	White	Heart disease, cerebrovascular disease, motor vehicle accidents	
	Nonwhite		
65 and up	White	Motor vehicle accidents	Cancer
	Nonwhite	Cerebrovascular disease	Cancer
All		Heart disease, cancer, cerebrovascular disease, respiratory-related, motor vehicle accidents, other accidents, other circulatory-related, perinatal-related, urinary-related.	Homicide

1. Mortality rate higher than expected.

2. SMSA = Standard Metropolitan Statistical Area.

Source: Steve Wright, Francois Champagne, G.E. Alan Dever, and F.C. Clark, "A Comparative Analysis of Rural and Urban Mortality in Georgia," *Journal of Community Health.*

worthwhile to quote at length from the investigators' report to examine how they went about trying to ascertain the place of occurrence:

> The place of exposure cannot be defined with certainty, but the most reasonable hypothesis is that exposure occurred within or in the immediate vicinity of Hotel A. Such a hypothesis is consistent with the observation that of delegates, those who stayed at Hotel A had a significantly

Figure 7-3 John Snow's Map of Cholera Deaths in the Soho District of London, 1848

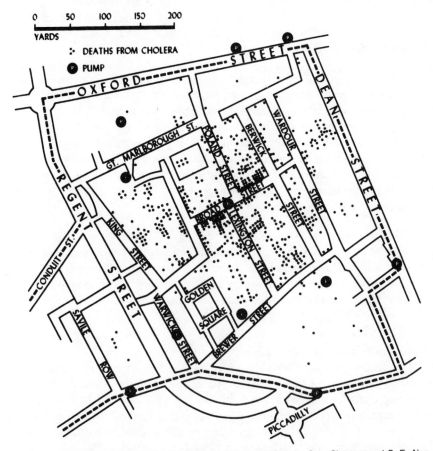

Source: Reprinted from *Health Care Delivery: Spatial Perspectives* by Gary Shannon and G. E. Alan Dever with permission of McGraw-Hill Book Company, ©1974, 3; based on *Some Aspects of Medical Geography* by L. D. Stamp with permission of Oxford University Press, ©1964, 16.

higher rate of illness than those who did not, and that of the delegates who did not stay at Hotel A, those who fell ill spent more time on the average in Hotel A than those who stayed well.

The fact that cases occurred in persons who had been near, but not in, Hotel A shows that in at least some cases, exposure occurred outside Hotel A, and suggests that exposure could have occurred on the streets or sidewalks around that hotel. Other evidence of exposure outside the hotel comes from the observation that serologically confirmed cases in delegates occurred more frequently in those who watched the parade from the sidewalk in front of Hotel A and that the length of time spent on the sidewalk was associated with illness. Exposure may well have occurred within Hotel A also. In the delegate group, there was a strong association between time spent in the lobby of Hotel A and risk of contracting the disease.

It is unlikely that the place of exposure was in any of the main convention function rooms in Hotel A because attendance at those functions was not associated with illness. Similarly, bedrooms were unlikely places of exposure since roommates of patients were not at increased risk of illness and because there was no geographic clustering of bedrooms of cases in Hotel A. Because no hospitality room was said to have been visited by more than half the patients and because there was no striking association between attendance or food consumption and illness, the rooms are unlikely to have been the sites of exposure.

If the exposure was airborne, the association of illness and time spent in the lobby might be explained. An airborne agent might also have affected non-Legionnaires who were in the hotel only transiently and had no other apparently noteworthy exposure; it might also have exposed persons who walked near the hotel but did not enter it.[32]

It was shown later that the main mode of transmission of the Legionnaires' disease bacterium was indeed through the air (airborne).

Noninfectious causes of death also can be analyzed and mapped on a local level. Figure 7-4 illustrates the excess mortality for diseases of the heart and of homicides in the regional planning districts of Baltimore (each planning district is an aggregate of approximately eight contiguous census tracts). Figure 7-5 shows the infant mortality rate, illegitimate birth rate, average number of children born per woman, and unemployment rate, per census tract, for Newport News, Va.

Health service managers can find it valuable to map a number of variables to help them analyze local situations.

Value, but with a Caution

The description of health and disease by place can help health services managers in identifying the problems of their population, in developing programs, and in focusing on high-risk areas for specific ailments. It also is used in epidemiology to study the etiology of disease.

Place may be associated with health and disease through physical and biological environmental variables. However, as the areas examined get smaller, the relationship of place and disease occurrence most often is caused by the clustering of personal characteristics (demographic, social, life style) of the inhabitants. In this sense, place is a good preliminary indicator of factors affecting health and disease.

An important corollary of locating health problems by geographic area is the spatial distribution of services.[33] As is described in Chapters 8 and 11, health services managers also can analyze the utilization of services by place, as well as the allocation of resources.

Figure 7-4 Excess Mortality Rates by Category of Excess

Regional Planning Districts, Baltimore, 1969-1977

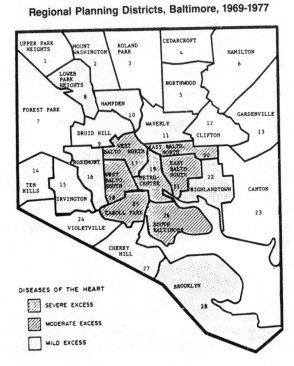

Figure 7-4 continued

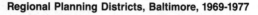

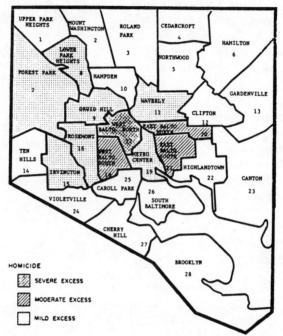

Source: Reprinted from "Data on Excess Mortality to Pinpoint Prevention Programs," by M. Lerner in *Proceedings of the 18th National Meeting of the Public Health Conference on Records and Statistics (1980),* U.S. Department of Health and Human Services, Public Health Service, 1980, 257-262.

A word of caution is necessary. Analysis by place can lead to ecological fallacy. As explained in Chapter 4, it is not possible to make assertions about individuals based only on examination of geographical areas. Analysis should be based on consistent factors. For example, the correlation between two attributes of a set of areas is not necessarily the same as that between the same attributes of individuals within the areas.[34]

TIME: WHEN DISEASE OCCURS

A final element in describing a disease is its time of occurrence. The distribution in time of a disease refers to trends in its incidence and prevalence as well as its fluctuations around this trend.[35] The variations in the incidence and prevalence of a

Figure 7-5 Plotting Vital Statistics

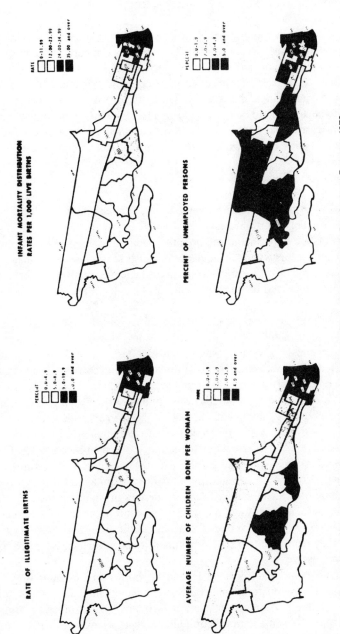

Newport News, Va., 1970

INFANT MORTALITY DISTRIBUTION
RATES PER 1,000 LIVE BIRTHS

PERCENT OF UNEMPLOYED PERSONS

RATE OF ILLEGITIMATE BIRTHS

AVERAGE NUMBER OF CHILDREN BORN PER WOMAN

Source: Reprinted from *Social Conditions and Services*, City of Newport News, Va., Community Development Program, 1973.

disease over time can be informative since they reflect temporal differences in the factors affecting health and disease (whether biological, environmental, life style, or medical care organization).

Time in epidemiology can be expressed either in hours, days, months, or years, depending on the disease studied. This analysis is in terms of three major kinds of time changes: short-term variations, secular trends, and cyclical trends. Although the focus is on time patterns of disease occurrence separate from person and place patterns, it is evident that to examine variations in time, the population of concern has to be defined previously at least by place. In other words, the variation in time of a disease cannot be examined without consideration of its place. The last section of this chapter examines a particular type of interaction—time-space clusters.

Short-Term Variations

Short-term variations are found mostly, although not exclusively, in infectious diseases. This short time may vary from hours to months. Several epidemiologic concepts are of particular importance when discussing short-term variations. An epidemic occurs when the incidence of a disease is unusually high at a given time. An epidemic therefore refers to an excess incidence of disease over what normally would be expected, no matter whether that incidence is, in absolute terms, high or low.

The level after which incidence can be considered in excess is called the epidemic threshold. When an epidemic is not restricted to a given place but occurs simultaneously at many points, such as often is the case with influenza, it is referred to as pandemic. The usual frequency of occurrence of a disease regularly and continuously present is referred to as its endemic level. The term outbreak is used when speaking of an epidemic, probably because it sounds less alarming, especially when dealing with an incidence that in absolute terms is not very high.

The two main types of epidemics are common source and propagated (or progressive). The difference is in the mode of transmission of the disease agent. Common source epidemics involve exposure of a group of persons to a common, noxious influence.[36] All noninfectious disease epidemics technically are from a common source. Infectious disease epidemics in which the mode of transmission of the causal agent is food, air, water, ice, tobacco, or alcohol are common source epidemics. When the mode of transmission is from person to person, or more generally from host to host (from animals to people), the epidemic is propagated, or progressive.

Another important concept related to short-term variations is the incubation period. This refers to the interval between involvement of an etiologic agent and onset of illness. Although this term most often refers to infectious diseases, it also can apply to noninfectious etiological agents as well. As discussed later, the incubation period is not necessarily short. For example, many chronic diseases are characterized by long latency (incubation) periods and indefinite onset. This is the case when life style, such as smoking, is the etiological factor, or when occupational or environmental exposure to hazardous substances (such as Agent Orange) lead to chronic illnesses years or decades later. The incubation period for some infectious diseases such as syphilis and tuberculosis also can be long.

Short-term variations are best analyzed with graphs by plotting (either on a histogram or a frequency polygon) the distribution of cases by time of onset. When dealing with epidemics, this distribution is referred to as the epidemic curve. Figure 7-6 shows the epidemic curve of an outbreak of food poisoning. In this case, the time units of importance are hours. Figure 7-7 shows the epidemic curve of the outbreak of Legionnaires' disease. The incubation period of that bacterium can be estimated from this graph as two to ten days.

As stated earlier, short-term variations are not limited to infectious diseases. Figure 7-8 shows the epidemic curve of deaths from heat-related illness in St. Louis in June and July 1980 when record-breaking high temperatures occurred. The epidemic threshold can be estimated from 1978 and 1979 data. As can be seen, a definite epidemic of deaths from heat-related illness occurred between July 7 and July 21, 1980.

In some other infectious diseases, months are the time units of interest. Figure 7-9 shows the time variation of cases of toxic-shock syndrome (TSS) between 1970 and 1982. This is an interesting example since little is known about the etiology of toxic shock syndrome, although it seems to be associated with the use of tampons. So few cases were reported between 1970 and 1978 that years are used as units of analysis (inset). The incidence increases continuously afterward, with a peak in August and September 1980, then a decline. Identification and reporting of cases probably is a major factor in the shape of the curve between 1970 and 1980. As the Centers for Disease Control report:

> Factors that might have affected [the subsequent decline in the incidence of toxic shock syndrome] include changes in the number of tampon users, in the way women use tampons, in the availability and frequency of use of different brands of tampons, in the rate of vaginal carriage of strains of staphylococcus aureus capable of causing TSS, or in other unrecognized factors in the maternal history of the disease. . . . The extent to which the observed change is due to a decrease in the incidence of TSS, as opposed to a decrease in the reporting of TSS is not known, although both factors are probably important.[37]

Cyclical Trends

Cyclical trends refer to recurring patterns of disease over time. This regular pattern may consist of cycles that last several years, as in the four-to-six-year cycle

Figure 7-6 Food Intoxication at a Military Base in Texas, October 8-9, 1968

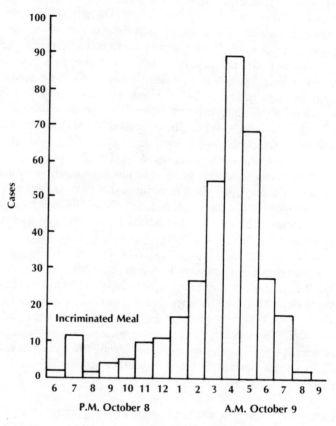

Source: Reprinted from *Epidemiology: An Introductory Text* by Judith S. Mausner and Anita K. Bahn with permission of W. B. Saunders Company, ©1974, 272; and from *Morbidity and Mortality Weekly Report* 18, no. 20, U.S. Department of Health Education, and Welfare, Public Health Service, Centers for Disease Control, ©1969.

of influenza Type B, or the two-to-three-year cycle of influenza Type A. A common cyclical pattern may be observed in the incidence of diseases or deaths related to seasonal changes. Seasonal variations have long been a favorite topic of epidemiologists. As a 1945 article reported:

> Seasonal fluctuation is not only a very general epidemiologic principle,
> but for a given disease is one of its most constant epidemiologic

Figure 7-7 Epidemic Curve of Legionnaires' Disease Philadelphia, July 1-
August 18,1976

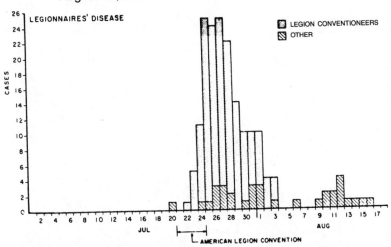

Source: Reprinted from "Legionnaires' Disease: Description of an Epidemic of Pneumonia;" by D. W. Fraser with permission of *The New England Journal of Medicine,* 297, no. 22, December 1, 1977, ©1977, 1193.

Figure 7-8 Heat-Related Illness—Deaths of St. Louis, Residents, by
Day, June and July, 1978, 1979, and 1980

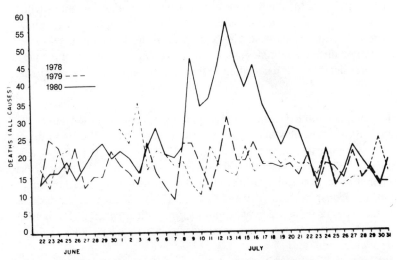

Source: Reprinted from *Mortality and Morbidity Weekly Report,* U.S. Department of Health and Human Services, Public Health Service, Centers for Disease Control, vol. 29, no. 54, September 1981, 109.

Figure 7-9 Confirmed Cases of Toxic-Shock Syndrome, U.S., January 1970-March 1982

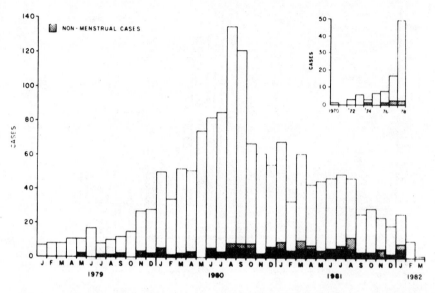

Source: Reprinted from *Mortality and Morbidity Weekly Report,* U.S. Department of Health and Human Resources, Public Health Service, Centers for Disease Control, vol. 31, no. 11, April 30, 1982, 201.

characteristics. Most infectious diseases exhibit marked variations with season and these are remarkably constant from year to year. The influence of season is most strikingly evident in the variation in seasonal curves at different latitudes amounting to a complete reversal of months of prevalence in corresponding latitudes in the northern and southern hemispheres.[38]

Many diseases, both infectious and noninfectious, exhibit seasonal fluctuations. Figure 7-10 demonstrates that even the overall death rate (all causes) fluctuates seasonally, higher in winter and lower in summer. Figure 7-11 shows clearly the seasonal pattern of encephalitis. The summer increase in 1975 definitely can be considered as an epidemic. Deaths attributed to pneumonia and influenza also exhibit a seasonal cyclical pattern (Figure 7-12), even though, as said earlier, particular types of influenza may exhibit longer cyclical patterns. The increase in drownings in the summer or skiing accidents in winter are other examples of seasonal fluctuations.

Finally, other diseases and causes of death show cyclical patterns over very short periods. For example, deaths from motor vehicle accidents exhibit weekly cycles,

Figure 7-10 Seasonal Fluctuations of the Death Rate, U.S. 1980-1982

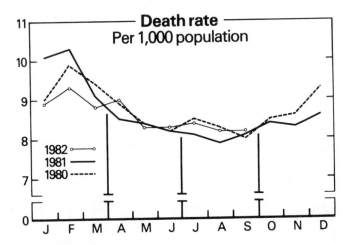

Source: Reprinted from *Monthly Vital Statistics Report,* U.S. Department of Health and Human Services, Public Health Service, National Center for Vital Statistics, vol. 30, no. 12, March 18, 1982, 2.

peaking on weekends. Folklore has it that births (or is it fecundity?) follow monthly (lunar) cycles, peaking on the full moon.

Several reasons may explain cyclical trends in disease incidence. There is no doubt that climate and other biometeorologic factors, including temperature and precipitation, affect both infectious and noninfectious diseases. Another factor is the length of the day: it has been shown, for example, that the incidence of neurosis increases during the long polar night in Norway.[39]

In a number of diseases, it is clear that seasonal variation is determined by corresponding changes in the opportunities for transmission of the infectious agent, as influenced by the bionomics of the vector.[40] In other words, the warm weather multiplication of insects, ticks, mites, etc., brings a corresponding increase in the incidence of infectious diseases transmitted to humans from those hosts.

Cyclical changes in activities, whether social, recreational, or even occupational/professional have an easily understandable impact on disease incidence. Swimming in summer and skiing in winter are obvious examples. In certain areas, hunting may bring people in unusual contact with some hosts such as rabbits. The seasonal increase in farming accidents is a factor. Similarly, an increase in the cholesterol level of accountants as the income tax deadline approaches has been reported.[41]

Figure 7-11 Encephalitis: Reported Cases by Month of Onset, U.S.,
1975-1982

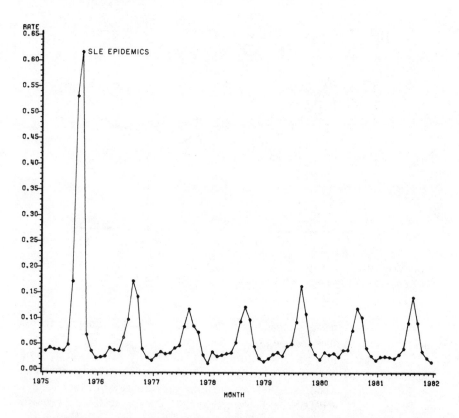

Source: Reprinted from *Morbidity and Mortality Weekly Report Annual Report 1981,* U.S. Department of Health and Human Services, Centers for Disease Control, vol. 29, no. 54, 33.

Secular Trends

Secular trends refer to changes that take place over a long period of time, such as years or decades, involving both infectious and noninfectious diseases. Figure 7-13 shows the trends in the overall death rate and the infant mortality rate between 1977 and 1981. As the preceding section noted, the death rate follows a yearly cyclical pattern. In such cases, secular trends are best shown in using moving averages so as to smooth out short-term variations. In Figure 7-13, this is done by using rates for successive 12-month periods, with the ending of each month

Figure 7-12 Deaths from Pneumonia and Influenza, U.S., 1979-1982

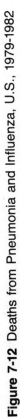

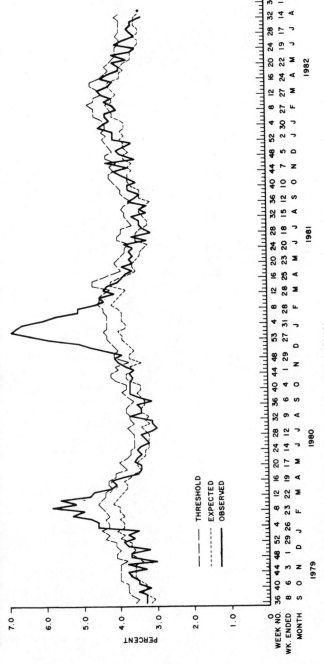

Source: Reprinted from *Morbidity and Mortality Weekly Report Annual Report 1981*, U.S. Department of Health and Human Resources, Public Health Service, Center for Disease Control, vol. 30, no. 54, September 1981, 117.

Figure 7-13 Secular Trends in Death and Infant Mortality Rates, U.S., 1978-1982

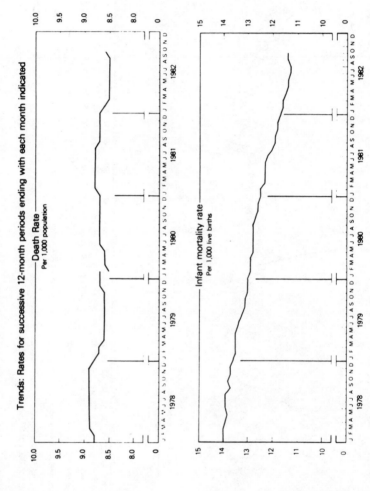

Source: Reprinted from *Monthly Vital Statistics Report,* U.S. Department of Health and Human Services, Public Health Service, National Centers for Health Statistics, vol. 30, no. 12, March 18, 1982, 3.

plotted. This shows that the death rate has been very stable between 1977 and 1981 while infant mortality has been declining.

Tracing secular trends in particular diseases and causes of death can be illuminating. Figure 7-14 shows the trends in some important causes of death. Most have been declining between 1950 and 1970, with the exception of lung cancer, which has been increasing steadily, and cirrhosis of the liver, which rose between 1950 and 1970 but has been slowly declining since.

Figure 7-15 illustrates secular trends in various cancers in females and males. In both sexes, stomach cancers have been declining substantially while lung cancer has been soaring since the 1930s in males and since the late 1960s in females. Uterine cancer in females and, to a smaller extent, liver cancer in both sexes also have been declining. The incidence of most other cancers has been fairly stable. Although not illustrated, deaths from all cancers have been slightly increasing.

As an example of secular trends in relation to person-characteristics (and place, of course); even though cancer death rates for the whole population have been increasing slightly, Figure 7-16 shows that they have been declining in both males and females ages 15-34.

Infectious diseases also evidence marked secular trends. Figure 7-17 shows the virtual elimination of anthrax, while Figure 7-18 indicates the increase in gonorrhea. A smaller increase also occurred following World War II.

Many factors may influence the secular trends in many diseases. One is whether the changes are real or artifactual—that is, resulting from errors in the numerator or the demoninator. Errors in the numerator may be caused by changes in the recognition of disease, in the rules and procedures for classifications of causes of death, or in accuracy of reporting, even in reporting age at death.[42] Errors in the denominator can stem from mistakes in the numeration of the population.

Real changes may result from shifts in the age distribution of the population (this can be controlled through the age-adjustment of rates), in survivorship and medical care organization, or from genetic, environmental, or life style factors.

Time-Place Clusters

The clustering in time and place of some diseases has been a topic of considerable interest in recent years among epidemiologists. A 1982 editorial in the *American Journal of Public Health* commented that "the greatest potential for geographic analysis of mortality lies in the examination of time-space interactions."[43]

The notions of time and place of occurrence of a disease are related conceptually. Although up to now they have been dealt with separately, the notion of time is always present in the consideration of place, and vice versa.

For example, the concept of epidemics is related not only to the time of occurrence but also to the place. An epidemic is in fact a clustering of a disease in

Figure 7-14 Secular Trends in Selected Causes of Death, U.S., 1950-1977

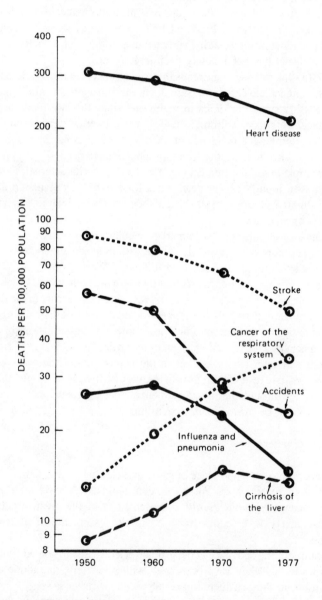

Source: Reprinted from *Health, United States, 1980,* U.S. Department of Health and Human Services, Public Health Service, December 1980, 291.

Figure 7-15 Secular Trends in Cancer Incidence: Age-Adjusted Cancer Death Rates* for Selected Sites

Females, U.S., 1930-1978

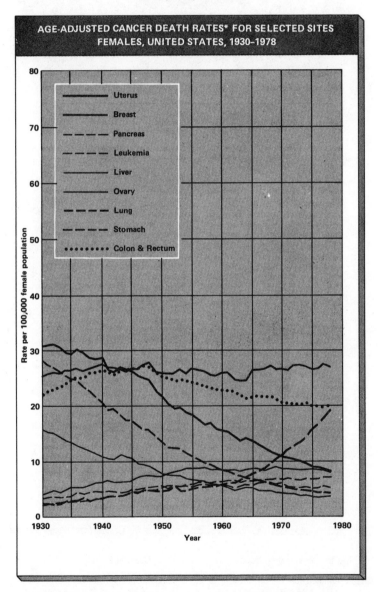

*Adjusted to the age distribution of the 1970 U.S. Census Population.

Figure 7-15 continued

Males, U.S., 1930-1978

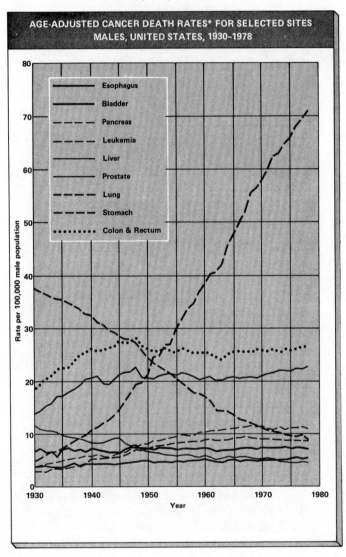

*Adjusted to the age distribution of the 1970 U.S. Census Population.

Source: Reprinted from *CA-Cancer Journal for Clinicians,* vol. 32, no. 1, January-February 1982, pp. 20, 21 with permission, ©1982. Sources of data: U.S. National Center for Health Statistics and U.S. Bureau of the Census.

Figure 7-16 Cancer Death Rates* by Sex, Ages 15-34, U.S., 1950-1978

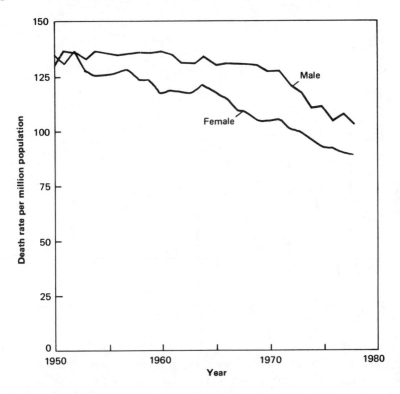

*Standardized for age on the 1970 U.S. population, ages 15-34.

Source: Reprinted from *CA-Cancer Journal for Clinicians,* vol. 32, no. 1, January-February 1982, 33, with permission, ©1982. Source of data: U.S. National Center for Health Statistics.

both time and place. When dealing with usual, classical infectious disease epidemics, the focus concentrates on the time variations, in a restricted place. This can be done because there are enough cases, even in such a restricted area, to demonstrate significant abnormally high levels of incidence.

When considering rare diseases, the additional information concerning the place of occurrence is vital. It is possible that some rare diseases might cluster in several different times and places in unusually high levels, but at too low levels for the usual consideration of time in a restricted place to be able to detect. Special techniques therefore have been developed to examine possible space-time clustering of rare diseases.

Figure 7-17 Secular Trend in Number of Cases of Anthrax, U.S., 1920-1980

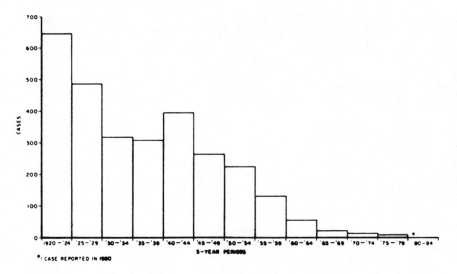

*i CASE REPORTED IN 1980

Source: Reprinted from *Morbidity and Mortality Weekly Report,* vol. 29, no. 54, September 1981, p. 21, U.S. Department of Health and Human Services, Public Health Service, Centers for Disease Control, 1981.

All of these techniques aim to answer the following question: When mapping a case of a rare disease, whose date and place of onset are known, will cases that follow it closely tend to be relatively nearby on the map compared with other cases that occur more distantly in time?[44] In other words, will there be a clustering in time and place of cases of the disease? If there is time-place clustering, those cases will be close both in time and space while unrelated cases will tend to have a larger average separation in time and space.[45]

The demonstration of time-space clusters is important since it indicates a common source, perhaps infectious, for disease. Such clusters have been demonstrated for rubella syndrome, thalidamide deformity, and tracheoesophageal fistula.[46] Some reports suggest that leukemia in children also may appear in time-space clusters.[47] Hodgkin's disease may follow this pattern,[48] although evidence is contradictory.[49]

SUMMARY

The distribution and variation in time of a disease is a fundamental feature of classical epidemiology. Short-term variations, cyclical and secular trends, and

Figure 7-18 Secular Trend in Incidence of Gonorrhea, U.S., 1976-1981

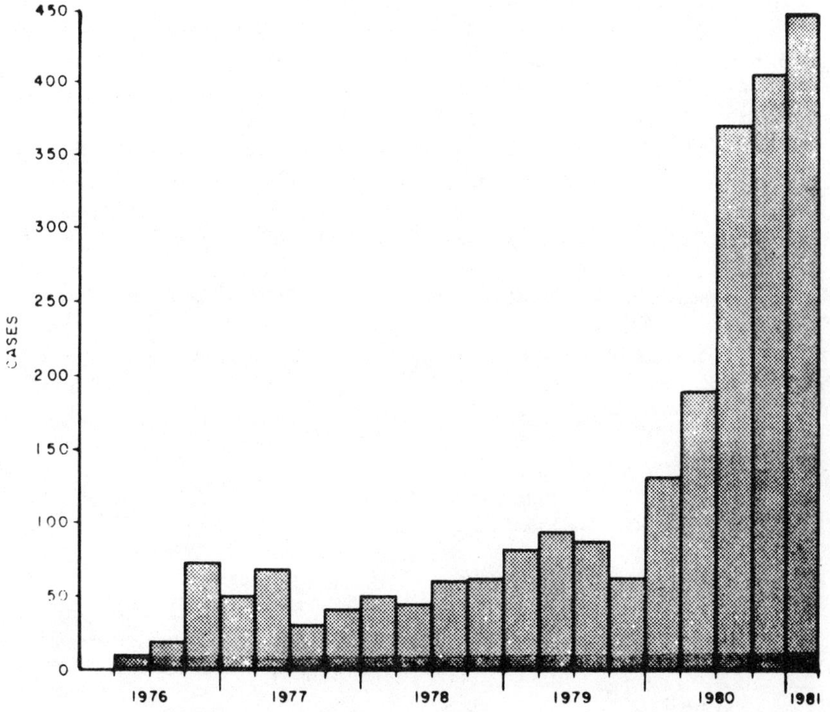

Source: Reprinted from *Morbidity and Mortality Weekly Report,* U.S. Department of Health and Human Resources, Public Health Service, Centers for Disease Control, vol. 29, no. 54, September, 1981, 35.

time-place clusters all provide important clues as to causation. Once again, however, the danger of ecological fallacy is ever present.

Time variations and trends are of major concern to health services managers. They are an essential part of the assessment and description of the health problems in a population. Trends can be extrapolated, so a knowledge of the irregular occurrence of a disease is essential to the provision of efficient standby capacity.[50] These trends also can assist health care managers in planning for future needs and identifying new markets for expansion.

NOTES

1. J.P. Fox, C.E. Hall, and L.R. Elveback, *Epidemiology—Man and Disease* (London: The Macmillan Company, 1970), 209.

2. Judith S. Mausner and Anita K. Bahn, *Epidemiology: An Introductory Text* (Philadelphia: W.B. Saunders Company, 1974), 64.

3. Ibid.

4. D.C. Poskanzer, "Neurologic Disease," in *Maxcy-Roseneau Public Health and Preventive Medicine*, 11th ed., ed. J.M. Last (New York: Appleton-Century-Crofts, Inc., 1980), 1258.

5. A. Donabedian, *Aspects of Medical Care Administration: Specifying Requirements for Health Care* (Cambridge, Mass.: Harvard University Press, 1973), 84.

6. Mausner and Bahn, *Epidemiology: An Introductory Text*, 66.

7. A.M. Lilienfeld, *Foundations of Epidemiology* (New York: Oxford University Press, 1976), 86.

8. Mausner and Bahn, *Epidemiology: An Introductory Text*, 65.

9. R.J. Shamberger, "Relationship of Selenium to Cancer. I. Inhibitory Effect of Selenium on Carcinogenesis," *Journal of the National Cancer Institute* 44 (1970): 931-936.

10. B. Janson et al., "Geographical Distribution of Gastrointestinal Cancer and Breast Cancer and Its Relation to Selenium Deficiency," in *Prevention and Detection of Cancer, Part I. Prevention, vol. 1, Etiology,* ed. H.E. Nieburgs (New York: Marcel Dekker Inc., 1977), 1161–1178.

11. B.E. Henderson, "Descriptive Epidemiology and Geographic Pathology," in *Cancer: Achievements, Challenges, and Prospects for the 1980s,* vol. 1, eds. J.H. Burchenal and H.F. Oettgen (New York: Grune & Stratton, Inc., 1980), 51-69.

12. P. Buell, "Changing Incidence of Breast Cancer in Japanese–American Women," *Journal of the National Cancer Institute* 51 (1973): 147.

13. W. Haenszel and M. Kurihara, "Studies of Japanese. I. Mortality From Cancer and Other Diseases Among Japanese in the United States," *Journal of the National Cancer Institute* 51 (1973): 1765-1779.

14. W. Haenszel et al., "Large-Bowel Cancer in Hawaiian Japanese," *Journal of the National Cancer Institute* 51 (1973): 1765-1779.

15. B. Armstrong and R. Doll, "Environmental Factors and Cancer Incidence and Mortality in Different Countries, With Special Reference to Dietary Practices," *International Journal of Cancer* 15 (1975): 617-631.

16. U.S. Department of Health and Human Services, *Geographic Patterns in the Risk of Dying and Associated Factors—Ages 35-74 Years—U.S., 1968-1972,* Vital and Health Statistics Analytical Studies series 3, no. 18 (Hyattsville, Md.: National Center for Health Statistics, September 1980), 120.

17. Ibid., 46-47.

18. Ibid., 43-44.

19. Fox et al., *Epidemiology—Man and Disease,* 233.

20. Steve Wright et al., "A Comparative Analysis of Rural and Urban Mortality in Georgia," *Journal of Community Health.*

21. T.H. Matthews, *Health Services in Rural America.* U.S. Department of Agriculture, Rural Development Service and Economic Research, Agricultural Information Bulletin No. 362 (April 1974), 102.

22. J.C. Kleinman, J.J. Feldman, and R.H. Mugge, "Geographic Variations in Infant Mortality," *Public Health Reports* 91 (1976): 423-432.

23. A.M. Lilienfeld, M.L. Levin, and I.I. Kessler, *Cancer in the United States* (Cambridge, Mass.: Harvard University Press), 1972.

24. U.S. Department of Health and Human Services, *Geographic Patterns,* 120.

25. P.C. Nasca et al., "Population Density as an Indicator of Urban-Rural Differences in Cancer Incidence, Upstate New York, 1968-1972," *American Journal of Epidemiology* 112 (1980): 362-375.

26. W.J. Blot and J.F. Fraumani, "Geographic Patterns of Lung Cancer: Industrial Correlations," *American Journal of Epidemiology* 103 (1976): 539-550.

27. W.J. Blot et al., "Geographic Patterns of Breast Cancer in the United States," *Journal of the National Cancer Institute* 59 (1977): 1407-1411.

28. P.E. Enterline et al., "Death Rates for Coronary Heart Disease in Metropolitan and Other Areas," *Public Health Reports* 75 (1960): 759-766.

29. I.M. Moriyama et al., *Cardiovascular Diseases in the United States* (Cambridge, Mass.: Harvard University Press, 1971).

30. U.S. Department of Health and Human Services, *Geographic Patterns*, 43-57.

31. J.R. McDonough, G.E. Garrison, and C.G. Hames, "Blood Pressure and Hypertensive Disease Among Negroes and Whites in Evans County, Georgia," in *Epidemiology of Hypertension*, J. Stamler, R. Stamler, and T.N. Pullman, eds. (New York: Grune & Stratton, Inc., 1967), 167-187.

32. D.W. Fraser et al., "Legionnaires' Disease: Description of an Epidemic of Pneumonia," *The New England Journal of Medicine* 297, no. 22 (December 1, 1977): 1189-1197.

33. Donabedian, *Aspects*, 86.

34. W. Robinson, "Ecological Correlations and the Behavior of Individuals," *American Sociological Review* 15 (June 1950): 351-357.

35. Donabedian, *Aspects*, 84.

36. Mausner and Bahn, *Epidemiology: An Introductory Text*, 273.

37. Centers for Disease Control, *Morbidity and Mortality Weekly Report* 31, no. 16 (April 30, 1982): 204.

38. W.L. Aycock, G.E. Lutman, and G.E. Foley, "Seasonal Prevalence as a Principle in Epidemiology," *American Journal of the Medical Sciences* 209 (March 1945): 396.

39. M. Jenicek, *Introduction à l'épidémiolojie* (St. Hyacinthe, Que.: Ediserne Inc., 1976), 106.

40. Aycock et al., "Seasonal Prevalence," 396.

41. Jenicek, *Introduction*, 106.

42. A.M. Lilienfeld, *Foundations of Epidemiology* (New York: Oxford University Press, 1976), 68.

43. J.C. Kleinman, "The Continued Vitality of Vital Statistics," *American Journal of Public Health* 72, no. 2 (February 1982): 126.

44. E.G. Knox, "Epidemics of Rare Diseases," *British Medical Bulletin* 27, no. 1 (1971): 45.

45. N. Mantel, "The Detection of Disease Clustering and a Generalized Regression Approach," *Cancer Research* 27, no. 2 (1967): 209.

46. Knox, "Epidemics," 47.

47. E.G. Knox, in *Current Research in Leukemia* ed. F.G.J. Hayhoe (Cambridge, England: Cambridge Unviersity Press, 1965), 274.

48. N.J. Vianna and A.K. Polan, "Epidemiologic Evidence for Transmission of Hodgkin's Disease," *The New England Journal of Medicine* 289 (1973): 532.

49. B. MacMahon, "Is Hodgkin's Disease Contagious?" *The New England Journal of Medicine* 289 (1973): 532.

50. Donabedian, *Aspects*, 84.

Chapter 8

The Epidemiology of Health Services Utilization

DETERMINANTS OF SERVICE UTILIZATION

Preceding chapters examined the relevance to health services management of the principles and techniques of epidemiology—the science concerned with the occurrence, distribution, and determinants of health and disease in a population. This chapter discusses how the occurrence of disease is translated into utilization of health services, focusing on determinants, recent trends, and the epidemiological (population-based) analysis of utilization for health services management.

The utilization of health services is an interaction between consumers and providers of care. It is a complex behavior determined by a wide range of factors.

There has been a great deal of research on this topic. A 1979 bibliography lists approximately 1,500 reports of studies related to the utilization of health services, most of them published between 1960 and 1976.[1] This discussion is based on the models by Donabedian[2] and by Andersen and Newman,[3] as well as on a critical review by McKinlay.[4]

Figure 8-1 illustrates the different types of determinants of health services utilization. This graphic representation is adapted from Donabedian's description of the medical care process and its environment. The set of interactions between health professionals and their clients takes place not within a vacuum but within an organizational environment that in turn is surrounded and penetrated by social and cultural features.[5] Health services utilization therefore is influenced by sociocultural, organizational, consumer-related, and provider-related factors. Although these categories are discussed as independent entities, it should be kept in mind that they often are indissociable.

Sociocultural Factors

Sociocultural determinants of health care utilization include technology and values.[6] Technology is considered a sociocultural as opposed to an organizational

Figure 8-1 Determinants of Health Services Utilization

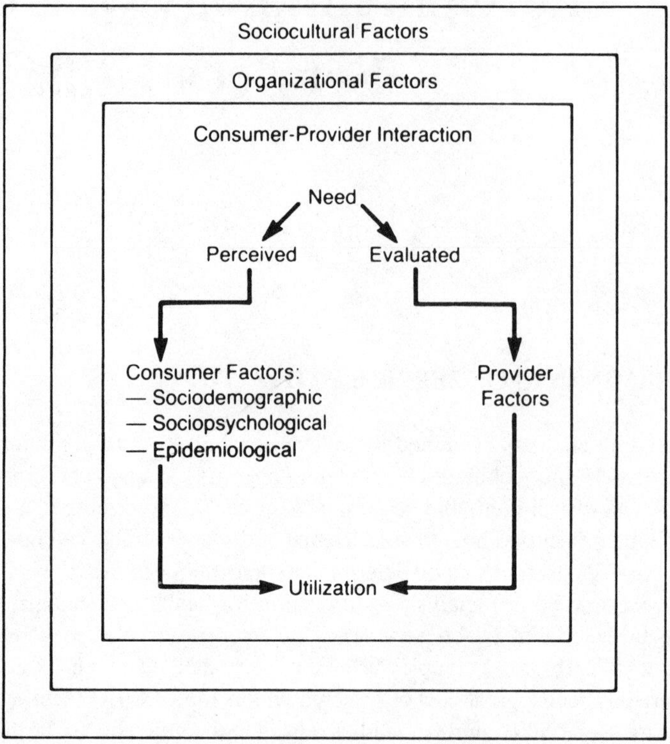

Source: Adapted from *Aspects of Medical Care Administration: Specifying Requirements for Health Care* by Avedis Donabedian with permission of Harvard University Press, © 1973, 61.

factor to denote the relatively little control health services managers have over it. Technology influences the utilization of services. In some cases, it reduces utilization by decreasing the illness levels or the need for medical care.

This is what Lewis Thomas calls the "genuinely decisive technology of modern medicine,"[7] exemplified by modern methods of immunization against diphtheria, pertussis, etc., and the contemporary use of antibiotics and chemotherapy for bacterial infections. For example, the use of tuberculosis hospitals has declined as a result of this high technology of medicine that has affected illness levels, which in turn have influenced utilization.

In other cases, technology increases the utilization of services. Thomas calls this "half-way technology," represented by such developments as transplantations of hearts, kidneys, and other organs, and by the invention of artificial organs. Progress in radiology and nuclear medicine also can be considered half-way technology. This technology is designed to compensate for the incapacitating effects of certain diseases that the medical profession is unable to do very much about—in other words, to "make up for disease" or to postpone death.

Societal values also influence the utilization of health services. Although this is a rather difficult field of study since societal values, norms, and beliefs influence all other aspects and determinants of the medical care process, some specific examples can be helpful.

In the United States, the use of the hospital as a place to be born and to die is almost totally determined by social norms, with technological factors of second importance.[8] This is attested by the fact that 98 percent of all live births in the United States in 1971 occurred in hospitals,[9, 10] while in the Netherlands, also a technologically advanced country, 70 percent of the births in 1968 took place in the home.[11] Another example is the financing of health care discussed in the next section on organizational determinants.

Several sociological studies have looked at the patterns of health services utilization by different subgroups of society.[12] Zola compares the presenting symptoms of Italian and Irish patients in the outpatient clinics of a Boston hospital.[13] He reports very different sets of complaints (more eye, ear, nose, and throat complaints from the Irish and more pain experienced by the Italians) and concludes that the particular symptoms individuals act upon—those for which they are going to use health services and seek medical care—are determined by their cultural, ethnic, or reference group.

Suchman, in a study of the effect of the social structure of various ethnic and cultural subgroups in New York on their utilization of health services,[14, 15] defines that structure as being either parochial or cosmopolitan. He finds that highly cosmopolitan groups tend to seek medical care more early and often while parochial groups rely more on other lay persons in their group (Friedson's lay referral system[16]). As McKinlay's later analysis points out, Suchman was crudely measuring the impact of "social networks" on health services utilization.[17] These social networks (family, kinship, and friendship) to which individuals belong probably determine, to a large extent, their health services utilization behavior.

Organizational Factors

The second category of determinants of health services utilization includes "the structures and processes that constitute medical care organization and which intimately surround and influence the medical care process"[18] (the patient-provider interaction). These organizational factors involve four factors: the availability of resources, the geographical accessibility, the social accessibility, and the characteristics of the structure (formal organization) and process of the delivery of care.

Availability of Resources

Availability refers to the relationship of the volume and type of existing resources to what are required to fill the population's health needs[19]—in other words, the adequacy of the supply of resources. A resource is available if it exists or is obtainable, without consideration of how easy or difficult it is to use. Availability of services obviously influences their utilization. A service can be used only if it is available. Availability usually is assessed on a relatively wide geographical basis (at least regional) and is expressed as volume of resources relative to the population served (personnel/population ratios, bed/population ratios).

Geographical Accessibility

Definitions of the concept of accessibility vary widely. Opinions differ concerning which factors should be included within this concept and whether access is a characteristic of the resources or of the clients.[20] Accessibility is considered here—following Donabedian's definition[21]—as referring to the characteristics of the resource that facilitate or obstruct use by potential clients. Two of these are related, geographical accessibility and temporal accessibility.

Geographical accessibility refers to spatial factors that facilitate or obstruct utilization. It is the relationship between the location of supply and the location of clients[22] (or of need). It can be measured by distance (mileage), travel time, or travel cost. These measures of accessibility have been studied extensively elsewhere.[23, 24, 25, 26]

The relationship between geographical accessibility and utilization of services, however, is less clear-cut than generally thought. The relationship between geographical accessibility and volume of services consumed seems to depend on the type of care and type of resource considered. Increased access (decreased distance, travel time, or travel cost) probably means increased use associated with milder complaints.

In other words, the use of preventive services is more highly associated with geographical accessibility than is the use of curative services, as is the use of generalist care as compared to specialists and of physician services as compared to hospital services. The more severe the illness or complaint, and the more sophisticated or specialized the resource or service, the less important or strong is the relationship between geographical accessibility and volume of services utilized.

There seems to be a stronger but still rather limited relationship between geographical accessibility and the choice of the site visited.[27] In a study of a prepaid group plan in an urban setting, in which equivalent services (internal medicine and pediatrics) are offered at three alternative clinics, Weiss, Greenlich, and Jones report that 69 percent of the visits were made to the clinic nearest to the patients' homes.[28] That 31 percent of the visits were not made at the closest clinic illustrates the point that other factors, such as prestige, also influence the choice of site.

However, as should be clear from the discussion of place in Chapter 7, investigation of place (and, therefore, of accessibility) should not be limited to place of residence. In the example just cited, place of work might explain some of the 31 percent of visits not made to the closest clinic. In fact, in performing an accessibility analysis, health services managers should always consider whether place of residence is the most appropriate indicator of the location of clients. In some instances, other indicators might be more useful.

The concept of temporal accessibility is closely related to geographical accessibility. Temporal accessibility refers to the limitations in the time the resources are available (as opposed to the space limitations in the case of geographical accessibility). As Donabedian puts it, "the hours during which the physician holds office sessions, or the ambulatory care facility remains open, influence the ability of clients, especially working people, to obtain care."[29] Penchansky and Thomas[30] refer to temporal accessibility as "accommodation," which they define as "the relationship between the manner in which the supply resources are organized to accept clients and the clients' ability to accommodate to these factors and the clients' perception of their appropriateness."

Social Accessibility

Social accessibility refers to the other nonspatial and nontemporal characteristics of resources that may facilitate or obstruct use of services. Social accessibility may be divided into two dimensions: acceptability and affordability. Acceptability refers to psychological, social, and cultural factors, affordability to economic factors.

Penchansky and Thomas define acceptability as "the relationship of clients' attitudes about personal and practice characteristics of providers to the actual characteristics of existing providers, as well as to provider attitudes about acceptable characteristics of clients."[31] Few studies have been done on acceptability of care. It seems, however, that consumers may be unwilling to use available and geographically accessible services because of provider attributes such as sex (reluctance of some men to see a woman physician), age, race, ethnicity, and religious affiliation.

Some of these same attributes may influence the willingness of providers to treat (or not want to treat) some patients. The refusal of certain providers to serve welfare patients is an example. Hospitals or other such facilities may have formal or informal admission policies that exclude patients. Donabedian even mentions exclusions on the basis of some diagnoses such as alcoholism, drug addiction, mental illness, tuberculosis, or contagious diseases as further examples of acceptability barriers to utilization.

On the other hand, the impact of affordability on utilization has been well documented. Affordability is "the relationship of prices of services and providers' insurance or deposit requirements to the clients' income, ability to pay, and existing health insurance."[32] Some authors consider affordability a characteristic pertaining to the individual. It is felt here, however, that affordability is a modality of the organization of health services, intimately linked to societal norms.

The relationship of affordability to health services utilization is best seen when comparing insured and noninsured patients where voluntary health insurance is available (in the United States) or, even better, when comparing utilization before and after the introduction of a universal (national) health insurance plan (in Canada).

In the United States, studies have shown that people with voluntary health insurance tend to consume more physician services than those who do not.[33] They also are admitted to hospitals more often and have higher rates of hospitalized surgery. In Canada, an analysis of the effects of the introduction of a universal health insurance plan in Quebec shows that when economic barriers are removed, lower income groups considerably increase their utilization of physician services.[34]

Characteristics of Care Structure and Process

Finally, the way services themselves are delivered may have an impact on utilization. The mode of remuneration of physicians definitely is a factor, as are fee-for-service, capitation, and salary (among others), which create their own incentives. Alternative forms such as solo practice, group practice, multispecialty group practice, comprehensive group plans (Kaiser Foundation), or others bring about different patterns of utilization.

In an insurance plan in which physicians are reimbursed on a fee-for-service basis, the fee structure influences the services provided (the utilization). Within limits, physicians tend to perform services for which they are advantageously remunerated as opposed to those that are not. A study of the practice profile of physicians after the introduction of health insurance in Quebec shows clearly that they adapt the type and quantity of their services in an effort to maximize their income under the fee structure.[35] For example, general practitioners performed nine times more allergy skin tests in 1973 than they did in 1971; anesthetists treated 14 times more varicose veins by injection. Home visits declined drastically. However, when the fee structure was altered in 1976 to make home visits more attractive financially, they increased sharply.

Consumer-Related Factors

As noted, health services utilization is an interaction between consumers and sources or providers of care in a social and organizational environment. Many characteristics and attributes of consumers (clients or patients) are related to utilization. The illness level or need for health care obviously is one. Others include such indicators of need as mobility status, perceived symptoms of illness, chronic activity limitation status, disability days, and diagnosis.

Perception of illness or of its probability of occurrence is almost always a necessary (although not sufficient) factor in the use of health services. More specifically, it is a factor in the decision to seek care. As the next section (on providers factors) shows, once care is sought, consumer factors become much less important in the subsequent utilization of services.

Other consumer-related factors can be divided into two categories: sociodemographic and sociopsychological. In the terminology of Andersen and Newman,[36] all of these are predisposing factors. Those authors also include in the individual determinants of utilization what they call enabling factors. These include family-related variables such as income, health insurance, type of and access to regular source of care, as well as community-related factors such as availability of care, price of health services, region of the country, and urban-rural character.

The opinion here is that these enabling factors pertain to the social and organizational environment of the medical care process, and were discussed as such.

Sociodemographic factors

The same demographic and social variables described in Chapter 5 as related to mortality and morbidity also are related to utilization of services. These variables include age, sex, race, ethnicity, marital status, and socioeconomic status (education, occupation, income). It often is difficult to know whether these sociodemographic variables really influence utilization; that is, whether they bring about differences in inclination toward use of health services or merely reflect differences in illness levels (mortality and morbidity patterns). Both of these aspects of the relationship between sociodemographic characteristics and use of services are important.

A descriptive epidemiological investigation for administrative, planning, or health policy purposes should describe the utilization of services specifically for each of the sociodemographic attributes (as was described in the mortality and morbidity patterns in Chapter 5). Analytical epidemiology is concerned with sociodemographic factors as determinants of health services use. For a given illness level, would certain age, sex, race, marital status, or socioeconomic groups tend to use more health services, assuming equal geographical and economic accessibility? Unfortunately, little research has been done on this topic.

The relationship between age and volume of physician visits is best described by a U-shaped curve.[37] Infants and older individuals consume more services than other age groups, a major factor for health services managers to consider when expanding or developing new services. This, too, seems simply to reflect the mortality and morbidity patterns described in Chapter 5. Hospital admission rates are lower for children and highest in the reproductive years, then decline until age 65, and peak again. Middle-aged adults have higher surgery rates. The length of hospital stay increases steadily with age, as does the consumption of prescribed and nonprescribed drugs.

The U curve for utilization of physician services is reversed for dental care, the youngest and oldest groups of clients being least likely to see a dentist. These data do not seem to indicate a direct (specific) influence of age on utilization. However, contradictory results have been reported. A 1981 Canadian survey states that the proportion of women having an annual pap smear test decreases markedly after age 45. So does the proportion of women conducting breast self-examinations, even though the risk of breast cancer continues to increase with age.[38]

Women utilize more health services than men, beginning with the child-bearing years (15 to 44) and continuing through old age.[39] Much of the difference involves obstetrical care. However, females also have more surgery, more dental care, more preventive physical examinations, and use more drugs and medications. Men outnumber women in mental hospitals. Since the need for dental care and preventive services is higher for females, their higher utilization seems to indicate that they do tend to seek more health services (or at least some types of services) than do men, regardless of morbidity patterns. Although various social scientists have long maintained this position, a 1982 study finds no support for it.[40] Once again, further studies seem indicated.

Income differences aside, whites consume more health services of all kinds than nonwhites, although the latter do have overall higher mortality and morbidity rates. This and the fact that nonwhites have longer average lengths of stay in hospitals[41] may indicate a racial/ethnic difference in the level of severity of symptoms and illnesses at which care is sought.

The literature does not report any specific effect of marital status on utilization; indeed, usage seems to reflect the expectable age and sex composition and morbidity status of the various marital status categories.[42]

It is not easy to examine the relationship of socioeconomic status to utilization since it is confounded by at least two important variables—health status and social accessibility (more precisely, affordability). Furthermore, the literature reports many contradictory results. Most studies say that the high socioeconomic groups traditionally have used more physician services.[43, 44] On the other hand, a 1973 study finds that "in the past, the lower income groups generally had lower hospital admission rates than the high income" ones[45] while a 1981 study by one of the same authors convincingly shows that "the poor have generally had higher rates of hospital admissions than the nonpoor over the past 25 years."[46]

In any case, all agree that the gap between the poor and the nonpoor has been narrowing since the introduction of Medicare and Medicaid. Data published in

Health U.S. 1980 show higher hospital admission rates and more physician visits per year among the poor than the nonpoor. A 1981 study relates this higher utilization to the fact that the poor tend to have more serious, especially chronic, illnesses compared to the nonpoor.[47] An analysis of the 1976-1978 National Health Interview Surveys shows that the poor have more physician visits than those with higher income but that after adjustment for age and health status, these differences are reversed.[48]

The variation in the results of all these studies may stem from two factors.

First, many studies have failed to distingish between different types of services. Different groups may utilize similar sources of care for entirely different reasons or, given the same need, may turn to different services.[49] For example, the 1981 Canada Health Survey[50] and a 1978 study in France[51] show that although those with higher levels of income consult health professionals somewhat more than those with lower incomes, these consultations frequently take place when no associated health problem is reported (for example, for preventive services).

In the United States, a 1980 study of children's utilization of medical care in a community with "generous Medicaid benefits and a university-sponsored pediatric project" shows that children in higher income families are taken to private practitioners more frequently but that youngsters below the poverty line go to health centers and clinics more often.[52]

The second factor in the wide variation in results is that, as McKinlay points out,[53] most researchers fail to consider that socioeconomic status may be associated only indirectly with utilization of health services. The relationship between that status and utilization may be ameliorated not only by the variables' affordability and health condition but also by participation in certain social institutions or social networks that dictate or suggest "acceptable" patterns of use. The studies mentioned earlier in regard to cultural factors in utilization patterns indirectly support such a hypothesis of "reference group" influence.

Sociopsychological Factors

Another set of consumer-related factors may be termed "sociopsychological." Researchers have long been aware that persons perceive illness symptoms differently. It is logical to propose that different persons therefore will behave differently in seeking care according to their perceptions. Some individuals may act on a set of symptoms while others may choose to totally disregard them or fail to act on them.[54] In addition to illness perception, attitudes or beliefs about medical care, physicians, and disease influence utilization.

Although it is easy to see, conceptually, how sociopsychological factors could have an impact on use of health services, past studies of these variables have shown little accuracy in predicting utilization. It should be pointed out, however, that these findings are far from conclusive.[55]

Researchers have failed to distinguish between different types of services. Psychosocial factors related to the use of care might be expected to have a different impact on the use of different services.

Researchers generally have looked at the relation between sociopsychological factors and total utilization of services. It would be much more appropriate to look at the initial visit per illness episode since the patient has much less control over the subsequent utilization of services.[56] In other words, perceptions, attitudes, and beliefs may have a high impact on the first decision to seek care but the relationship between sociopsychological factors and utilization may be obscured when looking at total use.

Finally, psychosocial factors are only some of the numerous factors related to utilization of services. Most studies have failed to control for the impact of these other variables. The relationship between sociopsychological variables and utilization thus may often have been masked by the impact of other variables.[57]

Provider-Related Factors

A last category of determinants of health services utilization consists of factors related to health care providers, mainly physicians. These factors can be divided into two groups: economic and provider characteristics.

Economic Factors

There has been a growing belief among health economists that the traditional interaction between supply and demand does not hold true in the medical marketplace. On the contrary, the alternative "demand-shift" or inducement hypothesis states that medical practitioners have the ability to generate demand for their services or (in economic terms) that they can shift the position of the consumers' demand curve.[58]

One of the first studies to suggest such an hypothesis was in 1972 by Fuchs and Kramer, who report that supply factors, technology, and number of physicians appear to be of decisive importance in determining the utilization of and expenditures for doctors' services.[59] Several studies have since reported similar findings[60, 61] although numerous criticisms also have been made:[62]

- Consumers of care are not really aware of their health services needs or, put another way, the professional and consumer definitions of need often differ. Furthermore, in many cases such as emergencies and mental illness, persons other than the consumer make decisions regarding the care to be received.
- Consumers often are not able to evaluate which providers may offer "better" care or which substitutes may be warranted.

- The occurrence of disease at a given point is a random, involuntary phenomenon, often of an urgent nature. Because of this and of the fact that the benefits that may be received from utilization of services are unknown before treatment actually occurs, consumers are unable to make "rational" decisions to utilize services.
- Consumers do not know which services to request. They simply demand to be treated and leave it up to the physicians to decide which services are appropriate. Consequently, the physicians are in the paradoxical position of being producers of services who must decide for the client what ones must be consumed.[63]
- Most treatments require full patient compliance over the episode of care.

As mentioned in the previous section, some of the contradictory results in the analysis of demand and utilization of medical care may come from the failure to distinguish between the first and subsequent visits. The utilization process could be viewed, for simplification purposes, as consisting of a patient-initiated stage (the initial visit) and a physician-generated stage (the subsequent visits). Some authors have suggested restricting the use of the term "demand" to the patient-initiated stage, with "utilization" referring to the physician-generated stage.[64] Such a distinction certainly would facilitate the investigation of the respective influence of provider-related factors and others on the use of health services.

Provider Characteristics

Provider characteristics also have been related to utilization of services. Physicians' behavior in generating utilization of services has been related to their degree of specialization, to the medical school from which they graduated, to the hospital of residency, and to the number of years that have elapsed since completion of residency training.

For example, it has been shown that physicians trained in medical schools and hospitals with a scientific-medical orientation generally use fewer clinical and technical resources; however, under conditions of uncertainty (when diagnosis is unknown), they tend to use more services.[65]

The setting in which physicians actually work also has an influence on their professional activity.[66] Furthermore, norms and rules develop and influence physicians' behavior. Finally, other factors such as number and types of auxiliary health personnel and other workers, equipment, and use of technological innovations are related to physicians' behavior.

TRENDS IN HEALTH SERVICES UTILIZATION

It is imperative to understand the trends in health services utilization if appropriate use is to be made of the ensuing epidemiological methods. This section describes trends in utilization at the turn of the 80s, first health resources in terms of personnel and facilities, then health care expenditures, and ambulatory and inpatient care.

Health Care Resources

In the United States, there were 19.7 professionally active physicians per 10,000 population in 1980. Their proportion has increased rapidly in recent years, since there were 14.0 per 10,000 population in 1950 and in 1960, with an increase only to 15.6 in 1970. It is projected that there will be 24.3 physicians per 10,000 population in 1990 and 27.1 in 2000.[67]

Table 8-1 shows the proportion of physicians in selected countries and continents. While the United States has many more physicians per population than most countries, including Canada and most European nations, it has fewer than the United Arab Emirates, the U.S.S.R., Israel, and Austria.

Within the United States, New York and New England have the highest rates (22.9 and 20.8), South Dakota and Mississippi the lowest (9.4 and 9.6), both in 1978. In 1979, 14.7 percent of American physicians were general practitioners, 85.3 percent were specialists. By comparison, in Canada, 50.7 percent were general practitioners, 49.3 percent were specialists.

There are far fewer registered nurses per population in the United States than Canada (respectively 45/10,000 and 85.5/10,000 in 1978); the ratios for licensed nursing assistants were 25.8/10,000 (U.S.) and 32.6/10,000 (Canada).

Table 8-1 Physicians per 10,000 Population, World and Selected Continents and Countries

Country	Phys./10,000	Country	Phys./10,000
World	8.08	Europe	18.12
Africa	1.84	France	16.32
Western, Eastern,		Austria	23.34
and Middle	0.60	Italy	20.62
Southern, Northern	4.65	Sweden	17.75
South America	6.26	Australia	15.37
Asia	3.48	Polynesia	4.99
Japan	11.83	U.S.S.R.	34.64
Canada	15.30	U.S.A.	20.20
Israel	28.60	United Arab	
		Emirates	41.21

Source: Adapted from *World Health Statistics Annual, Health Personnel and Hospital Establishments,* World Health Organization, Geneva, © 1980. Data for most areas are for 1977; for Canada and the United States, 1979.

It is difficult to compare the number of hospital beds in different countries since they are reported on the basis of dissimilar types of facilities. Of ten industrialized countries, nine (the U.S.A., Canada, Australia, Denmark, England, Wales, Finland, France, Scotland, and Sweden) had five or six short-term hospital beds per 1,000 population while the Federal Republic of Germany had eight.[68]

Health Services Utilization

In the United States, 75 percent of the population visited a physician in 1979, the same percentage as in 1974; in Canada, the proportion was 76.3 percent. Table 8-2 shows the utilization of physicians by age groups, sex, race, and family income. The variations obviously are not wide, although females see physicians more often than males (78.9 percent and 70.8 percent), as do persons over 65 years (79.8 percent).

Table 8-2 Percent of Population Having Consulted a Physician at Least Once, U.S., 1979

Age	%
Under 17	75.6
17-44	74.2
45-64	73.6
65 and over	79.8
Sex	
Male	70.8
Female	78.9
Race	
White	75.3
Black	74.7
Family Income	
Less than $ 7,000	75.7
$ 7,000 - $ 9,999	73.5
$10,000 - $14,999	74.4
$15,000 - $24,999	76.2
$25,000 or more	76.9
Total Population	75.1

Source: Reprinted from *Health, United States, 1981*, U.S. Department of Health and Human Services, Public Health Service, National Center for Health Statistics, 1981, 158.

When people who are high utilizers are the subjects, there is considerably more variation between demographic groups. For example, data from the 1981 Canada Health Survey (Table 8-3) show that the proportion of the population with ten or more consultations with a physician during 1979 varies from a low of 3.4 percent of the males 20-24 to a high of 22.4 percent of the females 65 and over.

Table 8-4 shows the utilization of short-term hospitals in the ten industrialized countries previously mentioned. Even though all countries have approximately the same number of beds per inhabitants, there is a wide variation in the number of discharges per 1,000 population and in the average length of stay. Except for Australia, the United States has the highest hospitalization rate but the lowest average length of stay. This could be an indication of the relative lack of severity of the cases for which hospitalization is considered to be required.

Table 8-5 presents the hospitalization (discharge) rate per 1,000 population in the United States (excluding deliveries) in 1974 and 1979 and the average length of stay in 1979, by population subgroups. Discharge rates show a decrease between 1974 and 1979 except for the elderly, blacks, and the very low and the higher income groups. The average length of stay is longer for blacks and for males and increases with age and decreases with income.

Health Care Expenditures

Between 1965 and 1980, health care expenditures in the United States rose an average of 12.8 percent per year. Of the main items in the Consumer Price Index, only energy costs grew more rapidly. Health care expenditures accounted for 9.4 percent of the gross national product in 1980, up from 8.6 percent in 1975, 7.5 percent in 1970, 5.3 percent in 1960, and 3.5 percent in 1929.[69]

Table 8-3 Percent of Population Having Consulted a Physician 10 Times or More, Canada, 1979

Age Group	Sex	%	Age Group	Sex	%
Less than 5	Male	6.9	20 - 24	Male	3.4
	Female	8.0		Female	11.3
5 - 9	Male	5.4	25 - 44	Male	4.2
	Female	3.6		Female	14.3
10 - 14	Male	4.0	45 - 64	Male	10.4
	Female	3.6		Female	15.1
15 - 19	Male	4.3	65 and over	Male	17.7
	Female	7.0		Female	22.4

Source: Reprinted from *The Health of Canadians—Report of the Canada Health Survey* by Health and Welfare Canada and Statistics Canada with permission of the Ministry of Supply and Services, © 1981, 169.

Table 8-4 Short-Term Hospital Utilization

Selected Industrialized Countries, Selected Years 1973-1977

Country and Year	Discharges per 1,000	Average Length of Stay (Days)
United States (1976)	168	7.7
Australia (1976-77)	182	7.6
Canada (1975)	163	8.3
Denmark (1977)	159	10.2
England and Wales (1975)	97	10.1
Federal Republic of Germany (1976)	141	16.4
Finland (1976)	154	9.5
Scotland (1976-78)	123	9.9
Sweden (1973-76)	145	10.6
France (1976)	119	13.2

Source: Reprinted from *Health, United States, 1980,* U.S. Department of Health and Human Services, Public Health Service, National Center for Health Statistics, 1981, 58.

This phenomenon of rising health expenditures has been occurring in virtually all of the Western world. A comparison of health care expenditures among nine industrialized countries for the period 1960-1976 shows that only the United States, Canada, and Sweden experienced average annual increases of less than 15 percent. In the six other countries (Australia, Finland, France, Germany, the Netherlands, and the United Kingdom), average annual increases range from 17 percent to 21 percent.[70] In 1975, the United States ranked fourth among these nine countries in the percentage of GNP devoted to health care; the Federal Republic of Germany spent 9.7 percent of its GNP, the United States 8.4 percent, Canada 7.1 percent, and the United Kingdom only 5.6 percent.

In 1980 in the United States, hospital care accounted for 40.3 percent of health expenditures, up from 30.4 percent in 1950, while physician services absorbed 18.9 percent, down from 21.7 percent in 1950.[71] However, in the 1975-1980 period, hospital and physician expenditures increased at approximately the same rate (13.8 percent and 13.4 percent respectively).

The three main components of the increase in health care expenditures are prices, population, and changes in use and/or services. It has been calculated that for the period 1965-1980, price increases accounted for 58 percent of the growth in health care expenditures, population growth for 9 percent, and increased consumption of health care 33 percent.[72] From 1979 to 1980, 75 percent of the increase in personal health expenditures could be attributed to prices, 8 percent to population growth, and 17 percent to intensity of utilization.

In 1980, two-thirds (67.6 percent) of health care payments in the United States were made through third parties (government, health insurance, industry, and

Table 8-5 Utilization of Short-Term Hospitals, U.S., 1974 and 1979

By Age, Sex, Race, and Family Income

	Discharges[1] per 1,000		Average Length of Stay, 1979 (Days)
	1974	1979	
Age			
Under 17	68.7	64.4	5.5
17-44	115.9	108.9	6.9
45-64	174.0	166.3	9.4
65 and over	254.1	269.9	10.8
Sex			
Male	123.3	117.2	8.9
Female	128.6	126.1	7.6
Race			
White	126.0	120.9	7.9
Black	127.8	137.3	10.4
Family income			
Less than $ 7,000	160.9	163.0	9.1
$ 7,000 - $ 9,999	141.8	139.2	9.2
$10,000 - $14,999	137.3	127.4	8.6
$15,000 - $24,999	118.7	110.1	7.3
$25,000 or more	102.7	107.2	7.6
Average	125.7	121.6	8.2

1. Excluding deliveries.

Source: Reprinted from *Health, United States, 1981,* U.S. Department of Health and Human Services, Public Health Service, National Center for Health Statistics, 1982, 168.

philanthropy).[73] Individuals paid directly for a third (32.4 percent) of health care expenditures. These proportions are exactly the reverse of what they were in 1950.

Table 8-6 shows that 11 percent of the nation's overall population had no coverage at all in 1976. This percentage decreases with age, with education, and with income. A lower proportion of whites has no coverage and there is a wide variation among the different areas of the country, with 14.6 percent of the Southern population having no coverage as compared to 7.6 percent in the Northeast. In addition, 16.4 percent of the population who did not consult a physician and 11.4 percent who were not hospitalized in 1975 had no coverage as

Table 8-6 Percent of Population with No Health Care Coverage, U.S., 1976

By Selected Characteristics

	% With No Coverage		% With No Coverage
All persons	11.0	**Family income**	
		Less than $3,000	21.8
Age		$3,000-$4,999	21.3
Under 6	13.0	$5,000-$6,999	21.0
6-18	11.6	$7,000-$9,999	15.1
19-54	12.6	$10,000-$14,999	7.7
55-64	9.7	$15,000 or more	4.1
over 65	2.0		
		Education	
Sex		0-11 years	14.3
Male	11.6	12 years	9.9
Female	10.5	13 years or more	7.1
Race		**Geographic region**	
White	10.2	Northeast	7.6
Black and other	16.3	North Central	7.9
		South	14.6
		West	13.7

Source: Reprinted from "Health Care Coverage: United States 1976," in U.S. Department of Health, Education and Welfare, Public Health Service, *Advance Data,* no. 44, September 29, 1979, 5.

compared to 9.2 percent who did visit a physician and 7.7 percent who were hospitalized.

It becomes obvious that these trends demonstrate major problems in the utilization of health services. If health care managers are to be able to have an impact on these trends, they must begin an epidemiological analysis of their data. This approach relates the epidemiology of a population group to its utilization of health services. Management has long ignored this most important association.

EPIDEMIOLOGICAL ANALYSIS OF UTILIZATION

As described in Chapter 3, analysis of utilization is part of the identification of needs and problems. As illustrated in Figure 3-5 (supra), analysis of health services utilization combines with the epidemiological analysis of health problems to help managers in determining needs. For management purposes, these health needs can be conceived of as market gaps and opportunities. This analogy between the combined epidemiological analyses of problems and utilization and the marketing process is developed in Chapter 10.

The Epidemiological Approach

Most organizations involved in health care delivery routinely compile and use utilization data, mostly for reporting purposes. An epidemiological approach to health services management, however, requires more than this simple accounting of the services provided. Figures such as number of admissions, length of stay, average occupancy rates, and so forth are poor indicators of the actual rate of health services utilization.[74]

An epidemiological analysis of such utilization is, by nature, population based. In other words, utilization data need to be related to the population at risk of using health services so that rates of use may be calculated. The denominator for rates— that is, the population at risk—often is unknown since the care provider rarely serves a defined population.[75]

This population at risk of using services was referred to earlier as the "surrounding community" or the "population of interest." It also has been called the "constituency"[76] or the "health services area." Several methods for the determination of health services areas are described in detail elsewhere.[77, 78, 79]

Organizational Services

The aim of an epidemiological analysis of health services utilization is to determine which of the problems previously identified in the area are not already being met and should be addressed by the organization.

The organization's existing services should be analyzed first. This should be done by specific service and program and should include a sociodemographic description of the users. It also should provide information on case mix—what types of morbidity (diagnosis) result in patients' seeking care. Analysis of patient origin (a detailed breakdown of where patients are coming from) should be included. Such an analysis of patient origin provides data on what has been called "organizational commitment," that is, the proportional distribution of all clients coming from given areas.[80]

Constituent Service Use

The second step is the analysis of the services used by the constituents (population of interest). This should include all the elements just described (sociodemographic characteristics, case mix, and patient origin). It will produce information on who uses health services, for what problems (diagnosis), and where. This will indicate the organization's market share for different services.

The proportion of a given area's admissions that go to one hospital as opposed to others has been called the "organizational relevance."[81] (The terms commitment and relevance in this context have been attributed to Robert Sigmand. Table 8-7 illustrates the relevance and commitment of an organization (Hospital A) whose constituency is composed of five census tracts. The commitment means that, for example, 30 percent of the inpatients of Hospital A came from census tract 02, and 25 percent came from census tract 04. These two areas are the major sources of inpatients for Hospital A. The relevance is an indicator of market penetration: what proportion of admissions from a given area is to Hospital A. In this example, it is census tract 05 that is the most relevant to Hospital A; although admissions from this area make up only 10 percent of its admissions, this still represents 90 percent of the total from the area. Overall, Hospital A receives 33 percent of the admissions from its constituency.

In performing this second step in the epidemiological analysis of health services utilization, data from all the providers used by people in the areas of interest (constituency) must be compiled. In many situations these may be almost impossible to gather unless a special survey can be done, except when the whole constituency is covered under a comprehensive health insurance plan such as in Canada or in prepaid settings.

When community-wide utilization data are not available, Medicare (Part B) data can be of value in describing utilization as well as listing variations in morbidity (diagnostic case mix).[82] Medicare data are available for virtually the total population over 65 so that utilization of health services for that subset can be described and analyzed fully. Some data such as patient origin (relevance) can be extrapolated to the whole population. Similarly, mortality and morbidity data from vital statistics are reasonable alternatives for estimating overall patient origin.[83, 84]

Table 8-7 Hospital A's Commitment and Relevance

Census Tracts	Total Admissions	Hospital A			Other Hospitals
		Admissions	Commitment: % of A's admissions	Relevance: % of admissions to A	Relevance: % admissions to others
01	5,000	2,000	20%	40%	60
02	5,000	3,000	30%	60%	40%
03	6,666	1,000	10%	15%	85%
04	12,500	2,500	25%	20%	80%
05	1,111	1,000	10%	90%	10%
Others	-----	500	5%	---	---
Total	30,277	10,000	100%	33%	---

Source: Adapted from *Determining Health Needs* by Robin E. MacStravic with permission of Health Administration Press, © 1978, 185-186.

The Epidemiological Process

Figure 8-2 illustrates the process of epidemiological (population-based) analysis of utilization. The purpose is to identify gaps in use of health services. This is done by comparing the institution's current utilization and constituents' overall use of health services with the previously identified needs and problems. As Figure 8-2 indicates, current utilization of services is a subset of overall constituency use, which in turn is a subset of the total (ideal, potential) that could result.

The sociodemographic characteristics of the users of the target organization can be compared to those of all the individuals from the constituency who used services (at this institution or elsewhere) and to the characteristics of all the constituents (users and nonusers). This will indicate which constituents the organization serves, which ones use health services, and which are not served by the institution and/or other facilities.

The health problems that resulted in utilization of the institution's services can be compared with those for which constituents sought care and with those identified previously—that is, all the health problems that potentially and ideally could result in consumption of services.

Figure 8-2 Epidemiological Analysis of Health Services Utilization

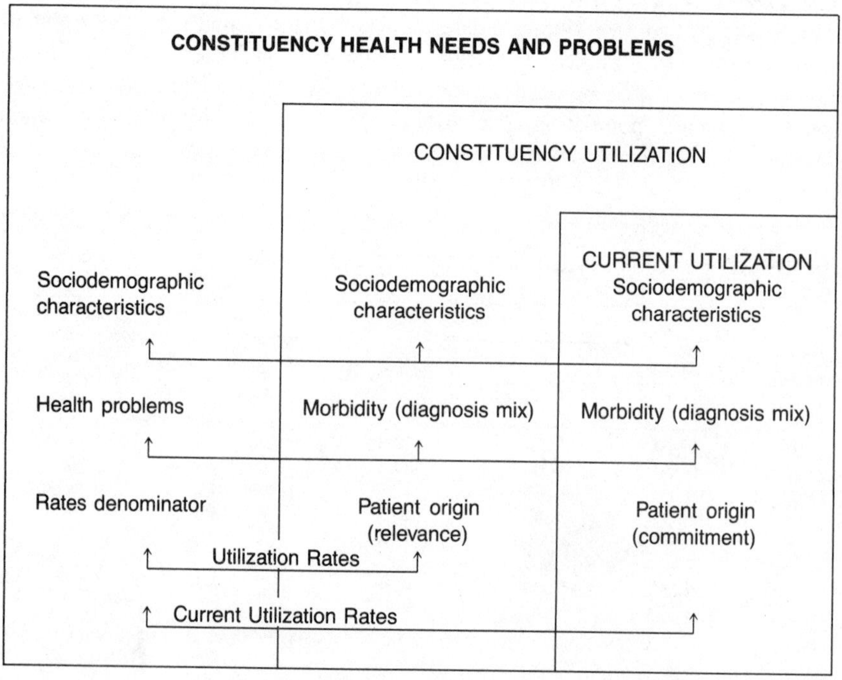

Current constituency rates also can be calculated. These rates should be made as specific as possible (age, race, sex, etc.) and should be calculated for specific services, programs, and diagnosis (i.e., morbidity and mortality). These rates can be adjusted (standardized) for comparison purposes. They then can be used to compare utilization from different areas of the constituency as well as from other areas, e.g., the county, the state, or the nation.

The Epidemiological Analysis: An Example

Through this epidemiological analysis of utilization, health services managers can identify underserved constituents as well as underserved problems. Table 8-8 presents a simplified epidemiological analysis of utilization for a hypothetical Hospital A. Hospital A's constituency is composed of five census tracts. Its commitment and relevance were described in Table 8-7. This example is limited to the distribution of three sociodemographic attributes (age, race, and sex) of the constituency population, of the constituents-users of services, and of the clients of Hospital A. It also presents a general analysis of health problems.

To simplify comparisons, a representation index (RI), adapted from Gerbner and Signorielli,[85] is used. This is defined as the ratio of the percentage of a population in a given sociodemographic group to the corresponding percentage in another population, multiplied by 100. When a group is overrepresented in a population, the index will be greater than 100, and vice versa. Thus, representation in the constituency user groups and in the current user groups can be measured, as well as constituency users among current users.

In Table 8-8, there are more than four times more males over 65 among the constituent users of services than among the overall constituency (representation index = 432.5) and even more among the hospital's patients (RI = 445.0). On the other hand, females under 20 are underrepresented (RI = 32.5). These relationships between age-sex and use of services are consistent with both morbidity patterns (Chapter 5) and determinants of utilization.

This is not true, however, for the race distribution of the users of services in this constituency. Whites are overrepresented both among constituency users and current users, blacks and others are underrepresented. Since this cannot be explained by morbidity patterns, it can be concluded that blacks and others definitely are underserved as compared to whites.

The last column in Table 8-8 compares the patients of Hospital A with the constituency users. This is similar to a measure of that facility's market share. That hospital thus serves proportionally fewer of the under-20 users and considerably fewer females ages 20 to 44. This indicates that a potential for expansion lies in obstetrical and pediatric services. Since Hospital A serves even fewer blacks and others than the other hospitals, they, too, offer a potentially larger market.

Similarly, the health problems of the constituency can be compared with the morbidity that resulted in use of services by constituents and by Hospital A's

Table 8-8 Age, Sex, and Race Distribution and Representation Indexes*

Age	Sex	Constituency %	Constituency Users %	Representation Index	Current Users %	Representation Index Constituency	Users
Under 20	Male	16.1	7.0	43.5	5.4	33.5	77.1
	Female	15.7	6.5	41.4	5.1	32.5	78.5
20-44	Male	19.0	4.3	22.6	4.9	25.8	114.0
	Female	18.3	15.1	82.5	9.2	50.3	60.9
45-64	Male	9.6	12.7	132.3	15.6	162.5	122.8
	Female	10.1	17.0	168.3	19.4	192.1	114.1
Over 65	Male	4.0	17.3	432.5	18.2	455.0	105.2
	Female	7.2	20.1	279.2	22.2	308.3	110.4
Race	White	72.3	80.2	110.9	88.4	116.2	110.2
	Black	24.2	17.1	70.7	10.3	42.6	60.2
	Other	3.5	2.7	77.1	1.3	37.1	48.1

*A representation index is the ratio of the percentage of population in a particular sociodemographic population to the similar percentage in any other population, multiplied by 100. When a group is overrepresented in a population, the index exceeds 100, and vice versa.

patients. However this can be done in only a relatively "soft" manner since utilization statistics relate to encounters, not to incidence of disease (for which many encounters may be necessary).[86]

The comparison of constituency and current utilization can be done in a more straightforward manner. The diagnosis distribution of constituency users and current users can be compared using representation indexes. For example, if 10 percent of the use of hospital services by constituents is attributed to deliveries while only 7 percent of Hospital A's patients were hospitalized for deliveries, the representation index would be 70, meaning that there are 30 percent fewer deliveries in Hospital A. Using fairly broad diagnostic groupings, Hospital A's market shares for different diagnosis (and services) also could be analyzed.

A final component of the epidemiological analysis of health services utilization involves Hospital A's commitment and relevance, using patient origin data. Table 8-7 (supra) indicates, for example, that the hospital is not doing well at serving patients from census tracts 03 and 05. It should investigate possible social and geographical accessibility barriers in these tracts.

Obviously, this type of epidemiological analysis in health services management is not limited to urban analysis; it can be accomplished just as easily in a rural setting.

SUMMARY

This chapter first examined the determinants of health services utilization. The translation of the occurrence of disease into use of health services was shown to be mediated by many sociocultural, organizational, consumer-related, and provider-related factors. Current trends in health services utilization were discussed, followed by description of an epidemiologic model for the analysis of health services utilization.

Health services managers should adopt an epidemiological population-based perspective of utilization, relating it to their constituency and to their health problems. Analysis of utilization is part of the identification of the needs of the population.

NOTES

1. L.C. Freeburg et al., *Health Status, Medical Care Utilization, and Outcome: An Annotated Bibliography of Empirical Studies*, 4 vols. (Washington, D.C.: National Center for Health Services Research, Publication No. PHS80-3263, November 1979).

2. A. Donabedian, *Aspects of Medical Care Administration: Specifying Requirements for Health Care* (Cambridge, Mass.: Harvard University Press, 1973), 61.

3. R. Andersen and J.F. Newman, "Societal and Individual Determinants of Medical Care Utilization in the United States," *Milbank Memorial Fund Quarterly* 51 (1973): 95-124.

4. J.B. McKinlay, "Some Approaches and Problems in the Study of the Use of Services—An Overview," *Journal of Health and Social Behavior* 13 (1972): 115-152.

5. Donabedian, *Aspects*, 60.

6. Andersen and Newman, "Societal Determinants," 99.

7. Lewis Thomas, *The Lives of a Cell* (New York: Bantam Books, Inc., 1975), 39.

8. Andersen and Newman, "Societal Determinants," 104.

9. Ibid., 104.

10. U.S. Bureau of the Census, *Statistical Abstract of the United States 1971*, 92nd ed. (Washington, D.C.: U.S. Government Printing Office, 1970), 34.

11. National Center for Health Statistics, *Infant Loss in the Netherlands*, NCHS publications series 3, no. 11 (1973): 2.

12. McKinlay, "Some Approaches," 128-132.

13. I.K. Zola, "Culture and Symptoms: An Analysis of Patients Presenting Complaints," *American Sociological Review* 31 (October 1966): 615-630.

14. E.A. Suchman, "Sociomedical Variations Among Ethnic Groups," *American Journal of Sociology* 70 (November 1964): 319-331.

15. E.A. Suchman, "Health Orientation and Medical Care," *American Journal of Public Health* 56 (January 1966): 97-105.

16. E. Friedson, *Patients' Views of Medical Practice* (New York: Russell Sage Foundation, 1961).

17. McKinlay, "Some Approaches," 131.

18. Donabedian, *Aspects*, 60.

19. R. Penchansky and J.W. Thomas, "The Concept of Access: Definition and Relationship to Consumer Satisfaction," *Medical Care* 19, no. 2 (February 1981): 127-140.

20. Ibid., 127.

21. Donabedian, *Aspects*, 419.

22. Penchansky and Thomas, "Concept of Access," 128.

23. G.E. Alan Dever, *Community Health Analysis* (Rockville, Md.: Aspen Systems Corporation, 1980), 251-261.

24. G.W. Shannon and G.E. Alan Dever, *Health Care Delivery: Spatial Perspectives* (New York: McGraw-Hill Book Company, 1974), 141.

25. Donabedian, *Aspects*, 425-463.

26. E.M. Bosanac et al., "Geographic Access to Hospital Care: A 30-Minute Travel Time Standard," *Medical Care* 14, no. 7 (July 1976): 616-624.

27. L.A. Aday and R. Eichhom, *The Utilization of Health Services: Indices and Correlates. A Research Bibliography* (Washington, D.C.: U.S. Public Health Service, Health Services and Mental Health Administration, DHEW Publication No. (HSM) 73-3003, 1973), 27.

28. J.E. Weiss, M.R. Greenlich, and J.F. Jones, "Determinants of Medical Care Utilization: The Impact of Spatial Factors," *Inquiry* 8 (December 1971): 50-57.

29. Donabedian, *Aspects*, 425.

30. Penchansky and Thomas, "Concept of Access," 128.

31. Ibid., 129.

32. Ibid.

33. Aday and Eichhom, *Utilization*, 24.

34. P.E. Enterline, A.D. McDonald, and J.C. McDonald, *Some Effects of Quebec Health Insurance* (Washington D.C.: U.S. Public Health Service, National Center for Health Services Research, DHEW Publication No. PHS 79-3238, January 1979).

35. A.P. Contandriopoulos, "Stimulants économiques et utilisation des services médicaux," *Actualité Economique* (Avril-Juin 1980): 264-296.

36. Andersen and Newman, "Societal Determinants."

37. Aday and Eichhom, *Utilization*.

38. Health and Welfare Canada and Statistics Canada, *The Health of Canadians—Report of the Canada Health Survey* (Ottawa: Minister of Supply and Services, 1981), 167.

39. Aday and Eichhom, *Utilization*, 18-19.

40. P.D. Cleary, D. Mechanic, and J.R. Greenly, "Sex Differences in Medical Care Utilization: An Empirical Investigation," *Journal of Health and Social Behavior* 23 (June 1982): 106-119.

41. Aday and Eichhom, *Utilization*, 20.

42. Ibid.

43. Ibid., 22-23.

44. L.A. Aday and R.M. Andersen "Equity of Access to Medical Care: A Conceptual and Empirical Overview," *Medical Care* 19, no. 12 (December 1981): Supplement, 14.

45. Aday and Eichhom, *Utilization*, 23.

46. Aday and Andersen, "Equity of Access," 13.

47. Ibid., 14.

48. J.C. Kleinman, M. Gold, and D. Makuc, "Use of Ambulatory Medical Care by the Poor: Another Look at Equity," *Medical Care* 19, no. 10 (October 1981): 1011-1022.

49. McKinlay, "Some Approaches," 120.

50. Health and Welfare Canada, *Health of Canadians*, 167.

51. P. Flamme and J.C. Portonnier, "Le système de santé face aux risques graves," *Revue Française des Affaires Sociales* (October-December 1978): 352-361.

52. L.B. Wolfe, "Children's Utilization of Medical Care," *Medical Care* 18, no. 12 (December 1980): 1196-1207.

53. McKinlay, "Some Approaches," 120.

54. Ibid., 126.

55. J.B. McKinlay and D.B. Dutton, "Social-Psychological Factors Affecting Health Service Utilization," in *Health Care Consumers, Professions and Organizations*, ed. J.B. McKinlay, Milbank Reader Series #2 (New York: Milbank Memorial Fund, 1978), 118-170.

56. R.M. Battistella, "Factors Associated with Delay in the Initiation of Physicians' Care Among Late Adulthood Persons," *American Journal of Public Health* 61 (July 1968): 1348-1361.

57. R.M. Battistella, "Limitations in the Use of the Concept of Psychological Readiness to Initiate Health Care," *Medical Care* 6 (July-August 1968): 308-319.

58. J. Richardson, "The Inducement Hypothesis: That Doctors Generate Demand for Their Own Services," in *Health, Economics, and Health Economics*, ed. J. Van Der Gaag and M. Perlman (Amsterdam: North Holland Publishing Company, 1981), 189-214.

59. Victor P. Fuchs and M.J. Kramer, *Determinants of Expenditures for Physicians' Services in the United States 1948-1968*. DHEW Publication No (HSM) 73-3013 (Washington, D.C.: U.S. Government Printing Office, December 1972).

60. R.G. Evans, "Supplier-Induced Demand: Some Empirical Evidence and Implications", in *The Economics of Health and Medical Care*, ed. M. Perlman (New York: John Wiley & Sons, Inc., 1974), 162-173.

61. Richardson, "Inducement Hypothesis," 189-214.

62. J.P. Newhouse, "The Demand for Medical Care Services: A Retrospect and Prospect," in Van der Gaad and Perlman, *Health, Economics,* 85-102.

63. A.P. Contandriopoulos, *Un modèle de comportement des médecins en tant que producteurs de services*. Ph.D. diss., Université de Montréal, 1976, 295.

64. G.L. Stoddart and M.L. Bares, "Analysis of Demand and Utilization Through Episodes of Medical Service," in Van Der Gaag and Perlman, *Health Economics,* 149-170.

65. R. Pineault, "The Effect of Medical Training Factors on Physicians' Utilization Behavior," *Medical Care* 15, no. 1 (January 1977): 51-67.

66. R. Pineault, "The Effect of Prepaid Group Practice on Physicians' Utilization Behavior," *Medical Care* 14, no. 2 (February 1976): 121-137.

67. U.S. Public Health Service, *Health, United States, 1981* (Washington, D.C.: U.S. Department of Health and Human Services, National Center for Health Statistics, December 1981), 177.

68. *Health, United States, 1980*, 57.

69. *Health, United States, 1981*, 81.

70. J.G. Simanis and J.R. Coleman, "Health Care Expenditures in Nine Industrialized Countries, 1960-1976," *Social Security Bulletin* 43, no. 1 (January 1980): 3-8.

71. *Health, United States, 1981*, 203.

72. Ibid., 82, 196.

73. Ibid., 202.

74. J.E. Wennberg, "A Small Area, Epidemiological Approach to Health Care Data" (Paper presented at the 16th National Meeting of the Public Health Conference on Records and Statistics, St. Louis, 14-16 June 1976).

75. P.E. Sartwell and J.M. Last, "Epidemiology," in *Maxcy-Rosenau Public Health and Preventive Medicine*, 11th ed., ed. J.M. Last (New York: Appleton-Century-Crofts, Inc. 1980), 29.

76. Robin E. MacStravic, *Determining Health Needs* (Ann Arbor, Mich.: Health Administration Press, 1978), 186-187.

77. Ibid.

78. G.E. Alan Dever, *Community Health Analysis* (Rockville, Md.: Aspen Systems Corporation, 1980), Chapter 8.

79. G.W. Shannon and G.E. Alan Dever, *Health Care Delivery Spatial Perspectives* (New York: McGraw-Hill Book Company, 1974), 14.

80. Dever, *Community Health Analysis*, Chapter 8.

81. Ibid.

82. Wennberg, "A Small Area Approach."

83. MacStravic, *Determining*, 186-187.

84. P.K. New, "Use of Birth Data in Delineation of Medical Service Areas," *Rural Sociology* 20 (September-December 1955), 272-281.

85. George Gerbner and N. Signorielli, "The World According to Television," *American Demographics* (October 1982): 15-17.

86. Sartwell and Last, *Epidemiology*, 29.

Chapter 9

Demographics: Epidemiological Tools

THE STUDY OF POPULATIONS

Proceeding from the fundamentals of epidemiology as essential tools of health services management, this chapter examines demography. This topic often is neglected in the training of health administrators and community health specialists. For that reason, the chapter is somewhat longer.

Demography, or the study of human populations, is a scientific discipline closely related to epidemiology. It is the study of the size, composition, distribution, density, growth, and other demographic and socioeconomic characteristics of the population as well as of the causes and consequences of changes in those factors.[1]

As discussed in Chapter 3, the contributions of epidemiology to health services management start with a description of the population of interest to the institution. Demographic data almost always are prerequisites for epidemiological measurements. Analysis of utilization (current, ideal, or expected) also requires demographic information. (As Chapter 10 explains, so does marketing.) Finally, demographic trends directly influence health and disease patterns as well as need for and use of services.

Accompanying any demographic trend is a public and health policy implication. A basic understanding of demographic principles and techniques thus is required for the use of epidemiology in health services management. This chapter therefore reviews the basic tools of demography necessary in health services management and presents examples of their use by describing demographic trends in world, United States, and Canadian populations and their impact on utilization of the health care system.

TOOLS OF DEMOGRAPHIC MEASUREMENT

The principle tools of demographic measurement are the same as those of epidemiological measurement as described in Chapter 4: crude counts, rates, ratios, proportions, cohort measures, and point and period measures. Demography includes an analysis of population statics and dynamics.[2] Population statics refers to the discipline involving the size, geographical distribution, and composition of a population at a fixed point in time. Population dynamics covers population change and components of change.

Population Statics

Population statics were examined in part in Chapter 7 on descriptive epidemiology. The demographic study of the geographical distribution of the population is similar to the place description of health and disease patterns. The person characteristics used by demographers to describe the population composition are the same as those used in Chapter 5 (age, sex, race, marital status, and socioeconomic status).

This analysis therefore concentrates on population statics reflecting the most basic characteristics of population—its age-sex composition—and only briefly reviews the other components. Only a few examples of the use of these data in epidemiology and health services management are included because previous chapters have extensively demonstrated the relationship between sociodemographic attributes and health, disease patterns, and service utilization.

Age and Sex Composition

As noted earlier, both age and sex influence disease patterns and utilization of health services. Analysis of the age-sex composition of the population of interest thus is a fundamental prerequisite of health planning and management.

A population's age and sex composition at any point is dependent on the dynamics or changes that took place earlier. As the next section indicates, births, deaths, and migration all influence population dynamics and, consequently, the composition of the group at any given time.

Median Age

The median age—that is, the age at which half the population is older and half is younger—is an indicator of the age composition of a population. For example, the median age of the United States population in 1980 was 30.2 years while Syria's was 15 (in 1975) and the German Democratic Republic's 36.[3]

Age-Dependency Ratio

Another indicator is the age-dependency ratio. This is the ratio of persons in what are termed the dependent ages (under 15 and over 64) to those in the economically productive ages (15-64). It usually is expressed as the number of persons in the dependent ages for every 100 persons in the productive ages:

$$\text{Age-dependency ratio} = \frac{\text{Population under 15} + \text{Population over 64}}{\text{Population Aged 15-64}} \times 100$$

The age-dependency ratio indicates (with questionable validity) the economic burden the productive portion of a population must carry. The higher the ratio, the heavier the burden. The United States age-dependency ratio in 1976 was 54, meaning that there were 54 persons in the dependent ages for every 100 persons in the working ages. By contrast, Syria's was 114.

The age-dependency ratio can be divided into old-age dependency (the ratio of those over 64 to those 15-64) and child dependency (the ratio of those under 15 to those 15-64).[4]

Sex Ratio

The sex ratio, describing the sex composition of the group, is the ratio of males to females in a given population, also usually expressed per 100 (males per 100 females). As discussed in Chapter 5, the sex ratio at birth in any population is approximately 106 males per 100 females. Because of different mortality and migration patterns, however, this ratio subsequently varies between places and between age groups. The ratio can be particularly useful when analyzing small areas since they might have more significant variations in sex distribution.

Population Pyramids

The best way to illustrate age and sex composition graphically is the population pyramid. It shows the numbers or proportions of males and females in each age group and is a vivid picture of a population's composition. As discussed later, it also is useful in projecting future trends.

The age-sex composition tends to fall into one of three general profiles,[5] as illustrated in Figure 9-1. Expansive populations have larger numbers of people in the younger ages, with each age cohort larger than the one born before it. Constrictive populations have smaller numbers of people in the younger ages while stationary ones have roughly equal numbers in almost all age groups, tapering off gradually at the older levels.

The most important factor influencing the shape of the population pyramid is the fertility rate.[6] The larger the number of children for each parent, the broader the base of the pyramid (and the younger the median age). Mortality has a somewhat less simple influence on the age distribution. Contrary to what might be assumed, a population with lower mortality rates will have a slightly younger age distribu-

Figure 9-1 The Three General Profiles of Age Composition, 1976

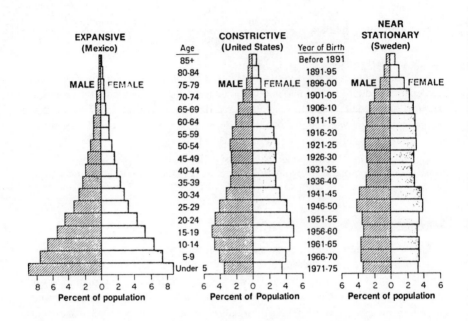

Source: Reprinted from *Population Handbook,* Int'l. Ed. by A. Haupt and T.T. Kane with permission of Population Reference Bureau Inc., 1980, 24.

tion,[7] since differences in those rates are much more likely to result from variances in younger age groups (mostly infants and children).[8]

Other Variables to Describe Composition

Other variables commonly used by demographers to describe the composition of a population include race, socioeconomic status, marital status, and other family-related variables. Race ratios similar to sex ratios can be calculated by (for example) dividing the number of whites by the number of blacks; in sex ratios, the race ratio usually is expressed as the number of whites per 100 blacks.

Income, occupation, and education data indicate socioeconomic status. These variables can be used individually or combined into a socioeconomic index.

In addition to marital status, several other related characteristics can be examined. Marital history refers to the number of times a person married, when each marriage occurred, and when and how each previous one ended. Age at first marriage can be a good demographic and social indicator. The mean (average) size[9] of household (based on the United Nations *Principles and Recommendations for the 1970 Population Census*[10]) and the mean size of family,[11] as well as the number of children of dependent ages, also are used as demographic indicators.

All of these social indicators may be used by health services managers to describe their population. As Chapters 4, 5, and 8 demonstrate, these social characteristics are closely associated with morbidity and health services utilization patterns.

Population Distribution

The last component of these statics to be considered is the distribution of the population. This refers to patterns of settlement and dispersal of population within a country or other area.[12] The main descriptive concepts are urban vs. rural, metropolitan status, population density, and population size.

There is surprisingly little agreement on the definition of urban. Various authors and publications offer different definitions based on any one or combination of the following criteria: population size, density, concentration, structure, types of occupation, sociocultural distinctions, ways of life, states of mind.

In the United States census, urban areas as defined as incorporated and unincorporated places of 2,500 or more inhabitants, including the contiguous areas around cities of 50,000 or more. In Canada, the minimum size is 1,000 inhabitants, with a population density of at least 1,000 persons per square mile. In both the United States and Canada, as in most countries, the rural population is simply the residuals—those living outside urban areas. The population in urban areas can be expressed as a percentage of the total population (percent urban). For example, in 1970, the population of the United States was 74 percent urban while Singapore was 100 percent urban and Burundi was only 2 percent.[13]

The concept of metropolitan area also is used often in the description of population distribution. In general, a metropolitan area is defined as a large concentration of population (i.e., a large urban area), usually with 100,000 or more inhabitants and at least one city of 50,000 or more. Administrative areas bordering the city that are socially and economically integrated with it are included.[14]

In some countries, the term "large urban agglomerations" is used. In Canada, these are called Census Metropolitan Areas (CMAs). In the United States, they are referred to as Standard Metropolitan Statistical Areas (SMSAs). These are defined by the Office of Management and Budget, using a large list of criteria supplied by the Bureau of the Census, including size, density, type of employment, and volume of commuting.[15]

Population density is a concept much used in the study of distribution. Its usual measure is the number of people per unit of land area (population per square mile or kilometer). This is not always satisfactory, however, since it assumes that the population is dispersed evenly over the entire area considered.[16]

In some cases where the inhabitants are concentrated in a small portion of an area, the population density will be very low, even though the people live in high-density areas. For example, Canada has a density of only 2 per square kilometer, the United States 23.2. Consequently, other measures of population density have been used: percent of population in multifamily dwellings, and population per square mile for urbanized areas only.[17]

Population size also is used in analyzing distributions. The main advantage of crude size of locality is that a classification by multiple size categories can be used instead of the dichotomous urban-rural or SMSA-non-SMSA classifications. Population distribution therefore can be examined on a continuum of urbanization.

Interaction among Variables

It is important for health services managers to analyze the demographic makeup of their population since, as discussed in earlier chapters, the variables of age, sex, race, marital status, and socioeconomic position are related to health, disease, and utilization of services. When performing such analysis, however, managers should be aware that some demographic variables may interact with each other in such a way that a composite analysis (a combination of variables) may be more appropriate and yield results different from a study of the components alone.[18] In other words, the relationship between one demographic variable and health, disease, or utilization may depend in part on another demographic variable.

For example, an analysis of utilization of health services may show no difference among age groups or incomes. However, a composite analysis by age and income may show that utilization is higher among both older age-lower income groups and younger age-higher income groups. This would indicate that utilization is related not to age and income separately but to the composite age/income variable.

Data to perform such a composite analysis are not always available (for example, when using published census data). However, when possible, it is always better to check for interaction between variables.[19]

Population Dynamics

In addition to the description of population composition (population statics), demography is concerned with population dynamics, or the changes in composition over time. Population change involves three components: births, deaths, and migration. Mortality measures were described in Chapter 4. This section reviews basic measures of mortality and migration and examines global measures of population change.

Natality

The term natality refers to the role of births in population change. Although some authors use the term fertility in this same broad sense, that most often is restricted to actual birth performance,[20] that is, to the intensity and tempo of births that actually occur in a population.[21] Fertility, therefore, refers to the production of live born young and fecundity to the physiological capacity to reproduce (to give birth to a live child). Fecundity is a prerequisite of fertility. Infertile persons may either be infecund (sterile) or may use some form of birth control.

Although this was not always the case, natality, fertility, and births have come to refer only to live births. Stillbirths, fetal deaths, and abortions are not included.

Crude Birth Rate: The most common measure of natality is the crude birth rate (CBR). It is simply the number of births in a year per 1,000 midyear population (the population as of July 1):

$$CBR = \frac{\text{Number of Births}}{\text{Total Midyear Population}} \times 1,000$$

The crude birth rate is a valid measure of the number of babies a population is producing in a given year. However, it is not very useful for temporal or spatial comparisons since it does not eliminate the impact of differential population structures.[22] In other words, it does not tell much about the reproductive experience or about the intensity or tempo of births since it does not account for the age-sex composition of the population.

General Fertility Rate: The general fertility rate (GFR) is a more refined measure than the crude birth rate because it relates the number of births to the population at risk of giving birth—that is, the female population aged 15-44.[23] The general fertility rate is defined as the number of live births per 1,000 women aged 15-44:

$$GFR = \frac{\text{Total Births}}{\text{females Aged 15-44}} \times 1,000$$

It should be noted that the total number of births, regardless of age of mother, is used in the numerator.[24] Some authors suggest using the population of women 15-49 but since those 45 to 49 contribute relatively few births to the total number, the general fertility rate usually is limited to those up to age 44. Contrary to the crude birth rate, the general fertility rate can be used for comparison purposes since it controls for the age and sex composition of the populations involved. It thus is much more indicative of differences in reproductive behavior than is the crude birth rate.

The difference between these two rates is illustrated by the situation in the United States: although the crude birth rate has been increasing in recent years, the general fertility rate has remained constant. In other words, there are more babies born but not because women are having more babies but because there now is a large number of women in reproductive years because of the baby boom after World War II.

Age-Specific Fertility: As described for mortality rates (Chapter 4), fertility rates can be made specific for any population subgroup. For example, it is possible to calculate the fertility rate for the black urban population of Georgia, and so on. Age-specific fertility rates are used for comparison over time and to detect differences in fertility behavior at different ages. An age-specific fertility rate (ASFR) is defined as the number of live births to women in an age group in one year per 1,000 women in that age group (at midyear):[25]

$$ASFR \ (15\text{-}19) = \frac{\text{Live Births to Women Aged 15-19 in the Year}}{\text{Midyear Population of Women Aged 15-19}}$$

The calculation of the age-specific rates for every five-year age group between 15 and 49 gives a complete picture of the fertility differences. The rates provide a specific indication of the population at risk, which can be valuable for planning purposes. Fertility behavior of different populations can be examined. A standardized fertility rate can be calculated involving the same methods (direct or indirect adjustment) used to standardize mortality rates (Chapter 4).

These standardized rates indicate how many births per 1,000 there would have been in the population of interest if its age and sex composition was the same as in the standard (arbitrarily chosen) population. Fertility rates also can be adjusted (standardized) for other demographic variables such as marital status, race, urban-rural residence, duration of marriage, etc.

It should be noted that some authors refer to specific and standardized fertility rates as specific and standardized birth rates.[26, 27] The use of the term fertility, however, seems more appropriate since the denominators always are limited to the female population at risk of childbearing while the denominator of the crude birth rate is the total population. Furthermore, the general fertility rate is in fact a weighted average of these age-specific rates.

Total Fertility Rate: The total fertility rate (TFR) is a hypothetical measure (a synthetic estimate) of the average number of children that would be born alive to a woman during her lifetime if she were to pass through all her childbearing years conforming to the age-specific fertility rates of a given year.[28] The TFR is one of the most important fertility measures since it indicates as nearly as possible how many children women are having.

Contrary to the general fertility rate, the total fertility rate is adjusted for the age and sex composition of the population. The TFR is in fact a summary measure of the age-specific fertility rates over all ages of the childbearing period:

$$TFR = \frac{5 \left(\sum\limits_{a=15\text{-}19}^{a=45\text{-}49} \right) fa}{1,000}$$

where: fa = is an age specific fertility rate per 1,000

Table 9-1 illustrates the calculation of a total fertility rate. A TFR of 1.78 means that if the 1979 age-specific fertility rates were to continue, Quebec women on the average would have 1.78 children during their childbearing years.

A good example of the usefulness of the TFR is the comparison of the fertility rates for the United States and Canada.[29] In 1973, the general fertility rate was 60.9 per 1,000 in the United States and 60.1 in Canada. However, age-specific fertility rates show that fertility is really higher in the United States only at ages under 25 while in Canada it is higher for all age groups over 25.

Furthermore, the total fertility rates (which control for the age and sex composition) are essentially identical (1.896 in the United States and 1.890 in Canada). Thus it can be concluded that in 1973, Americans had their children at earlier ages than Canadians but over their lifetime, women in both countries have the same number. The difference in the general fertility rate was caused by the fertility calendar, not by real differences in total fertility.

It should be noted that areas (two or more countries, districts, states, etc.) can be compared in the same manner. This information would be most important if a health services manager or administrator were thinking of building or expanding obstetrical services for the institution. The demographic trend becomes critical to the needs for and success of such ventures.

Although this now seems somewhat less relevant, demographers used to make a distinction between illegitimate and legitimate births.[30, 31, 32] An illegitimate birth was defined as one to a single, widowed, or divorced woman. The illegitimacy rate (IR) is the number of illegitimate live births per 1,000 unmarried women (single, widowed, divorced) aged 15 to 44 in a given year. The illegitimacy ratio is the number of illegitimate live births per 1,000 live births (not women) in a given year. It is a measure of the proportion of births that are illegitimate. It may now be

Table 9-1 Calculation of a Total Fertility Rate

Data for Quebec, 1979

Age Group	Age-Specific Fertility Rate per 1,000 Women
15–19	17.3
20–24	95.8
25–29	143.9
30–34	74.3
35–39	20.8
40–44	3.0
45–59	0.2

$$\Sigma\ fa\ =\ 355.3$$

$$TFR\ =\ \frac{5\ \times\ \Sigma\ fa}{1,000}$$

$$TFR\ =\ \frac{5\ \times\ 355.3}{1,000}\ \times\ 1.777$$

Where: TFR = Total fertility rate
  Σ = Summation
  fa = Age-specific fertility
  Σfa = Sum of all age-specific fertility rates

Note: In the formula, 5 is used because each group encompasses five years.

preferable simply to use fertility rates specific to marital status (as in Table 9-2) or to study teenage fertility rates separately (as in Table 9-11, infra).

The most useful fertility measures for health services managers remain the age-specific fertility rates and the total fertility rates. As illustrated in Table 9-2, these can be made specific for any population subgroups. Such specific data provide valuable information for health services management, for example in the planning of obstetrical services or family planning programs.

Migration

Migration is the third basic process that alters the size and composition of a population (with births and deaths). It refers to the geographic or spatial movement of population involving a change of usual residence between clearly defined geographic units.[33] This change of residence should not be temporary (for visiting,

Table 9-2 General Fertility Rates and Total Fertility Rates, U.S., 1980

Selected Regions

Characteristics	General Fertility Rate per 1,000 women	Total Fertility Rate per 1,000 women
Total, 18-44 years old	71.1	2.059
Age		
18-24 years old	96.6	2.023
25-29 years old	114.8	2.022
30-34 years old	60.0	2.150
Race		
White	68.5	2.036
Black	84.0	2.227
Spanish origin*	106.6	2.363
Marital Status		
Currently married**	95.0	2.187
Widowed, divorced, and separated	27.5	2.035
Single	28.4	1.807
Years of School Completed		
Not a high school graduate	91.9	2.427
High school, 4 years	71.5	2.018
College, 1 to 3 years	58.4	2.018
College, 4 years	65.9	1.857
College, 5 or more years	52.1	1.765
Labor Force Status		
In labor force	40.9	1.901
Employed	37.4	1.882
Unemployed	75.0	2.053
Not in labor force	130.1	2.370
Family Income		
Under $5,000	94.3	2.190
$5,000 to $9,999	86.8	2.071
$10,000 to $14,999	83.9	2.099
$15,000 to $19,999	77.1	2.048
$20,000 to $24,999	69.8	2.015
$25,000 and over	48.5	2.014

Table 9-2 continued

Selected Regions

Characteristics	General Fertility Rate per 1,000 women	Total Fertility Rate per 1,000 women
Region of Residence		
Northeast	62.4	2.061
North Central	70.8	2.122
South	71.7	1.984
West	80.2	2.098

*Persons of Spanish origin may be of any race.
**Except separated women.

Source: Adapted from "Who's Having those Babies?" by Cheryl Russell with permission from *American Demographics,* January 1982, vol. 4, no. 1, 37.

vacation, or business) but should be intended as permanent (for the purpose of residing).

Demographers usually distinguish between international and internal migration. The former refers to moves between countries and is designated as emigration from the nation left and as immigration to the receiving nation.[34] A country receives immigrants and loses emigrants. Internal migration refers to movements between different areas within a country. The terms in-migration and out-migration are used instead of immigration and emigration, respectively. In the United States and Canada, interstate (interprovincial) migration and intrastate (intraprovincial) migration also could be dealt with separately.

The immigration (or in-migration) rate is the number of immigrants (in-migrants) arriving at a destination per 1,000 population at that destination in a given year:[35]

$$\text{Immigration Rate} = \frac{\text{Number of Immigrants in a Year}}{\text{Total Midyear Population at Destination}} \times 1,000$$

Similarly, the emigration (out-migration) rate is the number of emigrants departing an area of origin per 1,000 population at that area of origin in a given year.

$$\text{Emigration Rate} = \frac{\text{Number of Emigrants in a Year}}{\text{Total Midyear Population at Area of Origin}} \times 1,000$$

Immigration and emigration (in-migration and out-migration) are more correctly referred to as gross immigration and gross emigration (gross in-migration and gross out-migration). The balance of the two for a given area during a given time (usually a year) is called net immigration or net emigration, depending on which is larger.[36] The net migration rate shows the net effect of immigration and emigration on an area's population, expressed as increase (+) or decrease (−) per 1,000 population of the area in a given year.[37]

$$\text{Net Migration Rate} = \frac{\text{Number of Immigrants} - \text{Number of Emigrants}}{\text{Total Midyear Population}} \times 1,000$$

For example, in 1976, the United States had a net migration rate of +1.7 per 1,000 population—a net increase of 1.7 persons per 1,000 population.

Measures of Population Change

The relationship among the three components of population change—births, deaths, and migration—and population change over time can be expressed by the balancing equation:[38]

$$P_2 = P_1 + (B - D) + (I - E)$$

Where: P_2 = Population at the later date

P_1 = Population at the earlier date

B = Births

D = Deaths between the two dates

I = Immigration or in-migration

E = Emigration or out-migration between the two dates

(I-E) thus is the net migration. The difference between the number of births and deaths is the natural increase *(NI = B-D)*. The rate of natural increase is the one at which a population is increasing (or decreasing) in a given year because of a surplus (or deficit) of births over (or under) deaths, expressed as a percentage of the base population:[39]

$$\text{Rate of Natural Increase} = \frac{\text{Births} - \text{Deaths}}{\text{Total Midyear Population}} \times 100$$

Or:

$$\text{Rate of Natural Increase} = \frac{\text{Birth Rate} - \text{Death Rate}}{10}$$

For example, the rate of natural increase in the United States in 1976 was 0.6 percent.

The growth rate is the rate at which a population is increasing (or decreasing) in a given year because of a natural increase and net migration, expressed as a percentage of the base population:

$$\text{Growth Rate} = \frac{(B-D) + (I-E)}{\text{Total Midyear Population}} \times 100$$

Or:

$$\text{Growth Rate} = \text{Rate of Natural Increase} + \text{Net Migration Rate}$$

The growth rate takes into account all components of population change (births, deaths, and migration). It should not be confused with the rate of natural increase, which considers only births and deaths, nor with the birth rate, which involves only births.

Another common way of measuring population change is to calculate the intercensus change (IC). It is simply the difference between the population indicated in a previous census (P_1) and a subsequent census (P_2) of the same area.

$$IC = P_2 - P_1$$

The intercensus change in percent (IC%) can be used to compare the growth of different populations.

$$IC\% = \frac{P_2 - P_1}{P_1} \times 100$$

These rates related to population dynamics are of importance to health services managers. The increased need for services, the marketing of new ones, expansion into a new location, and the demand for care in the institution are dependent on a changing population structure. However, concepts of preventive medicine applied to these areas require knowledge about the life styles and environment in the existing structure. It certainly will behoove health managers to use these techniques and tie them in directly with the material in earlier chapters.

POPULATION ESTIMATES

In most countries, the most reliable and complete source of information on population composition is the national census. However, since population is changing constantly, population data for many purposes can soon be considered out of date. For this reason, demographers have developed several methods and techniques for estimating intercensus and postcensus (current) populations.

This section examines how to estimate current or postcensus population. The following one deals with population projections, i.e., the computation of future changes in population. Both of these topics can be complex and beyond the scope of this book, so this analysis is limited. Demography textbooks offer a more complete discussion. (The U.S. Bureau of the Census publication, *The Methods and Materials of Demography,* offers an excellent discussion of population estimates in Chapter 23 and population projections in Chapter 24.)

Estimation of population is of special importance for an epidemiological approach to health services management. As noted throughout this book, epidemiology offers various principles and methods for relating the occurrence of health and disease, as well as the utilization of health services, to the population. Valid estimates of population thus are needed constantly for the denominators of rates.

Techniques for estimating population fall in two broad categories (Table 9-2a): demographic and statistical. Demographic techniques use data on any or all of the components of population change (births, deaths, migration). Statistical techniques, on the other hand, rely on predictors of population change, even though they may not be directly related to the three components of population change.[40]

The Component Method

Component methods estimate the three components of population change separately. The estimating formula therefore is exactly the same as what was referred to previously as the balancing equation.

$$P_2 = P_1 + (B-D) + (I-E)$$

The population is estimated by adding natural increase and net immigration for the period since the last census to the latest census count. When data are available,

---

Table 9-2a Methods for Estimating Population

Demographic Methods	Statistical Methods
Component Methods	Ratio-Correlation Methods
Housing Unit Methods	Census Censal Ratio Methods
Composite Methods	Extrapolation of Past Growth
Death Rate Method (ASDR)*	Sample Surveys

*ASDR = Age-Specific Death Rate

Source: Adapted from "Estimating Population" by M.J. Batitus with permission of *American Demographics,* © April 1982, 3.

this is without doubt the easiest way of estimating population. There usually is no problem getting data on births and deaths from vital statistics reports.

Net migration data may be much more difficult to obtain. Sometimes it may be necessary to assume that the net migration rate for the years since the last census was the same as that reported in the last census, or to extrapolate from past trends. If the net migration data are not available from the last census, they can be estimated by using figures from the two previous censuses (P_2 and P_1) and from vital statistics:

$$(I-E) = P_2 - P_1 - (B-D)$$

The Housing Unit Method

A second technique for estimating population relies on the net addition of housing. The housing unit method consists of looking first at the new additions to the housing stock and the loss of units from demolition. These data usually are available from municipal records of building permits. Next, the vacancy rate has to be determined. This usually is available from the last census or, again, from municipal building authorities. Finally, data on the average household size and on the number of households at the last census date are assembled from census data. The estimating formula is a follows:[41]

$$P_2 = [HH \text{ Census} + ((NHH-DHH) \times OR)] \times AHS$$

Where: P_2 = Population estimate

HH = Number of household units at last census date

NHH = New additions of housing units

DHH = Number of household units lost through demolition

OR = Occupancy rate (1 − vacancy rate)

AHS = Average household size

The Composite Method

Composite methods refer to a mixture of techniques to estimate population by broad age groups. For example, school enrollment can be used to estimate or measure changes in the population under age 18, income tax returns for the population 18 to 64, and Medicare enrollment for the population over 65. The total population estimate is calculated by adding the estimates for the different age groups.[42]

The Age-Specific Death Rate Method

A short-cut method for estimating population is the age-specific death rate method (ASDR).[43, 44] This simple method consists of dividing the number of deaths in the postcensus year by the corresponding age-specific death rates for the census year. The result is an estimate of population in the post-census year (P_2).

$$P_2 = \sum_{a}^{f} \left(\frac{\text{deaths}}{fa} \times 1,000 \right)$$

where: fa = age-specific death rate per 1,000

This method of course has several limitations. First, it assumes that the death rates have remained stable between the census year and the postcensus year of estimate. Furthermore, death rates in small areas tend to undergo considerable yearly fluctuations. Using an average of the death rates for a period of several years (see Chapter 4) may alleviate this problem. In any case, the populations by age group that are computed to obtain the total estimate should not be used as estimates of individual age groups. Overall, this method has been quite accurate even for relatively small areas (county level).[45] However, it should be used with great caution for very small areas (for example, less than 30,000 population).

The Statistical Methods

Several statistical methods also can be used to estimate population. The ratio-correlation methods use regression techniques to relate changes in indirect indicators (such as automobile registration and school enrollment) to population change itself. The census-ratio methods project the ratio of such indirect indicators to the total population.[46] This ratio is calculated from the last census. Another statistical technique consists of simply extrapolating past growth—for example, the growth between the last three or four censuses. Finally, sample surveys are used sometimes.

Thus, many techniques for estimating population, mainly the statistical ones, can be complex and time consuming to apply for making estimates of small areas. Health services managers should try first to obtain estimates for their population from outside sources such as federal, state, county, or municipal governments. When these are not available, the component methods and the housing unit method could be used. The age-specific death rate method can be used, with caution, to estimate county or metropolitan population.

POPULATION PROJECTIONS

While population estimates are used to determine the current number of people in a target area, population projections aim at determining what their total will be in the future. A distinction also can be made between projections and forecasts.[47] Population projections are based on certain assumptions about future trends in the rates of fertility, mortality, and migration. Demographers therefore usually make low, medium, and high projections of the same population based on different assumptions as to how these rates will change.[48] A forecast is a guess as to which of these projections is the most likely. To put it another way, all forecasts are projections but not all projections are forecasts.[49]

There are five broad categories for projecting population:

1. mathematical extrapolation methods
2. ratio methods
3. component and cohort-component methods
4. economy-based methods
5. land-use methods.

These categories are far from mutually exclusive and a mix of principles and techniques from each often is used. Once again, these are described only briefly here; several specialized textbooks can provide further details.[50, 51]

As with population estimates, past growth can simply be extended into the future. These mathematical extrapolations usually are not considered very valid, although large-scale applications of this method can become quite complex mathematically.[52] In general, however, mathematical extrapolation methods should be used only when rough approximation is required and only over a relatively short future.

Ratio Method—An Example

The ratio methods use an existing projection for a larger (parent) area and the ratio of the current population of the subareas to this parent group. The historical trend of the ratios is determined, projected into the future, and multiplied by the projection for the parent population.[53]

Table 9-2b illustrates the calculation of the ratio projection for a hypothetical County A. The projection of the future ratio is simply an extension of historical trends. As can be seen, the ratio of county population to state population has been

Table 9-2b Calculation of a Ratio Method of Population Projection for County A

County A's Historical Population Ratio with the State

	State Population	County A Population	County A as a Ratio of State
1960	696,092	27,690	.0398
1965	722,245	29,863	.0413
1970	755,103	31,643	.0419
1975	780,994	33,130	.0424
1980	817,220	34,902	.0427

Ratio Projection of County A's Population

	State Projection	County A's Ratio	County A's Projection
1985	873,089	.0430	37,542
1990	917,457	.0432	39,634
1995	956,085	.0433	41,398
2000	986,195	.0433	42,702
2005	1,008,547	.0433	43,670

Source: Adapted from *How Communities Can Use Statistics* by Statistics Canada, © June 1981, 54.

increasing but at a slowing rate. This trend has simply been extended to project that after 1995, the county will maintain its share of the state population. This ratio method is used often by government agencies and should be easy for health services managers to apply when population projections for larger (parent) areas are available.

Cohort Component Method—An Example

The component method and the cohort component method are essentially similar except that the former uses total population while the latter subdivides the population into age groups (cohorts). In both methods, the components of population change (births, deaths, migration) are projected separately. In the cohort component method (also called cohort survival method), the population is carried forward by cohort, taking into account the survival rate and the migration rate of that age-specific group. The population of each age group is projected individually.

For example, the population aged 10 to 14 in 1980 is projected forward five years to 1985 by adjusting for deaths and migration. In 1985, this cohort will be 15 to 19. The process is repeated for every age group and for each future date desired.

Table 9-3 Calculation of a Cohort Component Population Projection

Cohorts / Females	Col. 1 1971 Actual Population	Col. 2 1971-1975 Survival Rates per 1,000	Col. 3 1971-1975 Fertility Rates per 1,000	Col. 4 1971-1975 Births	Col. 5 1971-1975 (Estimated 1976 Population)	Col. 6 1976 Actual Population	Col. 7 1971-1975 Estimated Net Migration	Col. 8 1976-1980 Births	Col. 9 1981 Survivors	Col. 10 1981 Projection Estimate	Col. 11 1981-1985 Births	Col. 12 1986 Survivors	Col. 13 1986 Projection Estimate
0 - 4	1,290	982.2		1,044	1,025	1,115	+ 90	1,326	1,302	1,392	1,542	1,514	1,604
5 - 9	1,750	998.5			1,288	1,355	+ 67		1,113	1,180		1,390	1,457
10 - 14	1,870	998.5			1,747	1,730	- 17		1,353	1,336		1,178	1,161
15 - 19	1,610	997.5	204.5	329	1,865	1,750	-115	357	1,726	1,611	352	1,337	1,222
20 - 24	1,135	997.5	599.0	680	1,606	1,390	-216	833	1,746	1,530	916	1,607	1,391
25 - 29	955	997.0	661.0	631	1,132	1,480	+348	978	1,386	1,734	1,146	1,525	1,873
30 - 34	980	996.0	340.0	333	951	1,160	+209	394	1,474	1,683	572	1,727	1,936
35 - 39	1,130	994.0	125.5	142	974	1,070	+ 96	134	1,153	1,249	157	1,673	1,769
40 - 44	1,220	990.1	28.0	34	1,119	1,190	+ 71	33	1,059	1,130	32	1,237	1,308
45 - 49	1,145	984.2	1.5	2	1,201	1,155	- 46	2	1,171	1,125	2	1,112	1,066
50 - 54	850	975.9			1,117	1,125	+ 8		1,127	1,135		1,098	1,106
55 - 59	605	962.4			818	760	- 58		1,083	1,025		1,092	1,034
60 - 64	420	943.0			571	565	. 6		716	710		967	961
65 - 69	350	912.4			383	425	+ 42		516	558		648	690
70 - 74	270	862.6			302	340	+ 38		367	405		481	519
75 - 79	225	780.2			211	280	+ 69		265	334		316	385
80 - 84	140	648.1			146	190	+ 44		181	225		216	260
85 +	95	435.3			102	150	+ 48		148	196		183	231
	16,040			2,151 (x .4855)	17,063	17,230	+672	2,731 (x .4855)	17,886	18,558	3,177 (x .4855)	19,301	19,973

Table 9-3 continued

Footnotes:

Column 2: Calculated using death rates. This is done by taking the average annual death rate for the five-year period compounded at a declining rate, the result of which is multiplied by 1,000. In mathematical terms:

$$SR = 1,000 \times \frac{1}{(1 + i)^n}$$

where: SR = Survival rate
i = annual average death rate
n = number of years

In essence, this rate states the probability that a person who is in a certain age bracket will live from the beginning to the end of the particular time period. Published life tables are often used to calculate survival rates.

Column 4: Column 3 times Column 1. The entry opposite 0-4 indicates the total of all births factored by the number who will be female (48.55 percent). An alternative approach for this calculation would have been to apply the same fertility rates to the average midyear population:

$$\frac{\text{Population 1971 + Population 1976}}{2}$$

Column 5: Column 2 times Column 1 with its cohorts dropped one age bracket, that is, the survival rate for the next succeeding age bracket is applied to the number in the cohort. For example, the 955 women ages 25 to 29 in 1971 are multiplied by the survival rate for the age bracket 30-34 to obtain the 1976 estimate (migration held aside for the moment). The births calculated in Column 4 are factored by the 0-4 survival rate.

Column 7: Column 6 minus Column 5. The result is assumed to be net migration since Column 5 includes births and deaths of persons in 1971. This calculation also includes any error in census counts, fertility rate, and survival rate calculations of Columns 2 and 3. These errors are ignored, largely because they are impossible to measure. The calculation also includes births and deaths of migrants. With more work, the net migration could be recalibrated to extract these components, but [it was] decided to disregard this aspect.

Column 8: Column 3 times Column 6. The entry opposite 0-4 indicates the total of all births factored by the number who will be female (48.55 percent). Alternative calculation is possible, as noted for column 4.

Column 9: Column 2 times Column 6 as for Column 5.

Column 10: The projection estimate calculated by taking Column 9 and adding Column 7. No survival rate or fertility rate calculations are made with the migration estimates since these are assumed to be part of the residually derived estimates. If the estimates had been derived using another method, then it might have been necessary to apply separate fertility rate and survival rate calculations (usually at half the rate).

Column 11: Column 3 times Column 10. The entry opposite 0-4 indicates the total of all births factored by the number who will be female (48.55 percent). Alternative calculation is possible, as noted for Column 4.

Column 12: Column 2 times Column 10 as for Column 5.

Column 13: Column 12 plus Column 7 with same assumptions as in Column 10.

Source: Reprinted from *How Communities Can Use Statistics* by Statistics Canada, © June 1981, 57.

Table 9-3 illustrates the calculation of a cohort component projection for a hypothetical county. Only calculations for females are shown. Projections for the male population would be done the same way except that the fertility rate columns would be excluded. Total population projections would be obtained by summing the two.

The calculations in the table are based on the assumption that the fertility rates, survival rates, and net migration between 1971 and 1975 all remain unchanged in the succeeding time periods. If the person doing the projections had reason to believe that this would not be so, the rates could be altered accordingly.

The main advantage of the cohort component method is that it allows a detailed, age-specific analysis of future population trends. Births, deaths, and migration all are calculated and can be examined readily for each age group. An alternative would be simply to calculate the overall growth rate for each cohort between two censuses and apply that rate to the new cohort for the same age group, and so on. The procedure is essentially the same except that births, deaths, and net migration are not considered separately but are combined into a single measure, the growth rate.

Economy-based methods of population projection use projected economic data for the projection of migration. Births and deaths are projected using other methods, and immigration and emigration are projected in relation to the future economy of an area (creation or loss of jobs). The land-use methods are similar to the housing unit methods of population estimates. By calculating how many housing units could be built and with a knowledge of the average household size, the likely additions to the population can be estimated, given a presumed rate of building to reach the saturation point.[54]

The ratio and the cohort component methods thus are probably the easiest population projection measures that health services managers can use. It always is advisable to use more than one method and to project the population under several different assumptions of birth, death, and migration rates.

THE UNITED STATES CENSUS

Most of the data required for demographic analysis of the population comes from vital and health statistics and from the census. Census publications contain an enormous wealth of information that too often is ignored by hospitals and other health institutions.[55]

To illustrate the kind of information collected in the census, the 1980 United States census questionnaire is reproduced as Exhibit 9-1. All of this information is compiled and easily available for every area of the United States. (Equivalent data are available in Canada from Statistics Canada.) There also exist private firms that supply demographic data (from the census).[56] These "demographic supermarkets" can compile all kinds of information for any given area and can provide computer graphics and population forecasts.

Health services managers thus can use the basic tools of demography to describe, estimate, and project their population of interest. Demographic characteristics are related not only to health and disease patterns but also to utilization of services. Demographic principles and techniques also can be used, for example, to analyze physician or nurse populations.

The purpose of the preceding section is to serve as a basic reference on demography. In the rest of the chapter, many of these techniques are applied in examining population trends and their impact on the health care system.

POPULATION TRENDS

The World Population

In mid-1981, the world population was approximately 4.5 billion and growing at 1.7 percent a year. This growth rate means that, if it remains constant, the world population will double in 41 years. This is quite amazing when it is considered that it took two to five million years for the world to reach its first billion. Table 9-4 shows that it will take only until 1987 for the total population to reach five billion.

Most of the current growth is taking place in the less developed regions of the world. Table 9-5 lists the ten largest cities in the world in 1950, 1980, and (projected) 2,000. As can be seen, there will be a clear shift in their ranking.

The difference in the growth rate (mainly because of a difference in fertility behavior) also is evident when comparing the age pyramids of the developed and the developing regions of the world (Figure 9-2). The age profile of the developing nations clearly is expansive while the developed regions are nearly stationary.

Table 9-6 summarizes many demographic indicators for the world's continents. Asia is by far the most populous, although its current rate of natural increase is third to Africa and Latin America. Europe and North America have low rates of natural increase and the percentage of their population over age 64 is correspondingly high. They also have the highest life expectancy at birth and the highest percent urban population. Per capita gross national product is highest in North America, Oceania, and Europe, while the crude death rate is lowest in Oceania, followed by North America, Latin America, Europe, and the U.S.S.R.

Exhibit 9-1 The 1980 U.S. Census Questionnaire (Annotated)

2. provides information on type of household (husband/wife, other type of family, or single person households) and the number of persons in the household. Because of changes in society since 1970, the concept of household "head" has been replaced with that of a reference person in whose name the dwelling unit is owned or rented. This person is identified in column one. This key change means data will not be exactly comparable to "male-headed" or "female-headed" household data from the 1970 Census, but it will be easy to identify families and other types of households. In many tabulations characteristics will be shown for both husband and wife where they were shown previously only for the head of family households.

The questionnaire has space for up to seven household members to provide answers. We show only column 1. The other columns are identical except for question 2, which asks relationship. In question 2, columns 2 through 7 have the following language instead of the "Start in this column" language: "If relative of person in column 1: Husband/wife; Son/daughter; Brother/sister; Father/mother; Other relative (specify). If not related to person in column 1: Roomer, boarder; Partner, roommate; Paid employee; Other nonrelative (specify)."

Two of the categories are new: "Partner, roommate" and "Paid employee." The first was added to obtain statistics on the growing number of people who live together without being married.

3. same as in 1970.

4. expands the possible answers about race from nine in 1970 to 15. As a result we can expect a few Samoans to turn up in places like Kansas City, just ~~because~~ that alternative is listed. The expansion is the result of growing ethnic ~~awareness, but note~~ that the word "race" does not appear.

5. same as in 1970.

6. same as in 1970.

7. for the first time asks all Americans a single question about Spanish origin. These data will not be comparable with previous censuses. In 1970, this question was asked of a maximum of 15 percent of the population, and the data were tabulated differently for different regions of the country. This question ends the population questions asked of all Americans. The next three questions appear on the long form questionnaire only.

8. similar to 1970, but what was previously called "parochial" schools is now called "church related."

9. similar to 1970, but the highest college level asked for then was six or more years.

10. same as in 1970.

Note: Because of our format we have reduced the size of the questionnaire by about 40 percent and omitted certain instructions to respondents and Census Bureau use boxes. The census questionnaire also will have blue shading, not gray.

Read across two pages

Exhibit 9-1 continued

Here are the QUESTIONS ↓	These are the columns for ANSWERS ➡ Please fill one column for each person listed in Question 1.	PERSON in column 1	PEI
		Last name First name Middle initial	Last name First name
2. How is this person related to the person in column 1? Fill one circle. If "Other relative" of person in column 1, give exact relationship, such as mother-in-law, niece, grandson, etc.		_START_ in this column with the household member (or one of the members) in whose name the home is owned or rented. If there is no such person, start in this column with any adult household member.	If relative of pers O Husband O Son/dau O Brother/s If not related to p O Roomer, I O Partner, n O Paid emp
3. Sex Fill one circle.		○ Male ■ ○ Female	O Male
4. Is this person — Fill one circle.		○ White O Asian Indian ○ Black or Negro O Hawaiian ○ Japanese O Guamanian ○ Chinese O Samoan ○ Filipino O Eskimo ○ Korean O Aleut ○ Vietnamese O Other — _Specify_ ○ Indian (Amer.) _Print tribe_ ➡ _ _ _ _ _ _ _ _	O White O Black or I O Japanese O Chinese O Filipino O Korean O Vietname O Indian (A _Print tribe_ ➡

5. Age, and month and year of birth
 	
a. Print age at last birthday.
b. Print month and fill one circle.
c. Print year in the spaces, and fill one circle below each number.
		a. Age at last c. Year of birth
		birthday
		        1 ● 8 O 0 O 0 O
		        9 O 1 O 1 O
		b. Month of 2 O 2 O
		birth 3 O 3 O
		            4 O 4 O
		         ■ 5 O 5 O
		O Jan.—Mar. 6 O 6 O
		O Apr.—June 7 O 7 O
		O July—Sept. 8 O 8 O
		O Oct.—Dec. 9 O 9 O
			a. Age at last
			birthday
			
			b. Month of
			birth
			
			O Jan.—Ma
			O Apr.—Jur
			O July—Se
			O Oct.—De

6. Marital status Fill one circle.		O Now married Separated O Widowed Never married O Divorced	O Now mar O Widowed O Divorced
7. Is this person of Spanish/Hispanic origin or descent? Fill one circle.		O No (not Spanish/Hispanic) O Yes, Mexican, Mexican-Amer., Chicano O Yes, Puerto Rican ■ O Yes, Cuban O Yes, other Spanish/Hispanic	O No (not S O Yes, Mex O Yes, Pue O Yes, Cub O Yes, othe
8. Since February 1, 1980, has this person attended regular school or college at any time? Fill one circle. Count nursery school, kindergarten, elementary school and schooling which leads to a high school diploma or college degree.		O No, has not attended since February 1 O Yes, public school, public college O Yes, private, church-related O Yes, private, not church-related	O No, has r O Yes, publ O Yes, priva O Yes, priva
9. What is the highest grade (or year) of regular school this person has ever attended? Fill one circle. If now attending school, mark grade person is in. If high school was finished by equivalency test (GED), mark "12."		Highest grade attended: O Nursery school O Kindergarten Elementary through high school _(grade or year)_ 1 2 3 4 5 6 7 8 9 10 11 12 O O O O O O O O O O O O College _(academic year)_ ■ 1 2 3 4 5 6 7 8 or more O O O O O O O O Never attended school — _Skip question 10_	Highest grade at O Nursery : Elementary throu 1 2 3 4 5 O O O O C College _(academi_ 1 2 3 4 5 O O O O C O Never att
10. Did this person finish the highest grade (or year) attended? Fill one circle.		O Now attending this grade _(or year)_ O Finished this grade _(or year)_ O Did not finish this grade _(or year)_	O Now atter O Finished O Did not fi

Exhibit 9-1 continued

H1. Did you leave anyone out of Question 1 because you were not sure if the person should be listed — *for example, a new baby still in the hospital, a lodger who also has another home, or a person who stays here once in a while and has no other home?*

○ Yes — *On page 20 give name(s) and reason left out.*
○ No

H2. Did you list anyone in Question 1 who is away from home now — *for example, on a vacation or in a hospital?*

○ Yes — *On page 20 give name(s) and reason person is away.*
○ No

H3. Is anyone visiting here who is not already listed?

○ Yes — *On page 20 give name of each visitor for whom there is no one at the home address to report the person to a census taker.*
○ No

H4. How many living quarters, occupied and vacant, are at this address?

○ One
○ 2 apartments or living quarters
○ 3 apartments or living quarters
○ 4 apartments or living quarters
○ 5 apartments or living quarters
○ 6 apartments or living quarters
○ 7 apartments or living quarters
○ 8 apartments or living quarters
○ 9 apartments or living quarters
○ 10 or more apartments or living quarters

○ This is a mobile home or trailer

H5. Do you enter your living quarters —

○ Directly from the outside or through a common or public hall?
○ Through someone else's living quarters?

H6. Do you have **complete** plumbing facilities in your living quarters, that is, hot and cold piped water, a flush toilet, and a bathtub or shower?

○ Yes, for this household only
○ Yes, but also used by another household
○ No, have some but not all plumbing facilities
○ No plumbing facilities in living quarters

H7. How many rooms do you have in your living quarters?
*Do **not** count bathrooms, porches, balconies, foyers, halls, or half-rooms.*

○ 1 room   ■ ○ 4 rooms   ○ 7 rooms
○ 2 rooms   ○ 5 rooms   ○ 8 rooms
○ 3 rooms   ○ 6 rooms   ○ 9 or more rooms

H8. Are your living quarters —

○ Owned or being bought by you or by someone else in this household?
○ Rented for cash rent?
○ Occupied without payment of cash rent?

H9. Is this apartment (house) part of a condominium?

○ No
○ Yes, a condominium

H10. If this is a *one-family house* —

a. Is the house on a property of **10 or more acres?**

○ Yes   ■   ○ No

b. Is any part of the property used as a commercial establishment or medical office?

○ Yes   ○ No

H11. If you live in a one-family house or a condominium unit which you own or are buying —

What is the value of this property, that is, how much do you think this property (house and lot or condominium unit) would sell for if it were for sale?

Do not answer this question if this is —
■ • A mobile home or trailer   ■
  • A house on 10 or more acres
  • A house with a commercial establishment or medical office on the property

○ Less than $10,000   ○ $50,000 to $54,999
○ $10,000 to $14,999   ○ $55,000 to $59,999
○ $15,000 to $17,499   ○ $60,000 to $64,999
○ $17,500 to $19,999   ○ $65,000 to $69,999
○ $20,000 to $22,499   ○ $70,000 to $74,999
○ $22,500 to $24,999 ■ ○ $75,000 to $79,999
○ $25,000 to $27,499   ○ $80,000 to $89,999
○ $27,500 to $29,999   ○ $90,000 to $99,999
○ $30,000 to $34,999   ○ $100,000 to $124,999
○ $35,000 to $39,999   ○ $125,000 to $149,999
○ $40,000 to $44,999   ○ $150,000 to $199,999
○ $45,000 to $49,999   ○ $200,000 or more

H12. If you pay rent for your living quarters —
What is the monthly rent?
If rent is not paid by the month, see the instruction guide on how to figure a monthly rent.

○ Less than $50   ○ $160 to $169
○ $50 to $59   ○ $170 to $179
○ $60 to $69   ○ $180 to $189
○ $70 to $79   ○ $190 to $199
○ $80 to $89   ○ $200 to $224
○ $90 to $99   ■ ○ $225 to $249
○ $100 to $109   ○ $250 to $274
○ $110 to $119   ○ $275 to $299
○ $120 to $129   ○ $300 to $349
○ $130 to $139   ○ $350 to $399
○ $140 to $149   ○ $400 to $499
○ $150 to $159   ○ $500 or more

FOR CENSUS USE ONLY

A4. Block number	A6. Serial number	B. Type of unit or quarters	For vacant units	D. Months vacant	F. Total persons
		Occupied	**C1.** Is this unit for —	○ Less than 1 month	
		○ First form	○ Year round use	○ 1 up to 2 months	
		○ Continuation	○ Seasonal/Mig. — *Skip C2, C3, and D.*	○ 2 up to 6 months	
0 0 0	0 0 0 0	**Vacant**	**C2.** Vacancy status	○ 6 up to 12 months	0 0 0
1 1 1	1 1 1 1	○ Regular	○ For rent ■	○ 1 year up to 2 years	1 1 1
2 2 2	2 2 2 2	○ Usual home elsewhere	○ For sale only	○ 2 or more years	2 2 2
3 3 3	3 3 3 3		○ Rented or sold, not occupied		3 3 3
4 4 4 ■	4 4 4 4	**Group quarters**	○ Held for occasional use	**E. Indicators** ■	4 4 4
5 5 5	5 5 5 5		○ Other vacant	1. ○ ○ Mail return	5 5 5
6 6 6	6 6 6 6	○ First form	**C3.** Is this unit boarded up?	2. ○ ○ Pop./F	6 6 6
7 7 7	7 7 7 7	○ Continuation			7 7 7
8 8 8	8 8 8 8		○ Yes ○ No	○ ○	8 8 8
9 9 9	9 9 9 9				9 9 9

Read across two pages

Exhibit 9-1 continued

H1-H3. the housing part of both the 100 percent and sample question- naires starts with these three questions to make sure that everyone in the household was counted.

H4. same as in 1970. This question is asked so that census personnel can be sure that all units at an address are enumerated. Question H13 provides superior data on the number of dwell- ing units in the structure. Like the first three housing questions, H4 is intended to check coverage.

H5. has the objective of making certain the respondent occupies a bona fide dwelling unit, not just a few rooms in someone else's house.

H6. one of the few questions left from a series of questions in the 1970 Census which attempted to measure housing quality.

H7. same as in 1970.

H8. same as in 1970.

H9. for the first time poses a sepa- rate question on condominiums. The term "cooperative" also appeared on the test questionnaires but was misun- derstood by many respondents.

H10. separates farmhouses, es- tates, and partly commercial structures from single family dwelling units. Value is not tabulated for these types of units.

H11. asks value. There are 24 categories instead of the 11 in 1970, when the highest value was only $50,000 or more.

H12. also shows the impact of in- flation. The highest interval in 1970 was $300 or more. It is now $500 or more, and 24 categories appear instead of the former 14.

H12 ends the housing questions asked of all Americans. The Census Bureau estimates it takes 15 minutes to answer the 19 population and housing questions on the short questionnaire, while the remaining questions add another 30 minutes.

Exhibit 9-1 continued

H13. Which best describes this building?

Include all apartments, flats, etc., even if vacant.

- ○ A mobile home or trailer
- ○ A one-family house detached from any other house
- ○ A one-family house attached to one or more houses
- ○ A building for 2 families
- ○ A building for 3 or 4 families
- ○ A building for 5 to 9 families
- ○ A building for 10 to 19 families
- ○ A building for 20 to 49 families
- ○ A building for 50 or more families

- ○ A boat, tent, van, etc.

H14a. How many stories (floors) are in this building?

Count an attic or basement as a story if it has any finished rooms for living purposes.

- ○ 1 to 3 — *Skip to H15*
- ○ 4 to 6
- ○ 7 to 12
- ○ 13 or more stories

b. Is there a passenger elevator in this building?

- ○ Yes
- ○ No

H15a. Is this building —

- ○ On a city or suburban lot, or on a place of less than 1 acre? — *Skip to H16*
- ○ On a place of 1 to 9 acres?
- ○ On a place of 10 or more acres?

b. Last year, 1979, did sales of crops, livestock, and other farm products from this place amount to —

- ○ Less than $50 (or None)
- ○ $50 to $249
- ○ $250 to $599
- ○ $600 to $999
- ○ $1,000 to $2,499
- ○ $2,500 or more

H16. Do you get water from —

- ○ A public system *(city water department, etc.)* or private company?
- ○ An individual drilled well?
- ○ An individual dug well?
- ○ Some other source *(a spring, creek, river, cistern, etc.)*?

H17. Is this building connected to a public sewer?

- ○ Yes, connected to public sewer
- ○ No, connected to septic tank or cesspool
- ○ No, use other means

H18. About when was this building originally built? *Mark when the building was first constructed, not when it was remodeled, added to, or converted.*

- ○ 1979 or 1980
- ○ 1975 to 1978
- ○ 1970 to 1974
- ○ 1960 to 1969
- ○ 1950 to 1959
- ○ 1940 to 1949
- ○ 1939 or earlier

H19. When did the person listed in column 1 move into this house (or apartment)?

- ○ 1979 to 1980
- ○ 1975 to 1978
- ○ 1970 to 1974
- ○ 1960 to 1969
- ○ 1950 to 1959
- ○ 1949 or earlier
- ○ Always lived here

H20. How are your living quarters heated?

Fill one circle for the kind of heat used most.

- ○ Steam or hot water system
- ○ Central warm-air furnace with ducts to the individual rooms
  (Do not count electric heat pumps here.)
- ○ Electric heat pump
- ○ Other built-in electric units *(permanently installed in wall, ceiling, or baseboard)*

- ○ Floor, wall, or pipeless furnace
- ○ Room heaters with flue or vent, burning gas, oil, or kerosene
- ○ Room heaters without flue or vent, burning gas, oil, or kerosene *(not portable)*
- ○ Fireplaces, stoves, or portable room heaters of any kind
- ○ No heating equipment

Read across two pages

Exhibit 9-1 continued

	CENSUS USE

H21a. Which fuel is used most for house heating?

- ○ Gas: from underground pipes serving the neighborhood
- ○ Gas: bottled, tank, or LP
- ○ Electricity
- ○ Fuel oil, kerosene, etc.
- ○ Coal or coke
- ○ Wood
- ○ Other fuel
- ○ No fuel used

b. Which fuel is used most for water heating?

- ○ Gas: from underground pipes serving the neighborhood
- ○ Gas: bottled, tank, or LP
- ○ Electricity
- ○ Fuel oil, kerosene, etc. ■
- ○ Coal or coke ■
- ○ Wood
- ○ Other fuel
- ○ No fuel used

c. Which fuel is used most for cooking?

- ○ Gas: from underground pipes serving the neighborhood
- ○ Gas: bottled, tank, or LP
- ○ Electricity
- ○ Fuel oil, kerosene, etc.
- ○ Coal or coke
- ○ Wood
- ○ Other fuel
- ○ No fuel used ■

H22. What are the cost of utilities and fuels for your living quarters?

a. Electricity

$ _____ .00 OR
- ○ Included in rent or no charge
- ○ Electricity not used

Average monthly cost

b. Gas

$ _____ .00 OR
- ○ Included in rent or no charge
- ○ Gas not used

Average monthly cost ■

c. Water

$ _____ .00 OR
- ○ Included in rent or no charge

Yearly cost

d. Oil, coal, kerosene, wood, etc.

$ _____ .00 OR
- ○ Included in rent or no charge
- ○ These fuels not used

Yearly cost

H23. Do you have **complete** kitchen facilities? *Complete kitchen facilities are a sink with piped water, a range or cookstove, and a refrigerator.*

Yes ■   ○ No

H24. How many bedrooms do you have?
Count rooms used mainly for sleeping even if used also for other purposes.

| No bedroom | ○ 2 bedrooms | ○ 4 bedrooms |
| 1 bedroom | ○ 3 bedrooms | ○ 5 or more bedrooms |

H25. How many bathrooms do you have?
A complete bathroom is a room with flush toilet, bathtub or shower, and wash basin with piped water.

A half bathroom has at least a flush toilet or bathtub or shower, but does not have all the facilities for a complete bathroom.

- ○ No bathroom, or only a half bathroom
- ○ 1 complete bathroom
- ○ 1 complete bathroom, plus half bath(s)
- ○ 2 or more complete bathrooms

H26. Do you have a telephone in your living quarters?

○ Yes ■   ○ No ■

H27. Do you have air conditioning?

- ○ Yes, a central air - conditioning system
- ○ Yes, 1 individual room unit
- ○ Yes, 2 or more individual room units
- ○ No

H28. How many automobiles are kept at home for use by members of your household?

| ○ None ■ | ○ 2 automobiles |
| ○ 1 automobile | ○ 3 or more automobiles ■ |

H29. How many vans or trucks of one-ton capacity or less are kept at home for use by members of your household?

| ○ None | ○ 2 vans or trucks |
| ○ 1 van or truck | ○ 3 or more vans or trucks |

Census Use columns:

H22a.
0 0 0
1 1 1
2 2 2
3 3 3
4 4 4
5 5 5
6 6 6
7 7 7
8 8 8
9 9 9

H22b.
0 0 0
1 1 1
2 2 2
3 3 3
4 4 4
5 5 5
6 6 6
7 7 7
8 8 8
9 9 9

H22c.
0 0 0
1 1 1
2 2 2
3 3 3
4 4 4
5 5 5
6 6 6
7 7 7
8 8 8
9 9 9

H22d.
0 0 0 0
1 1 1 1
2 2 2 2
3 3 3 3
4 4 4 4
5 5 5 5
6 6 6 6
7 7 7 7
8 8 8 8
9 9 9 9

PH ○ ○
0 0 0 0
1 1 1 1
2 2 2 2
3 3 3 3
4 4 4 4
5 5 5 5
6 6 6 6
7 7 7 7
8 8 8 8
9 9 9 9

0 0 0 0
1 1 1 1
2 2 2 2
3 3 3 3
4 4 4 4
5 5 5 5
6 6 6 6
7 7 7 7
8 8 8 8
9 9 9

Exhibit 9-1 continued

Please answer H30—H32 If you live in a one-family house
which you own or are buying, unless this is —

- A mobile home or trailer..............
- A house on 10 or more acres...........
- A condominium unit...................
- A house with a commercial establishment
  or medical office on the property.......

If any of these, or if you rent your unit or this is a
multi-family structure, skip H30 to H32 and turn to page 6.

H30. What were the real estate taxes on this property last year?

$ _____ .00   OR   ○ None

H31. What is the annual premium for fire and hazard insurance on this property?

$ _____ .00   OR   ○ None

H32a. Do you have a mortgage, deed of trust, contract to purchase, or similar debt on this property?

○ Yes, mortgage, deed of trust, or similar debt
○ Yes, contract to purchase
○ No — Skip to page 6

b. Do you have a second or junior mortgage on this property?

○ Yes   ○ No

c. How much is your total regular monthly payment to the lender?
Also include payments on a contract to purchase and to lenders holding second or junior mortgages on this property.

$ _____ .00   OR   ○ No regular payment required — Skip to page 6

d. Does your regular monthly payment (amount entered in H32c) include payments for real estate taxes on this property?

○ Yes, taxes included in payment
○ No, taxes paid separately or taxes not required

e. Does your regular monthly payment (amount entered in H32c) include payments for fire and hazard insurance on this property?

○ Yes, insurance included in payment
○ No, insurance paid separately or no insurance

FOR CENSUS USE ONLY

H13. boats, vans, and tents have been added to the possible answers. Otherwise, it is the same as a question asked in 1970.

H14. same as in 1970.

H15. same as in 1970.

H16. a slight variation from the 1970 question in that the respondent is asked to differentiate a drilled well from a dug well

H17. same as in 1970.

H18. same as in 1970.

H19. asked in 1970, but of each person in the household, and appeared in the population section.

H20. same as in 1970 except that the choice "electric heat pump" has been added, and an open-ended "other" choice has been eliminated.

H21. same as in 1970.

H22. asked only of renters in 1970. Now all sampled households are expected to answer. Census tests show that respondents almost always overstate their utility costs.

H23. asked in 1970, but on the short form.

H24. same as in 1970.

H25. asked in 1970, except the highest category was "3 or more" bathrooms.

H26. on the 100 percent questionnaire in 1970 and asked differently: Is there a telephone on which people in your living quarters can be called?" If the answer was yes, the respondent was asked to write down the phone number. The simpler form for 1980 may produce better results.

H27. same as in 1970.

H28. same as in 1970.

H29. a new question reflecting the substantial increase in the number of vans and trucks.

H30-H32. all new. Their purpose is to obtain a measure of total shelter costs for one-family owner-occupied units. The Census Bureau does not plan to tabulate these questions separately, but to combine them with H22 for a single tabulation of "total shelter costs."

Exhibit 9-1 continued

Name of
Person 1
on page 2: _____
                Last name   First name   Middle initial

11. In what State or foreign country was this person born?
*Print the State where this person's mother was living
when this person was born. Do not give the location of
the hospital unless the mother's home and the hospital
were in the same State.*

_____
Name of State or foreign country; or Puerto Rico, Guam, etc.

12. *If this person was born in a foreign country —*
**a. Is this person a naturalized citizen of the
United States?**

- ○ Yes, a naturalized citizen
- ○ No, not a citizen
- ■ ○ Born abroad of American parents   ■

**b. When did this person come to the United States
to stay?**

- ○ 1975 to 1980
- ○ 1965 to 1969
- ○ 1950 to 1959
- ○ 1970 to 1974
- ○ 1960 to 1964
- ○ Before 1950

**13a. Does this person speak a language other than
English at home?**

- ○ Yes   ○ No, only speaks English — *Skip to 14*

b. What is this language?

_____
(For example — Chinese, Italian, Spanish, etc.)

c. How well does this person speak English?

- ○ Very well   ■
- ○ Well
- ○ Not well
- ○ Not at all

14. What is this person's ancestry? *If uncertain about
how to report ancestry, see instruction guide.*

_____
*(For example — Afro-Amer., English, French, German, Honduran,
Hungarian, Irish, Italian, Jamaican, Korean, Lebanese, Mexican,
Nigerian, Polish, Ukrainian, Venezuelan, etc.)*

**15a. Did this person live in this house five years ago
(April 1, 1975)?** *If in college or Armed Forces in
April 1975, report place of residence there.*

- ○ Born April 1975 or later — *Turn to next page for
next person*
- ○ Yes, this house — *Skip to 16*
- ○ No, different house

**b. Where did this person live five years ago
(April 1, 1975)?**
**(1) State, foreign country,
Puerto Rico,
Guam, etc.:** _____

(2) County: _____

**(3) City, town,
village, etc.:** _____

**(4) Inside the incorporated (legal) limits
of that city, town, village, etc.?**

- ○ Yes   ○ No, in unincorporated area

Read across two pages

Exhibit 9-1 continued

16. When was this person born?
- ○ Born before April 1965 —
  Please go on with questions 17-33
- ○ Born April 1965 or later —
  Turn to next page for next person

17. In April 1975 *(five years ago)* **was this person —**

a. On active duty in the Armed Forces?
- ○ Yes   ○ No

b. Attending college?
- ○ Yes   ○ No

c. Working at a job or business?
- ○ Yes, full time   ○ No
- ○ Yes, part time

18a. Is this person a veteran of active-duty military service in the Armed Forces of the United States?
If service was in National Guard or Reserves only, see instruction guide.
- ○ Yes   ○ No — *Skip to 19*

b. Was active-duty military service during —
Fill a circle for each period in which this person served.
- ○ May 1975 or later
- ○ Vietnam era *(August 1964–April 1975)*
- ○ February 1955—July 1964
- ○ Korean conflict *(June 1950–January 1955)*
- ○ World War II *(September 1940–July 1947)*
- ○ World War I *(April 1917–November 1918)*
- ○ Any other time

19. Does this person have a physical, mental, or other health condition which has lasted for 6 or more months and which . . .

	Yes	No
a. **Limits** the kind or amount of work this person can do at a job?	○	○
b. **Prevents** this person from working at a job?	○	○
c. **Limits or prevents** this person from using public transportation?	○	○

20. *If this person is a female —*
How many babies has she ever had, not counting stillbirths?
Do not count her stepchildren or children she has adopted.

None 1 2 3 4 5 6
○ ○ ○ ○ ○ ○ ○
7 8 9 10 11 12 or more
○ ○ ○ ○ ○ ○

21. *If this person has ever been married —*

a. Has this person been married more than once?
- ○ Once   ○ More than once

b. Month and year of marriage?   **Month and year of first marriage?**

(Month) (Year)   (Month) (Year)

c. *If married more than once* — Did the first marriage end because of the death of the husband (or wife)?
- ○ Yes   ○ No

22a. Did this person work at any time last week?
- ○ Yes — *Fill this circle if this person worked full time or part time. (Count part-time work such as delivering papers, or helping without pay in a family business or farm. Also count active duty in the Armed Forces.)*
- ○ No — *Fill this circle if this person did not work, or did only own housework, school work, or volunteer work.*

Skip to 25

b. How many hours did this person work last week (at all jobs)?
Subtract any time off; add overtime or extra hours worked.

Hours

23. At what location did this person work last week?
If this person worked at more than one location, print where he or she worked most last week.
If one location cannot be specified, see instruction guide.

a. Address *(Number and street)*

If street address is not known, enter the building name, shopping center, or other physical location description.

b. Name of city, town, village, borough, etc.

c. Is the place of work inside the incorporated (legal) limits of that city, town, village, borough, etc.?
- ○ Yes   ○ No, in unincorporated area

d. County

e. State   **f. ZIP Code**

24a. Last week, how long did it usually take this person to get from home to work (one way)?

Minutes

b. How did this person usually get to work last week?
If this person used more than one method, give the one usually used for most of the distance.

- ○ Car
- ○ Truck
- ○ Van
- ○ Bus or streetcar
- ○ Railroad
- ○ Subway or elevated
- ○ Taxicab
- ○ Motorcycle
- ○ Bicycle
- ○ Walked only
- ○ Worked at home
- ○ Other — *Specify*

If car, truck, or van in 24b, go to 24c.
Otherwise, skip to 28.

FOR CENSUS USE ONLY

11. similar to a 1970 question, but the wording has been changed from "Where was this person born?"

12. similar to 1970, but the word "alien" has been changed to "not a citizen."

13. replaces one that asked about language other than English spoken in the home when the respondent was a child.

The 1980 question should be more useful for determining how many Americans speak a language other than English and for determining how many persons do not speak English at all.

14. replaces two questions in 1970 on where the respondent's parents were born. The new approach is more subjective than the previous approach to ancestry.

Exhibit 9-1 continued

c. When going to work last week, did this person usually —

- ○ Drive alone — *Skip to 28*
- ○ Share driving
- ○ Drive others only
- ○ Ride as passenger only

d. How many people, including this person, usually rode to work in the car, truck, or van last week?

- ○ 2
- ○ 3 ▪
- ○ 4
- ○ 5
- ○ 6
- ○ 7 or more ▪

After answering 24d, skip to 28.

25. Was this person temporarily absent or on layoff from a job or business last week?

- ○ Yes, on layoff
- ○ Yes, on vacation, temporary illness, labor dispute, etc.
- ○ No

26a. Has this person been looking for work during the last 4 weeks?

- ○ Yes ▪
- ○ No — *Skip to 27*

b. Could this person have taken a job last week?

- ○ No, already has a job
- ○ No, temporarily ill
- ○ No, other reasons *(in school, etc.)*
- ○ Yes, could have a job ▪

27. When did this person last work, even for a few days?

- ○ 1980
- ○ 1979
- ○ 1978
- ○ 1975 to 1977
- ○ 1970 to 1974
- ○ 1969 or earlier
- ○ Never worked

} *Skip to 31d*

28–30. Current or most recent job activity

Describe clearly this person's chief job activity or business last week. If this person had more than one job, describe the one at which this person worked the most hours. If this person had no job or business last week, give information for last job or business since 1975.

28. Industry

a. For whom did this person work? *If now on active duty in the Armed Forces, print "AF" and skip to question 31.*

(Name of company, business, organization, or other employer)

b. What kind of business or industry was this?
Describe the activity at location where employed.

(For example: Hospital, newspaper publishing, mail order house, ▪ *auto engine manufacturing, breakfast cereal manufacturing)*

c. Is this mainly — *(Fill one circle)*

- ○ Manufacturing ▪
- ○ Wholesale trade
- ○ Retail trade
- ○ Other — *(agriculture, construction, service, government, etc.)*

29. Occupation

a. What kind of work was this person doing?

(For example: Registered nurse, personnel manager, supervisor of order department, gasoline engine assembler, grinder operator)

b. What were this person's most important activities or duties?

(For example: Patient care, directing hiring policies, supervising ▪ *order clerks, assembling engines, operating grinding mill)*

30. Was this person — *(Fill one circle)*

Employee of private company, business, or individual, for wages, salary, or commissions ..... ○

Federal government employee .... ○
State government employee .... ○
Local government employee *(city, county, etc.)*...... ○

Self-employed in own business, professional practice, or farm — ▪
Own business not incorporated .... ○
Own business incorporated .... ○

Working without pay in family business or farm ..... ○

31a. Last year (1979), did this person work, even for a few days, at a paid job or in a business or farm?

- ○ Yes ▪
- ○ No — *Skip to 31d*

b. How many weeks did this person work in 1979?
Count paid vacation, paid sick leave, and military service.

---------- Weeks

c. During the weeks worked in 1979, how many hours did this person usually work each week?

---------- Hours

d. Of the weeks not worked in 1979 (if any), how many weeks was this person looking for work or on layoff from a job?

---------- Weeks

32. Income in 1979 —
Fill circles and print dollar amounts.
If net income was a loss, write "Loss" above the dollar amount.
If exact amount is not known, give best estimate. For income received jointly by household members, see instruction guide.

During 1979 did this person receive any income from the following sources?

If "Yes" to any of the sources below — How much did this person receive for the entire year?

a. Wages, salary, commissions, bonuses, or tips from all jobs ... *Report amount before deductions for taxes, bonds, dues, or other items.*

- ○ Yes → $ _____ .00
- ○ No
(Annual Amount – Dollars)

b. Own nonfarm business, partnership, or professional practice ... *Report net income after business expenses.*

- ▪ ○ Yes → $ _____ .00
- ○ No
(Annual Amount – Dollars)

c. Own farm ...
Report net income after operating expenses. Include earnings as a tenant farmer or sharecropper.

- ○ Yes → $ _____ .00
- ○ No
(Annual Amount – Dollars)

d. Interest, dividends, royalties, or net rental income ...
Report even small amounts credited to an account.

- ○ Yes → $ _____ .00
- ○ No
(Annual Amount – Dollars)

e. Social Security or Railroad Retirement ...

- ▪ ○ Yes → $ _____ .00
- ○ No
(Annual Amount – Dollars)

f. Supplemental Security (SSI), Aid to Families with Dependent Children (AFDC), or other public assistance or public welfare payments ...

- ○ Yes → $ _____ .00
- ○ No
(Annual Amount – Dollars)

g. Unemployment compensation, veterans' payments, pensions, alimony or child support, or any other sources of income received regularly ...
Exclude lump-sum payments such as money from an inheritance or the sale of a home.

- ▪ ○ Yes → $ _____ .00
- ○ No
(Annual Amount – Dollars)

33. What was this person's total income in 1979?
Add entries in questions 32a through g; subtract any losses.

$ _____ .00
(Annual Amount – Dollars)

If total amount was a loss, write "Loss" above amount.

OR ○ None

Read across two pages

Exhibit 9-1 continued

15. same as in 1970.

16. same as in 1970.

17. same as in 1970.

18. same as in 1970.

19. resembles a question asked in 1970, but then it was asked only of persons less than 65 years old and was concerned only with a work disability. The 1980 question tested poorly, but so many public agencies need disability data that the question will appear anyway.

20. same as in 1970.

21. same as in 1970.

22. asked in 1970, but in 1980 respondents are also asked to write in the number of hours worked.

23. same as in 1970.

24a. a new question which attempts to measure average time spent getting to work.

24b. same as in 1970 but with the additional categories of truck, van, motorcycle, or bicycle.

24c & d. a new series of questions to measure the extent of carpooling.

25. same as in 1970.

26. same as in 1970.

27. same as in 1970.

28. resembles a question asked in 1970, but the words "...this person" have been substituted for the pronoun "he" in the questions on occupation, industry, and income.

29. same as in 1970.

30. same as in 1970.

31a & b. same as in 1970.

31c & d. new questions to measure part-time workers and the extent of unemployment in the previous year.

32. similar to 1970 except that the question has been recast as "income" instead of "earnings" and "interest, dividends ..." and "unemployment compensation ..." have been separated.

33. appeared in 1970 in slightly different form as part of the earnings question. This is the last question. The questions about population characteristics are repeated for up to seven persons in the household. If there are more than seven persons in a household an enumerator calls and tabulates responses of the additional persons.

Source: Reprinted from *The 1980 Census: The Counting of America* by Peter K. Francese with permission of Population Reference Bureau, vol. 34, no. 4 (September 1979), 18-23.

Table 9-4 Estimated Timing of Each Billion of World Population

	Time taken to reach	Year attained
First billion	2-5 million years	About 1800 A.D.
Second billion	Approx. 130 years	1930
Third billion	30 years	1960
Fouth billion	15 years	1975
Projections:		
Fifth billion	12 years	1987
Sixth billion	11 years	1998

Sources: United Nations and "Historical Estimates of World Population" by John D. Durand, *Population and Development Review,* vol. 3, no. 3, September 1977, 253-296; reprinted, by permission, from *World Population: Toward the Next Century,* November 1981, 3.

The United States and Canada

In both the United States and Canada, the most striking recent demographic trend is the aging of the population. In 1980, the median age of the United States population was 30.2 years, Canada's slightly below 29.9. This median age is the same as in 1950, before the postwar baby boom. The baby boom cohort is now 20 to 34 and it is those age groups that show the largest relative increases between 1970 and 1980. The number of young adults aged 20-24 increased by 30.1 percent during this period, the 25-29 and 30-34 groups 44.7 percent and 53.5 percent, respectively. The over-55 bloc also rose rapidly, with a greater relative gain for females than for males.[57]

On the other hand, the number of children under 15 declined by 4.5 percent, with 4.8 percent fewer under 5, 16.4 percent fewer in ages 5-9 and 12.3 percent fewer 10-14. The Depression cohort (babies born in the Depression years of low birth rates) is now 40 to 49, so this group also decreased between 1970 and 1980. Table 9-7 shows the 1970 and 1980 distribution of the population by age group in the United States. Canada's population is slightly younger, with 9.5 percent over 64 (up from 7.6 percent in 1961), 61.7 percent 18-64 (up from 53.5 percent in 1961), and 28.8 percent under 17 (down from 38.9 percent in 1961).

The changing age structure in both the United States and Canada is a result of changing fertility behavior. Both the crude birth rate and the general fertility rate decreased dramatically between 1950 and 1975 but increased slightly thereafter (Table 9-8). These changes in fertility can be observed at every age (Figure 9-3).

Table 9-5 Ten Largest Cities in the World in 1950, 1980, 2000

1950	Population (in millions) 1980		Population (in millions) 2000		Population (in millions)
1. New York-N.E. New Jersey	12.3	1. New York-N.E. New Jersey	20.2	1. Mexico City	31.0
2. London	10.4	2. Tokyo-Yokohama	20.0	2. Sao Paulo	25.8
3. Rhine-Ruhr	6.9	3. Mexico City	15.0	3. Shanghai	23.7
4. Tokyo-Yokohama	6.7	4. Shanghai	14.3	4. Tokyo-Yokohama	23.7
5. Shanghai	5.8	5. Sao Paulo	13.5	5. New York-N.E. New Jersey	22.4
6. Paris	5.5	6. Los Angeles-Long Beach	11.6	6. Peking	20.9
7. Greater Buenos Aires	5.3	7. Peking	11.4	7. Rio de Janeiro	19.0
8. Chicago-N.W. Indiana	4.9	8. Rio de Janeiro	10.7	8. Greater Bombay	16.8
9. Moscow	4.8	9. Greater Buenos Aires	10.1	9. Calcutta	16.4
10. Calcutta	4.6	10. London	10.0	10. Jakarta	15.7

Source: Reprinted from *World Population: Toward the Next Century* with permission of Population Reference Bureau, Inc., Washington, D.C., November 1981, 2.

Figure 9-2 Population Age Pyramids

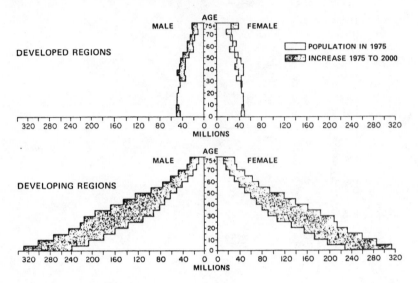

Source: Reprinted from *World Population: Toward the Next Century* (Washington, D.C.: Population Reference Bureau, 1981), 6.

The total fertility rate in the United States in the early 1980s was about 1.8 births per woman, in contrast to nearly 3.7 in the late 1950s. The average family size declined correspondingly, from a high of 3.67 in 1960 to 3.28 in 1980. The marriage rate decreased from 90.2 marriages per year per 1,000 unmarried women age 15 and older in 1950 to 64.6 in 1981.[58]

The divorce rate appeared to be leveling off at around 22.8 divorces per year per 1,000 married women aged 15 and over, after having more than doubled since 1967 and almost tripled since 1940.[59] The proportion of nonfamily households (individuals living alone or sharing living quarters with unrelated persons) increased from 18.8 percent in 1970 to 26.6 percent in 1980.

Although fertility rates in the United States are low, teenage rates are very high as compared to other industrialized countries (Table 9-9). There were 54.7 births per 1,000 women under 20 years of age in the United States in 1976, compared to 33.8 in Canada, 28.8 in France, 12.4 in Switzerland, and only 3.7 in Japan.

Only East Germany was higher than the United States—61.6. However, as shown in Table 9-10, teenage fertility in the United States decreased slightly after 1973, and even though the decline was more rapid for blacks than for whites, the fertility rates in 1978 remained three times higher for black teenagers than for whites.

Table 9-6 1981 World Population Data

	Population Estimate, Mid-1981 (millions)	Crude Birth Rate	Crude Death Rate	Rate of Natural Increase (annual, %)	Number of Years to Double Population (at current rate)	Population Projected for 2000 (millions)	Infant Mortality Rate	Total Fertility Rate	Population under Age 15 (%)	Population under Age 64 (%)	Life Expectancy at Birth (years)	Urban Population (%)	Persons per Sq. Kilometer of Arable Land	Per Capita Gross National Product (US$)
WORLD	4,492	28	11	1.7	41	6,095	97	3.7	35	6	62	41	98	2,340
MORE DEVELOPED	1,144	16	9	0.6	113	1,255	20	2.0	24	11	72	71	59	7,260
LESS DEVELOPED	3,348	32	12	2.1	34	4,840	109	4.3	39	4	58	30	128	560
LESS DEVELOPED (Excl. China)	2,363	38	14	2.4	29	3,640	120	5.3	42	3	54	32	103	710
AFRICA	486	46	17	2.9	24	833	142	6.4	45	3	49	28	50	620
ASIA	2,608	29	11	1.8	39	3,564	102	3.9	37	4	60	28	243	800
EUROPE	486	14	10	0.4	178	511	17	1.9	23	13	72	71	212	6,820
NORTH AMERICA	254	16	9	0.7	95	286	13	1.8	23	11	74	74	51	10,710
LATIN AMERICA	366	32	9	2.3	30	562	75	4.4	40	4	64	63	54	1,580
USSR	268	18	10	0.8	86	310	36	2.3	26	9	69	65	44	4,110
OCEANIA	23	21	8	1.3	54	30	51	2.7	30	8	69	71	5	7,080

Source: Reprinted from *World Population: Toward the Next Century*, with permission of the Population Reference Bureau, Inc., Washington, D.C., © November 1981, 8-11.

Table 9-7 United States Population by Age, 1970 and 1980

Age Group	1970	1980
Under 5	8.4%	7.2%
5-9	9.8	7.3
10-14	10.2	8.0
15-19	9.4	9.3
20-24	8.1	9.4
25-34	12.3	16.3
35-44	11.4	11.6
45-54	11.4	10.2
55-64	9.1	9.5
over 64	9.9	11.2
Median Age	28.1	30.2

Source: Reprinted from *American Demographics* with permission of *American Demographics*, © April 1980, Vol. 2, no. 4, 12.

DEMOGRAPHIC TRENDS' IMPACT ON UTILIZATION

As noted extensively throughout this book, many demographic characteristics of the population are related to health, disease, and service utilization. Therefore, it is obvious that demographic trends have definite health policy implications. This section briefly examines, for illustrative purposes, the impact on the health care

Table 9-8 Crude Birth Rates and General Fertility Rates, U.S., 1950-1980

	Crude Birth Rate per 1,000 population	General Fertility Rate per 1,000 women 15-44
1950	24.1	106.2
1955	25.0	118.3
1960	23.7	118.0
1965	19.4	96.6
1970	18.4	87.9
1975	14.8	66.7
1977	15.4	67.8
1978	15.3	66.6
1979	15.8	68.0
1980	16.2	69.2

Source: Health, United States, 1982, U.S. Department of Health and Human Services, Public Health Service, Publication No. (PHS) 83-1232 (Washington, D.C.: U.S. Government Printing Office, 1983), 42-44.

Figure 9-3 Age-Specific Fertility Rates, U.S., 1955-1978

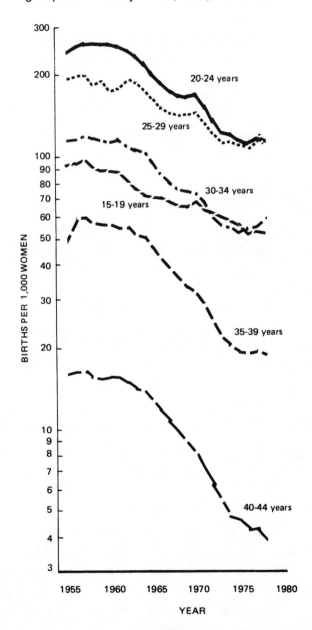

Source: Reprinted from *Health, United States, 1980,* U.S. Department of Health and Human Services, Public Health Service, National Center for Health Statistics, December 1980, 17.

Table 9-9 Fertility Rates and Percent of All Births for Women under 20 Years of Age

Selected Countries, Selected Years 1972-1976

Country and year	Births per 1,000 Women Under 20 years	Percent of All Births
Canada (1975)	33.8	11.0
United States (1976)	54.7	18.0
Sweden (1976)	25.0	6.6
England and Wales (1976)	32.4	9.9
Netherlands (1976)	11.3	3.7
German Democratic Republic (1975)	61.6	21.8
German Federal Republic (1976)	19.9	7.5
France (1972)	28.8	6.7
Switzerland (1976)	12.4	3.9
Italy (1974)	50.7	11.3
Israel (1975)	43.7	7.2
Japan (1976)	3.7	0.8
Australia (1975)	40.9	10.4

Source: Reprinted from Health, United States, 1980, U.S. Department of Health and Human Services, Public Health Service, National Center for Health Statistics, December 1980, 19.

Table 9-10 Race-Specific Teenage Fertility Rates, U.S., 1970-1978

Age Groups Years	TOTAL			WHITE			BLACK		
	10-14	15-17	18-19	10-14	15-17	18-19	10-14	15-17	18-19
1970	1.2	38.8	114.7	0.5	29.2	101.5	5.2	101.4	204.9
1971	1.1	38.3	105.6	0.5	28.6	92.4	5.1	99.7	193.8
1972	1.2	39.2	97.3	0.5	29.4	84.5	5.1	99.9	181.7
1973	1.3	38.9	91.8	0.6	29.5	79.6	5.4	96.8	169.5
1974	1.2	37.7	89.3	0.6	29.0	77.7	5.0	91.0	162.0
1975	1.3	36.6	85.7	0.6	28.3	74.4	5.1	86.6	156.0
1976	1.2	34.6	81.3	0.6	26.7	70.7	4.7	81.5	146.8
1977	1.2	34.5	81.9	0.6	26.5	71.1	4.7	81.2	147.6
1978	1.2	32.9	81.0	0.6	25.4	70.1	4.4	76.6	145.0

Source: Reprinted from Health, United States, 1981, U.S. Department of Health and Human Services, Public Health Service, National Center for Health Statistics, December 1981, 102.

system of two important demographics trends: (1) the post-World War II baby boom and (2) the aging of the population.

The Baby Boom

Between 1946 and 1964, 76.4 million babies were born in the United States, one-third of the present population. This postwar increase in the fertility rate occurred in many countries, including Canada, New Zealand, Australia, and the U.S.S.R. The baby boom created unusually large cohorts of births compared to those of the 1930s and early 1940s and to the baby bust years of the 1960s and 1970s.[60] As one author puts it, the boom generation can be thought of "as a moving bulge in the population that, like a pig swallowed by a python, causes stretch marks and discomfort along the way."[61]

The moving through time of the baby boom cohort (Figure 9-4) by the early 1980s was mostly between 20 and 30. The small proportion of the population 45 to 49 reflects the Depression cohort, while the drop in fertility in more recent years is shown in the baby bust cohort under 20. The population distribution over 50 resembles a pyramid as older age groups are thinned by death.

The fact that there was a great upsurge in fertility between 1945 and 1960 is affecting all aspects of people's daily lives. Contrary to the Depression or the "good times" cohort, which, "by virtue of this smaller number, upon encountering each inpatient life cycle event, have experienced relative abundance,"[62] the baby boom cohort has been experiencing and can expect problems and frustrations as it passes through the life cycle.[63] Problems of overcrowded classrooms and shortages of teachers through the 1960s and 1970s, and school closings and unemployment problems in the 1980s are all related directly to the baby boom.

The recent increase in the number of births and in the crude birth rate also is caused by the baby boom of the 1950s. This so-called "echo" effect of the baby boom simply results from the fact that the women of that era now are in the prime childbearing ages of 20 to 29. Thus, annual birth totals were expected to rise during the 1980s even if the fertility rate remained at around 1.8 births per woman.[64] Number of births will remain high during the early 1990s but, as Figure 9-4 projects, they should then decrease (fertility rates remaining constant) since the baby bust cohort will be in prime childbearing ages from 1995 to 2005. From then on, the number of births should remain constant at the early 1990s level since the age-sex pyramid will assume a stationary, rectangular profile.

As the baby boom generation ages and as fertility remains low, the median age of the population is pushed up, thus artificially raising the crude death rate.[65] When the baby boom cohort becomes elderly, starting in 2020, crude death rates will go up even more, as some 15 percent of the population then will be 65 or over compared to 11 percent in 1980.

Figure 9-4 Population Age-Sex Pyramids, U.S., 1960-2050

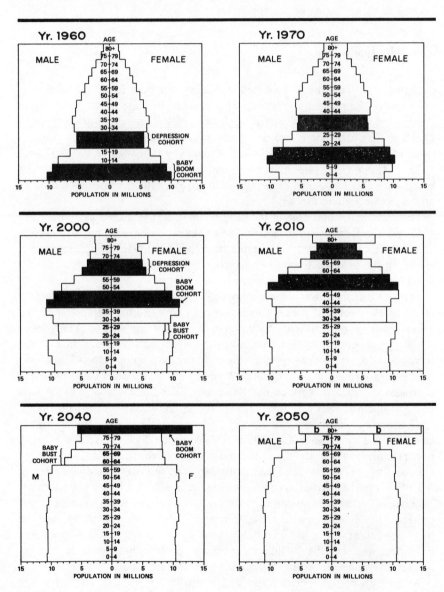

Read Figure 9-4 across two pages

Figure 9-4 continued

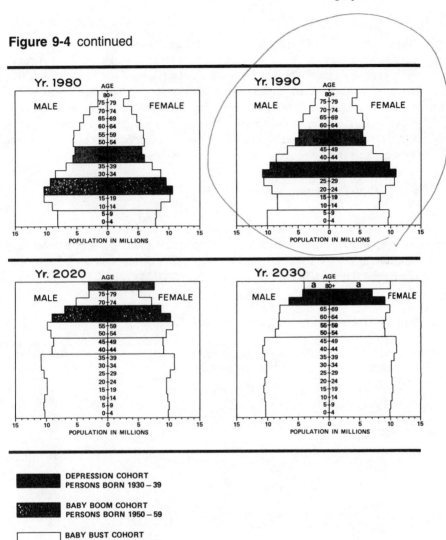

DEPRESSION COHORT
PERSONS BORN 1930 – 39

BABY BOOM COHORT
PERSONS BORN 1950 – 59

BABY BUST COHORT
PERSONS BORN 1970 – 79

Source: Reprinted From "America's Baby Boom Generation: The Fateful Bulge," by L.F. Bovrier with permission of *Population Bulletin,* 35, no. 1, © April 1980, 18-19.

Meanwhile, using the age-specific mortality and morbidity figures in Chapter 5, it can be projected that if rates for these factors remain constant, the number of motor vehicle accidents, homicides, suicides, depressions, and heart diseases will increase through the 1990s because the baby boom cohort then will be between 30 and 40. Similarly, morbidity rates remaining constant, the prevalence of cancers, heart diseases, stroke, and respiratory conditions should increase during the early 2000s if age was the only determinant. Obviously other factors operate to change disease patterns.

Aging of the Population—the Senior Boom

With declining birth rates and a progressively aging population, people 65 and over (particularly those 75 and over), are the fastest growing group in America.[66] As shown in Table 9-11, the proportion of the United States population 65 and over rose from 4.0 percent in 1900 to 11.2 percent in 1980. As a result of low birth rates

Table 9-11 Percent of Population 65 and Over, U.S., 1900–2040

Year	% of Total Population Aged 65 and Over	Median Age of Total Population
Estimates		
1900	4.1	22.9
1910	4.3	24.1
1920	4.7	25.3
1930	5.5	26.5
1940	6.9	29.0
1950	8.2	30.2
1960	9.3	29.5
1970	9.9	28.1
1980	11.2	30.2
Projections		
1990	12.1 (11.7–12.6)*	32.8 (31.4–33.7)*
2000	12.2 (11.3–12.9)	35.5 (32.5–37.3)
2010	12.7 (11.1–13.9)	36.6 (31.1–40.2)
2020	15.5 (12.7–17.8)	37.0 (31.4–41.7)
2030	18.3 (14.0–22.1)	38.0 (31.2–43.2)
2040	17.8 (12.5–22.8)	37.8 (30.7–43.9)

*High and low rates of population projection

Source: "America's Elderly in the 1980's," by Beth J. Soldo. Population Reference Bureau, Vol. 35, no. 4 (November 1980): 9.

and greater life expectancy, the proportion of elderly is expected to go up to 12 percent in 1990.

Because of the effects of the small Depression cohorts, this growth will slow in the 1990s and in the first decade of the 2000s. Thereafter, however, the baby boom of the 1950s will become a senior boom and the proportion of the population over 65 will grow rapidly to 15 percent in 2020 and 18 percent in 2030. After 2030, that group probably will fall sharply again as the baby bust cohorts of the 1960s and 1970s become 65 and over.[67]

In the United States, life expectancy at age 65 is more than 14 years for men and 18 years for women. Age-specific death rates for males 65 years and over declined by almost 30 percent between 1940 and 1978, for females approximately 40 percent.[68]

The leading causes of death in the elderly were the same in 1978 as in 1950, with heart disease, cancer, and stroke accounting for 75 percent.[69] Mortality trends from heart disease parallel the decline for all causes combined. Death rates from stroke have been falling even more rapidly than those from heart disease. However, death rates from cancer have been rising, with rapid increases in recent years resulting primarily from lung cancer.

Older people naturally require more health and social services than the general population, especially after age 75. Arthritis and rheumatism, followed closely by heart conditions, are the most common causes of activity limitation at ages 65 and over.[70] A study reported in early 1982 that 39 percent of more than 4,200 individuals age 65 and older had some form of hypertension and in 25 percent of these it was either untreated or poorly controlled.[71] Hearing disease affects 21 percent of the elderly population.[72]

These problems are important since they often lead to withdrawal, isolation, depression, further disability, and dependence.[73] Finally, approximately half the elderly individuals have no teeth, no dentures, or dentures that fit poorly, or that they do not wear,[74] predisposing them to malnutrition and increasing their already high susceptibility to disease and disability.[75]

Health services utilization is higher among the elderly population. In 1980 in the United States, persons at age 65 and over averaged 6.4 physician visits during the year as against 5.1 for those 45 to 64 and 4.4 for those under 45.[76] Rates of hospital utilization also are much higher for the elderly, who occupy more than 30 percent of acute care beds while comprising only 16 percent of the total population.[77] Although females in the general population have much higher rates of hospital utilization than males, elderly females have much lower rates.[78]

The impact of the aging on health care utilization is, of course, highly dependent upon this group's health. However, it is not easy to determine what changes are related to age and occur in everyone and which ones are pathologic and represent the development of disease.[79] Death, disease, and disability in the older population stem mostly from chronic conditions. These tend to originate early in life and develop gradually.

This does not mean, however, that the elderly population in the years to come will be a sicker one.[80] Fries predicts a continued decline in premature death resulting from chronic conditions and the emergence of a pattern of natural death at the end of a natural life span.[81] As he points out, some chronic illnesses definitely can be postponed. Elimination of cigarette smoking greatly delays the date of onset of emphysema and reduces the risk of lung cancer.

The decline in mortality rates, which is caused principally by a drop in arteriosclerosis and cerebrovascular disease, is the first demonstration of a national decrease in mortality rates from a major chronic disease. It is attributed by most observers to changes in life style (primary prevention) and to better treatment of hypertension (secondary prevention).[82] Fries suggests that through further life style changes, chronic illnesses may be postponed and morbidity may be compressed until near the end of the life span (which he calculates as, ideally, 85 years).

The impact the aging of the population will have on the health care system thus is dependent on present health policy. An effective health care policy for the elderly should stress health maintenance and promotion, disease prevention, comprehensive and integrated health and social services, and personal autonomy and social interaction.[83, 84, 85]

SUMMARY

Demography is one of the disciplines necessary for the use of epidemiology in health services management. It supplies the tools for the analysis of population composition and distribution, of changes in its components, and for the estimation and projection of its future.

All of these are essential for an epidemiological approach to health services management since health, disease, and utilization all are related to population characteristics. Furthermore, demographers supply health services managers with some of the tools, including methods for estimating and projecting population, needed to relate the delivery of health services to the population. Accompanying any trend in population demographics is a health care management implication.

NOTES

1. E.M. Murphy, *World Population: Toward the Next Century* (Washington, D.C.: Population Reference Bureau, Inc., November 1981), 7.

2. U.S. Bureau of the Census, *The Methods and Materials of Demography,* 4th ed., by Henry S. Shyrock, Jacob S. Siegel, and Associates (Washington, D.C.: U.S. Government Printing Office, June 1980), 91.

3. A. Haupt and T.T. Kane, *Population Handbook,* Int'l. ed. (Washington, D.C.: Population Reference Bureau, Inc. 1980), 76.

4. Ibid.

5. Ibid.

6. D. Ewbank and J.D. Wray, "Population and Public Health," in *Maxcy-Rosenau Public Health and Preventive Medicine,* 11th ed., ed. J.M. Last (New York, Appleton-Century-Crofts, Inc., 1980), 1512.

7. Ibid.

8. J. Coale, "How a Population Ages or Grows Younger," in *Population: The Vital Revolution,* ed. R. Freedman (New York: Anchor Press, 1964), 47-58.

9. U.S. Bureau of the Census, *Methods and Materials,* 284.

10. U.S. Bureau of the Census, *Methods and Materials,* 299.

11. U.S. Bureau of the Census, *Methods and Materials,* 300.

12. Haupt and Kane, *Population Handbook,* 51.

13. Ibid., 53.

14. Ibid., 51.

15. U.S. Office of Management and Budget, Office of Statistical Standards, *Standard Metropolitan Statistical Areas,* 1-3.

16. U.S. Department of Health and Human Services, Public Health Service, *Geographic Patterns in the Risk of Dying and Associated Factors,* Vital and Health Statistics Analytical Studies, Series 3, no. 18 (Public Health Service, 1980), 48.

17. G.C. Myers and K.G. Mantar, "The Structure of Urban Mortality: A Methodological Study of Hannover, Germany," *International Journal of Epidemiology,* 6 (September 1977): 203-213.

18. A.S. Boote, "How to Get More from Demographic Analysis," *American Demographics,* June 1981, 30-33.

19. H. Assael, "Segmenting Markets by Group Purchasing Behavior: An Application of the A.I.D. Technique," *Journal of Marketing Research* 7 (May 1970): 153-158.

20. U.S. Bureau of the Census, *Methods and Materials,* 462.

21. G.J. Wunsch and M.G. Termote, *Introduction to Demographic Analysis—Principles and Methods* (New York: Plenum Press, 1978), 143.

22. Wunsch and Termote, *Introduction to Demographic Analysis,* 143.

23. Haupt and Kane, *Population Handbook,* 28.

24. U.S. Bureau of the Census, *Methods and Materials,* 472.

25. Ewbank and Wray, "Population and Public Health," 1507.

26. U.S. Bureau of the Census, *Methods and Materials,* 473.

27. Haupt and Kane, *Population Handbook,* 29.

28. Ibid.

29. Ewbank and Wray, "Population and Public Health," 1508.

30. Haupt and Kane, *Population Handbook,* 31.

31. Ewbank and Wray, "Population and Public Health," 1509.

32. Haupt and Kane, *Population Handbook,* 32.

33. U.S. Bureau of the Census, *Methods and Materials,* 579.

34. Ibid.

35. Haupt and Kane, *Population Handbook,* 48.

36. U.S. Bureau of the Census, *Methods and Materials*, 603.

37. Haupt and Kane, *Population Handbook*, 50.

38. Ibid., 54.

39. Ibid., 55.

40. M.J. Batutis, "Estimating Population I," *American Demographics*, April 1982, 3-5.

41. M.J. Batutis, "Estimating Population II," *American Demographics*, May 1982, 38-40.

42. Batutis, "Estimating Population I," 3-5.

43. R.C. Atchley, "A Short-Cut Method for Estimating the Population of Metropolitan Areas," *Journal of the American Institute of Planners* 34 (1968): 259-262.

44. L.F. Bouvier, "Estimating Post-Censal Populations of Counties," *Journal of the American Institute of Planners* 37 (1971), 45-46.

45. Ibid.

46. U.S. Bureau of the Census, *Methods and Materials*, 752.

47. J.V. Grauman, "Population Estimates and Projections," in *The Study of Population*, ed. P.M. Hauser and O.D. Duncan (Chicago: The University of Chicago Press, 1959), 544-575.

48. Haupt and Kane, *Population Handbook*, 11.

49. U.S. Bureau of the Census, *Methods and Materials*, 771.

50. Ibid., Chapter 24.

51. D.B. Pittenger, *Projecting State and Local Populations* (Cambridge, Mass.: Ballinger Publishing Company, 1976), 246.

52. D.A. Kruekeberg and A.L. Silvers, *Urban Planning Analysis, Methods and Models* (New York: John Wiley & Sons, Inc., 1974), 259-273.

53. R. Irwin, "Methods on Data Sources for Population Projections of Small Areas," in *Population Forecasting for Small Areas*. Proceedings of a conference of Oak Ridge (Tenn.) Associated Universities, October 1977, 15-26.

54. Statistics Canada, *How Communities Can Use Statistics* (Ottawa: Minister of Supply and Services, June 1981), 53.

55. Statistics Canada.

56. *American Demographics*, February 1981, 15-21.

57. "Changes in the Age Profile of the Population," Metropolitan Life Insurance Company *Statistical Bulletin* 62, no. 3 (July-September 1981): 12.

58. Alvin P. Sanoff, "As Americans Cope With a Changing Population," *U.S. News & World Report*, 9 Aug. 1982, 27.

59. J.A. Weed, "Divorce: Americans' Style," *American Demographics*, March 1982, 12-17.

60. Haupt and Kane, *Population Handbook*, 26.

61. L.Y. Jones, *Great Expectations: America and the Baby Boom Generation* (New York: Ballantine Books, 1982), 512.

62. C.L. Harter, "The 'Good Times' Cohort of the 1930s," *Population Reference Bureau Report* 3, no. 3 (April 1977): 4.

63. L.F. Bouvier, "America's Baby Boom Generation: The Fateful Bulge," *Population Bulletin* 35, no. 1 (April 1980): 17.

64. Ibid., 15.

65. Ibid.

66. B.J. Soldo, "America's Elderly in the 1980s," *Population Bulletin* 35, no. 4 (November 1980): 3.

67. Ibid., 7.

68. U.S. Public Health Service, *Health, United States, 1981* (Hyattsville, Md: U.S. Department of Health and Human Services, National Center for Health Statistics, December 1981), 17.

69. Ibid.

70. "Health of the Elderly," Metropolitan Life Insurance Company, *Statistical Bulletin* 63, no. 1 (January-March 1982): 3.

71. W.E. Hale et al., "Screening for Hypertension in an Elderly Population: Report from the Dunedin Program," *Journal of the American Geriatrics Society* 29 (1981): 123-125.

72. A.R. Somers, "The High Cost of Care for the Elderly: Diagnosis, Prognosis, and Some Suggestions for Therapy," *Journal of Health Politics and Law* 3 (1978): 163-180.

73. J.G. Ouslander and J.C. Beck, "Defining the Health Problems of the Elderly," *Annual Review of Public Health* 3 (1982): 55-83.

74. M.G. Kovar, "Health of the Elderly and the Use of Health Services," *Public Health Reports,* no. 1 (1977): 9-19.

75. Ouslander and Beck, "Defining Health Problems," 65.

76. Kovar, "Health of the Elderly," 5.

77. Soldo, "America's Elderly," 18.

78. L.O. Stone and S. Fletcher, *A Profile of Canada's Older Population* (Montreal: The Institute for Research on Public Policy, 1980), 39.

79. Ouslander and Beck, "Defining Health Problems," 60.

80. *Health, United States, 1981,* 23.

81. J.F. Fries, "Aging, Natural Death, and the Compression of Morbidity," *The New England Journal of Medicine* 303, no. 3 (July 17, 1980): 130-135.

82. M.P. Stern, "The Recent Decline in Ischemic Heart Disease Mortality," *Annals of Internal Medicine* 91 (1979): 630-640.

83. A.R. Somers, "Demographics Can Help Guide Health Policy," *Hospitals,* JAHA 54 (May 16, 1980): 67-72.

84. Beth J. Soldo, "America's Elderly in the 1980's," Population Reference Bureau, *Population Bulletin* 35, no. 4 (November 1981).

85. Fries, "Aging, Natural Death," 130-135.

Chapter 10

Marketing, Epidemiology, and Management

MARKETING: A MANAGEMENT TOOL

The management of health services should be population-based; epidemiology offers principles and methods to guide such decision making. This chapter examines how marketing also can contribute to epidemiologically oriented health services management.

The marketing of health services may well be the most popular topic in the health care organization literature. Numerous textbooks[1, 2, 3, 4, 5] and literally hundreds of articles have been published on this topic in recent years. This chapter cannot hope to present all that could be discussed on this topic. Therefore, it is limited to a broad discussion of marketing and its application to health services delivery. The object is to show that the same basic principles lie behind both the marketing and epidemiological approaches to the management of health services and that the combination of the two can lead to optimal population-based management.

There is in fact a close affinity and complementarity between epidemiology and marketing as they relate to health services management. Both aim at strengthening the fit between the health services offered and the needs of the population. Both thus provide a set of principles and tools that can be used to manage the delivery of health services in a more equitable, appropriate, effective, and efficient way.

WHAT IS MARKETING?

Marketing can be conceived of as a set of methods aiming at reconciling the resources and production capacity of an organization with the needs and preferences of the consumers. Marketing theory is based on a systemic view of organizations in which their functioning is viewed in terms of exchanges.

An exchange relationship requires two things:[6] (1) a constituency—that is, some person, group, or organization with whom an exchange is to be accomplished; and (2) a value—that is, "something" that is exchanged by the organization and by the constituency.

In other words, an exchange relationship involves the offering of something of value, such as a product or service, to someone who is willing to exchange it for something else of value, such as money or time.[7] Marketing offers a structure to analyze, predict, and manage exchanges to the benefit of all concerned. In this usage, marketing is defined simply as the conscious, systematic approach to the planning, implementation, and evaluation of the exchange relationships of an organization.[8]

Marketing is based on the fundamental assumption that if each constituency can be identified and analyzed, and if each exchange can be examined and controlled, the organization will attain its objectives (profit or other) more effectively. An important corollary of the model is that exchanges are maximized if and only if supply is matched with demand—if the product (or service) of the organization coincides with the needs, wants, and desires of the consumers. As Peter Drucker writes, "the aim of marketing is to make selling superfluous."[9] Philip Kotler similarly states that "marketing is the philosophical alternative to force."[10]

The negative connotation often attached to this subject—that marketing creates needs—results from a misconception of its modern orientation. Although it may well be possible to find organizations with a product orientation, that is, entities in which production precedes marketing, they are likely to fail because they are trying to impose on a market a product (or service or idea) that is not matched to the consumer's needs or wants.

To the contrary, modern theory holds that marketing's only effective form involves consumer orientation through a strategic or integrated approach in which the marketing function precedes and embodies production and in which the product is matched to needs.

Another inherent feature of modern or strategic marketing is the identification and selection of specific subgroups of the constituency, or target markets. Any attempt at serving every possible market undoubtedly will be in vain. The correct marketing process is one that includes the decision as to which possible market segments can best be served and focuses on them.

Marketing thus is not selling or publicity. It is not an after-the-fact way of promoting a product. Rather, it is a planned activity aimed at achieving organizational objectives through the satisfaction of needs and wants of consumers (patients, in the health care field). Marketing takes place long before any selling, and precedes and directs production.

MARKETING TERMINOLOGY

Three particularly important marketing concepts need to be defined at some length: the organization's publics, its markets, and its marketing mix.

The Publics of an Organization

A public is any distinct group that has an actual or potential interest or impact on an organization—in this instance, the health care institution.[11] The sum of all the publics constitutes the entity's immediate environment. The publics are all of the internal and external individuals or groups that influence or potentially could influence the organization.[12]

The Markets of an Organization

A market is a public that is involved (or might realistically become involved) in an exchange relationship with the organization. It is composed of a distinct set of people and/or entities that have or will have resources (values) that they want to exchange (or might be willing to exchange) for something they want and that the organization has (or will have). In the health care marketing literature, markets often are referred to as constituencies.[13] Both of these terms are used interchangeably here.

As Kotler wrote:

> If the organization wishes to attract certain resources from that public through offering a set of benefits in exchange, then the organization is taking a "marketing viewpoint" toward that public. Once the organization starts thinking in terms of trading values with that public, it is viewing the public as a market.[14]

The markets of a health care organization can be of four types.[15]

1. the external markets, which may include supporters, suppliers, regulators, and the community at large
2. the internal markets, including the board of trustees, the employees, the physicians (including both those with hospital privileges and referring physicians), and the volunteers
3. the client markets, including patients and other consumers such as purchasers of services such as laboratory tests, radiology examinations, blood, etc. (Other publics that benefit indirectly from services provided by the hospital, such as relatives of patients and members of the constituency whose health is affected by environmental, occupational, prevention, and health education programs the institution undertakes, also can be considered as client markets.)
4. the competitors or colleagues markets—other health care providers or the producers of health-related services and products.

A marketing program can be developed for each of these constituencies. The hospital can engage in patient marketing, physician marketing, community marketing, donor marketing, public health marketing, etc. A hospital short of nurses can engage in nurse marketing, and so on. Although the focus here is on patient marketing, precisely the same process can be used to develop effective exchange relationships with any markets.

The Marketing Mix

The marketing process involves four distinct groups of elements, together referred to as the marketing mix. They represent forces or variables that the organization can control or influence to achieve its objectives in the target market.[16] The four groups of elements are known traditionally as the four Ps: product, place, price, and promotion. The organization can devise different combinations of these to optimize exchanges with a given target market. The marketing mix of course must be adapted to each target.

Marketing often has been regarded erroneously as involving only promotion; that is the genesis of the negative public attitude toward it. The marketing mix concept suggests that effective results will occur only through careful consideration and adaptation of the product, the place of exchange, the price, and finally the promotion, to the target market.

Under the term product are included all the characteristics of what the organization offers to exchange with the target market. These include quality, features, options, styles, brand names, packaging, sizes, warranties, returns, etc. Each of these should be carefully adapted to the needs, wants, and desires of the target.

In health services marketing, or more precisely in patient marketing, the products are the services to be delivered. These should be (1) geared to the health needs of the constituency, (2) of high quality, (3) adapted to the patients' social characteristics (culture, ethnicity, language, etc.), and so on. As part of the exchange process between the hospital and its patients, such services as nursing, dietary, housekeeping, etc., also are included. Clearly, this approach requires the knowledge of descriptive epidemiology–person.

Place refers to the location where the product or services are delivered (exchanged). Such variables as geographical and temporal accessibility and availability (see Chapter 7) are important place variables to be considered in patient health services marketing. Again, descriptive epidemiology—place and time—is an important aspect to marketing.

Price refers to what earlier was called financial accessibility (Chapter 8). It includes all direct and indirect costs that the patient must bear in the exchange of services.

Finally, promotion refers to the causal, informative, or persuasive communication by the organization to the target market. Persuasive communication occurs when the institution consciously develops its messages (publicity, advertising) to have a calculated impact on the attitude and/or behavior of the target market.[17] Promotion generally has four objectives:[18]

1. to inform and educate consumers as to the existence of a product (or service) and its capabilities
2. to remind present and former users of the product's continuing existence
3. to persuade prospective purchasers that the product is worth buying
4. to inform consumers of where and how to obtain and use the product.

THE MARKETING PROCESS

Strategic or integrated marketing (consumer oriented as opposed to product oriented) can be defined as a managerial process of identifying, analyzing, choosing, and exploiting marketing opportunities to fulfill the organization's mission and objectives.[19] Although no two authors describe the marketing process in exactly the same way, all definitions include three fundamental components or steps:

1. a research and analysis component in which the environment, the competition, and the potential markets are identified and analyzed and in which target markets are selected
2. an implementation or operational component in which programs are elaborated and the marketing mix is developed
3. an evaluation and control component in which the exchange relationship is monitored and appropriate corrective actions are taken as needed.

These three basic components are illustrated in Figure 10-1. As can be seen, the research and analysis component actually includes many different analyses: of the environment; of the market, including its structure, opportunities, and targeting; of the competition; and of the institution's resources. Furthermore, all of these serve as inputs into the analysis of the organization's portfolio. Programs then are set up and the marketing mix is developed. The last stage of the marketing process consists of the monitoring, control, and evaluation of the exchanges (delivery of services).

MARKETING'S CONTRIBUTIONS TO HEALTH SERVICES MANAGEMENT

The epidemiological approach to health services management requires that it be population based and that health be conceptualized as resulting from four broad

Figure 10-1 The Strategic Marketing Process

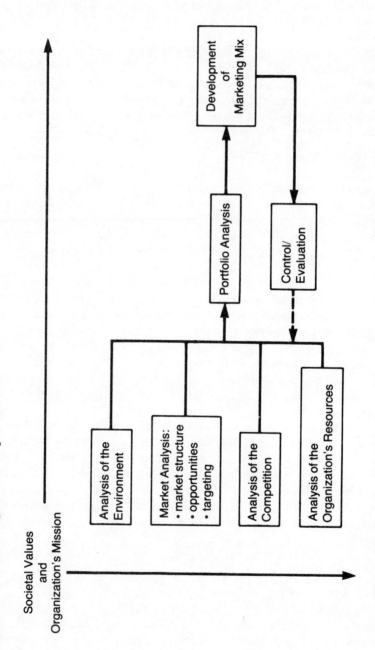

Source: Reprinted from "Le marketing et la planification des services de santé" by Francois Champagne with permission of *Administration Hospitalière et Sociale,* vol. 27, no. 5, September–October 1981.

determinants—human biology, life style, environment, and health care organization). Chapter 3 discussed how these two general epidemiological principles can be incorporated into the management process to guide what has been referred to as a global planning process (Figure 3-4 and Tables 3-1 and 3-3, supra.). Marketing is essentially a process complementary to this global (or strategic) planning process, in effect a set of principles and techniques that can be used to enhance planning.

Furthermore, since, as just discussed, strategic or integrated marketing is by definition consumer oriented and geared to the needs, wants, and desires of users, it can be adopted advantageously by managers in conjunction with epidemiology to achieve sound and effective population based operation of health services.

Figure 10-2 illustrates how the marketing process can be integrated with the global planning process described in Chapter 3 and consequently with epidemiologically oriented management. The marketing analyses of the environ-

Figure 10-2 Marketing's Contribution to Strategic Health Planning

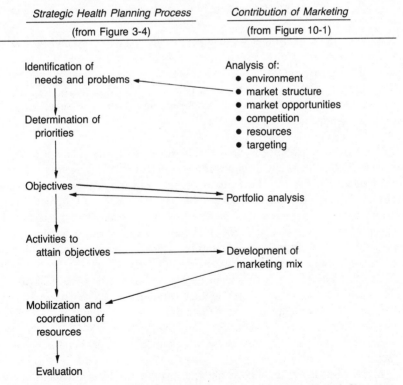

Source: Reprinted from "Le marketing et la planification des services de santé" by Francois Champagne with permission of *Administration Hospitalière et Sociale,* vol. 27, no. 5, September-October 1981,

ment, the market, the competition, and the resources, and the resulting identification of target markets, all contribute to the identification of health needs and problems. The planning process then moves on to the determination of priorities and the setting of objectives, after which portfolio analysis can be conducted. Activities and programs then are planned and the marketing mix devised.

Analysis of the Environment

The organization's thorough understanding and knowledge of its environment and its subsequent flexibility and adaptation is an essential prerequisite to the success of the marketing and planning effort.

A distinction can be made between an organization's macroenvironment and its microenvironment. Its microenvironment consists in what were described earlier as its publics. These include any distinct groups that have an actual or potential interest or impact on an institution. Since, as noted previously, the difference between a public and a market is that the organization is viewing the market as a potential exchange partner, the four categories that describe an institution's markets also can be used to define its publics (its microenvironment). These involve:

1. the external environment, including the general population, the news media, the interest groups, the regulatory agencies, etc.
2. the internal environment, consisting of the internal markets (board, employees, staff, volunteers)
3. the external market environment, including clients and suppliers
4. the competitive environment.

The macroenvironment consists of large-scale uncontrollable fundamental forces that may shape opportunities or pose threats to the organization.[20] These can be divided into five broad categories of factors: demographic, economic, technological, political/legal, and cultural/behavioral.[21, 22] It is through the microenvironment that the macroenvironment indirectly influences the organization. Each of the macroenvironmental factors influences every one of the publics. Detailed discussion of the impact of each dimension of the macroenvironment on the publics of a health care organization can be found elsewhere.[23, 24]

The analysis of the environment consists of forecasting the behavior of its different factors and their impact on the institution. Some categories of factors in the macroenvironment, such as demographic and economic, can be forecast quantitatively with some accuracy. A qualitative approach definitively is more appropriate in forecasting technological, political/legal, and cultural/behavioral factors.

In any case, several qualitative and quantitative forecasting methods have been developed in the social sciences[25, 26] and have been applied to the health field.[27, 28]

Techniques such as Delphi and nominal groups (see Chapter 3) can be used by any health care organization.

The analysis of the macroenvironment, or macroenvironmental audit, includes the following steps:[29, 30]

- The major factors in the five dimensions of the macroenvironment should be listed.
- The major trends in each factor should be determined and described.
- The impact and implications of these trends for the organization should be estimated.
- The environmental factors should be ranked as to the importance of the impact and implications of their trends on the organization.
  1. Environmental factors should be sorted into two groups: those with a potentially positive impact and those with potentially negative implications.
  2. The list of factors (both positive and negative) should be shortened as much as possible by eliminating those whose impact on the organization is not thought to be truly critical.

    It sometimes is recommended not to keep more than the two or three most important factors in each of the two subgroups (positive and negative). The question should always be raised whether too many factors have been included. The aim is to come up with a short list of truly critical factors.

- The potential organizational responses to the factors that have been kept in both sub-groups should be determined, i.e., the implications of the critical factors should be converted into specific opportunities and threats (negative trends). In which ways can the organization adapt itself to the major trends; that is, how can positive trends be translated into opportunities and how can the institution avoid threats? A specific evaluation of each potential response must be conducted. It should be noted that many environmental crises can represent opportunities for the organization. For example, a mandatory wage-control program may induce unions and management to negotiate for fringe benefits including prepaid health insurance plans rather than for pay increases.

Trends in the institution's publics or microenvironment can be analyzed in a similar manner. (Description of the trends in the different markets are considered in the next section.)

The remaining important parts of the microenvironmental audit are the analyses of competition and resources. Because of their special importance to the marketing process and to distinguish them from the macroenvironmental analyses, these are shown in Figures 10-1 and 10-2 as separate from environmental analyses. However, they are conducted in basically the same way.

Analysis of the competition involves the collection of basic information about other organizations or individuals providing comparable services.[31] Even if the notion of rivals may seem unbecoming to the health field, competition nevertheless does exist, even among nonprofit institutions. In any case, even if health services managers do not want to think of other providers in their area as competitors, they still must identify the needs of the population, specifically including what others are doing, in determining service gaps or market opportunities (see Chapters 3 and 8).

The institution also should conduct a resource analysis or resource audit.[32] This involves listing the major organizational resources—people, money, facilities, technology, and market assets. Each resource can be evaluated as constituting a strength (high, medium, low) or a weakness (low, medium, high). This resource audit also serves as an input in the determination of market opportunities since the facility should avoid getting involved in those for which its resources are weak or inadequate and concentrate on those for which it has distinctive competences.

Many organizations may hesitate to perform environmental analyses, and particularly macroenvironmental audits, since accuracy of prediction often is doubtful. The opinion here is that any environmental analysis, even if it is informal and tentative, will promote organizational flexibility and capacity of adaptation to environmental threats and opportunities.

The important point is that health services managers' adoption of the marketing approach, including the effort to forecast and predict the environment and analyze the competition and resources, can only increase the adaptation of the institution's services to the needs of its population.

Analysis of the Market

Analysis of the market consists of three distinct parts: the market structure analysis, the market opportunity analysis (or consumer analysis), and the target market selection.

Market Structure Analysis

This refers to the identification and analysis of the organization's markets. In the initial step, the publics who are (actual markets) and those who realistically might become (potential markets) involved in an exchange relationship with the institution must be defined and identified.

For a hospital, the actual markets can be determined with a patient-origin study, while the potential markets can be ascertained on a geographical/political basis or on a service capacity basis (see Chapter 8).

Actual and potential markets then should be broken down into distinct and homogenous subgroups. This is called market segmentation. Its aim is to facilitate the analysis of actual and potential exchanges in an effort to improve their effectiveness. Since each market is composed of a wide variety of individuals (or groups or organizations), and since on the other hand it is not realistic to consider each individual as a separate market, it is advisable to subdivide each market into separate groupings or segments of individuals with common characteristics.

The criteria of segmentation should be the homogeneity within each segment and the heterogeneity among the different segments. A market segment is a grouping of individuals who might be expected to behave differently than another market segment in the exchange relationship.

Three classes of variables can be used for market segmentation:

1. Geographic segmentation refers to the grouping of people according to their locations of residence or work. This can be done either on a simple geographic basis or by population density, climate, etc.[33]
2. Demographic segmentation is the grouping of individuals on the basis of such variables as age, sex, income, occupation, education, religion, race, etc.
3. Psychographic segmentation uses such criteria as personal values, attitudes, opinions, personality, behavior, and life style.[34, 35, 36]

It has long been known that psychographic segmentation often is the most useful. However, since psychographic data rarely are readily available and since their collection requires special market surveys, health services managers may prefer to use geographic and demographic segmentation. (Information in Chapters 6, 7, and 8 on the relationships among demographic and geographical variables, health status, and service utilization can be used as the basis of patient market segmentation.)

Market Opportunity Analysis

Once market structure analysis is completed, the needs, preferences, perceptions, and motivations of the individuals composing the various market segments must be determined.

Needs assessment techniques for the determination of a population's health needs already have been explained (Chapter 3). The same methods can be used for the determination of the needs of any market. Needs can be defined by the organization and/or by the markets. The institution can pinpoint the needs of its markets using any number of indicators, including trend analysis and forecasting of demand.

Epidemiological techniques and data should be used for the organizational (or professional) definition of health needs. All epidemiological principles and methods described earlier can thus contribute to the marketing effort by providing a scientific framework to determine the population's health needs. Needs also can be defined by the consumers themselves, either through the use of surveys or through participation in consensus-reaching approaches.

In marketing, three types of surveys are used:[37]

1. Direct surveys: Individuals are asked to describe their needs in answering either open-ended questions ("What services would you like to see added?" etc.) or closed-ended questions ("Rate the following services in terms of your level of interest," or "Rate the following services on a scale from one to ten").
2. Projective surveys: While the direct method assumes that consumers are aware of their needs and capable of expressing them, the projective method aims to identify needs that consumers are not really aware of or may be unable to verbalize. Psychometric techniques such as word associations, sentence completions, picture completions, and role playing are used.
3. Prototype surveys: The consumers are exposed to and asked to respond to a prototype of a real product or service. For example, instead of asking a group of elderly persons what they want in the way of housing, they can be shown alternative blueprints and asked to comment on what they like and dislike about each, why, what is missing, etc.

Although all of these factors are fairly well known to health planners, market opportunity analysis also calls for the identification of preferences, perceptions, and motivation, which rarely is done in health services management. Marketers use three methods for the identification of preferences: (1) simple route ordering, (2) paired comparison, (3) monadic (scale) rating.[38]

The simplest method is to ask the individuals to rank services in order of preference. Such simple ordinal ranking, however, does not provide for any indication of magnitude of preference or distance between services.

The second method is to present a set of services, two at a time, and ask which is preferred in each pair. From the analysis of each paired comparison, the marketer then can rank all of the services. Although this has the same disadvantages as the simple rank ordering, it often is considered a better method since people find it easier to state their preference between only two objects or services at a time and since they can concentrate better on differences and similarities.

The third method (monadic rating) consists of asking individuals to rate their liking of each service on a scale (usually of five or seven points). This method is considered easier to use (especially when there are numerous services to evaluate) and provides more information than the other methods.

The perceptions of the individuals composing the different market segments regarding the institution and its products (services) also significantly influence their "buying behavior." Therefore it is important for the facility to identify these perceptions so that it can either concentrate in the areas where they are deemed appropriate and favorable or do something to modify and improve its image.

Many methods can be used to measure perceptions. Multidimensional scaling[39] and semantic differentials[40, 41] are among the most sophisticated of such tools. For marketing purposes, Kotler proposes a simple "familiarity-favorability analysis."[42] Respondents are asked first how familiar they are with the organization (or, specifically, with one of its services) on a five-point scale from "never heard of" to "know very well." Those who have some familiarity then are asked how favorable they feel toward the institution, also on a five-point scale from "very unfavorable" to "very favorable." The results can be used to determine what further actions the organization should take.

For example, a hospital may find that members of its constituency (or some segments of it) are not very familiar with its obstetric service but that those who are familiar have a very favorable attitude toward it. The hospital's task then should be to bring itself to the attention of more people.

Of course, it also might find that many people are familiar with it but have an unfavorable attitude toward it. The hospital then should keep a low profile (avoid news and publicity), find out why people dislike it, mend its ways, and then seek public attention again. Similarly, situations of high familiarity-favorable attitude, and low familiarity-unfavorable attitude, also are possible and call for still different strategies.

The final component of market opportunity analysis is the evaluation of the motivation of the various segments. The exchange relationship for (for example, the utilization of a health service) depends not only on needs, preferences, and perceptions but also on some catalyst or trigger that will convert a potential user into an actual client.[43] Individuals may perceive a need for the service and have appropriate attitudes toward the organization, yet still not use it unless some specific stimulus or cue attracts them to do so.

For example, a reminder card (or phone call) informing a patient of a forthcoming appointment might be necessary to stimulate the individual to keep the appointment. Different market segments are likely to respond differently to various stimuli. The organization that can identify and predict these stimuli is likely to better plan for and influence desired exchanges.

Target Market Selection

The last component of market analysis is the selection of target segments with which the institution could or should try to establish an exchange relationship. A target market is a well-defined set of customers whose needs the organization plans to satisfy.[44] It must decide which market segments it will fit into its services. All of the analyses discussed earlier should serve as inputs in the decision as to which market segments will be targeted. This decision should be based on macroenvironmental analysis, resource analysis, market structure, market opportunity analysis, and competition analysis.

Still another element is market positioning, a method of examining one's product as compared to the competition's in relation to any number of characteristics.[45, 46]

The results and conclusions of the various analyses can be fed into the planning process (Figure 10-2, supra) where priorities can be determined (Chapter 3). It should now be clear how the use of these marketing principles and techniques can contribute, along with epidemiology, to population-based management of health services. Marketing also can make contributions to health services planning and management through portfolio analysis and expansion of the marketing mix. These are discussed next.

Portfolio Analysis

Once priorities have been determined and objectives set, management next must determine and set up the activities or strategies to attain the goals (Figure 10-2, supra). To this translation of objectives into activities/services/programs, marketing can contribute what is known as portfolio analysis.

As an analogy to the mix of shares and investments an investor may hold, the portfolio of an organization refers to the mix of services (or products) it offers. Portfolio analysis consists of a critical review of an institution's services to decide which ones should be developed, which should be maintained, which should be scaled down, and which should be eliminated. This analysis can be based on many criteria,[47] including the centrality of the service; the strategic position of the institution, and its market attractiveness in relation to its organizational strengths.

The centrality of the service refers to the degree to which it is central or pertinent to the objectives just established. Each service should be examined in relation to its contribution and usefulness in achieving the facility's objectives. This concept of centrality also can be used later in the evaluation of services and programs.

A second criterion that can be used in portfolio analysis is the institution's strategic position for every service. The development of this method involves rating all of the organization's services along two dimensions: market growth and market share.[48] Each service can be classified in one of the four categories: stars, cash cows, wildcats, and dogs.

Each category has a different strategic (and portfolio) implication.[49] Services for which the organization holds a high share of a fast-growing market are referred to as "stars." In other words, they are provided by relatively few organizations and are in increasing demand. Such services might include high-risk pregnancy units, life style counseling, and organ transplant (for which demand is increasing since the discovery of cyclosporin, an antirejection drug). "Star" services should be developed further to keep up with the market's growth and maintain the facility's leading position.

Services for which the facility's market share of a stagnant or decreasing market is high are called "cash cows" since they need only be maintained to reap (milk) as many benefits as possible without further investment. An example is tuberculosis treatment services: incidence of tuberculosis is low and not increasing but competition is most regions also is low. Hospitals providing special wards or units to treat tuberculosis probably should just maintain them. In other areas, "cash cow" services may include obstetrics.

"Wildcats" are services for which demand is increasing rapidly but for which competition also is high. The institution may only hold a small share of the market or may not even offer these services. It can decide either to invest resources and increase its market share or maintain or even reduce (or eliminate) its investment to concentrate resources on stars services (for which competition is less strong). An excellent example of a "wildcat" is the rapid increase in and demand for preventive medicine services. Furthermore, most new high-technology services fit into this "wildcat" category. Examples include computerized axial tomography (CAT) scanners or, more recently, nuclear magnetic resonance (NMR) scanners. The potential market for the NMR scanners is very promising. Furthermore, few hospitals had one in the early 1980s. On the other hand, the devices cost about 50 percent more than a CAT scanner and, with time, competition also could become high.

Finally, services for which the organization holds a small share of a slow-growth or declining market are called "dogs." Many organizations offer these services and, since demand is slackening, the institution probably should consider eliminating them. In most regions, pediatric services in general hospitals could be considered "dogs." In addition, hospitals devoted exclusively to pediatrics have a major impact on the viability of pediatric services in a general hospital.

A third approach to portfolio analysis has been formulated which uses two groups of variables: market attractiveness and organizational strength.[50] Market attractiveness is judged by indicators such as market size, market growth rate, competitive intensity, and profit margin, and is summarized for each service as being either low, medium, or high. Organizational strength also is evaluated for each service (or program) using indicators such as quality, efficiency, and market knowledge and summarized as either strong, average, or weak. Each service (or program) then can be classified in a 3 × 3 grid (Exhibit 10-1). The institution should invest in and develop services located in "A" cells while maintaining those in "B," and eliminating those in "C."

All of these methods of portfolio analysis may seem rather crude and insufficient for health services organizations. They are presented here as useful but far from the

Exhibit 10-1 Market Attractiveness and Organizational Strength Portfolio Analysis

Organizational Strength

		Strong	Average	Weak
Market Attractiveness	High	A	A	B
	Medium	A	B	C
	Low	B	C	C

Source: Adapted from *Marketing for Nonprofit Organizations,* 2nd ed., by Philip Kotler, Prentice-Hall, Inc., © 1982, 97, with permission of General Electric, Inc.

only tools that health services managers should use in deciding which activities and programs the organization should pursue. Other considerations such as the hospital's mission and role in the delivery of health care to a given constituency can and should predominate in managers' decisions.

Development of the Marketing Mix

Once the organization has decided upon which services it should and will offer, the marketing mix should be developed (Figure 10-2 supra). The four attributes (the four Ps) of the exchange should be designed specifically for each service and each target market segment. The characteristics of the services themselves, of the location of delivery, their price, and their promotion all should be studied and adapted to the target markets.

This is a critical component of the marketing process and, for that matter, of successful management. It suggests that, for example, a program or service not tailored to the characteristics and needs of the target market segment will not be effective even though the price might be right, the location of delivery accessible, and the publicity (promotion) effective. Similarly, a well-tailored, accessible, and well-promoted service at an inappropriately high price (direct and/or indirect) will not be as successful as could be expected. The same is true for accessibility and promotion.

Variables to be considered in each of the four components of the marketing mix were described earlier in this chapter.[51]

SOCIAL MARKETING: IDEAS AND BEHAVIORS

Since the early 1970s, there has been discussion of the potential of applying the marketing process to advance social causes, ideas, or behaviors. Is it possible to market such intangible ideas as energy conservation, a political candidate, good nutrition, smoking cessation, etc.?

Social marketing was introduced in 1971.[52] It is defined as "the design, implementation, and control of programs seeking to increase the acceptability of a social idea or cause in a target group(s)."[53] While business marketing aims at satisfying the needs and wants of target markets, social marketing seeks to change their attitudes or behavior.

Many articles have been published on social marketing[54, 55, 56] and, of more direct interest to health services managers, on the marketing of preventive health behaviors.[57, 58] One of the first books on social marketing was published in 1981.[59] The major message of this literature is that, although the marketing of intangible ideas, including preventive health behavior, is more complex and arduous, it is possible and feasible but only if the marketing process (as described in this chapter) is followed in its entirety.

The best way to explain this may be to analyze why past efforts at social marketing have been considered disappointing. There seem to be four major reasons for this (apparent) lack of success:

1. attitudes and behavior are much more difficult to change
2. the marketing process is misunderstood
3. the promotion or communication strategies are misunderstood
4. there is inadequate measurement of performance.

Attitudes and Behavior: Difficult to Change

There is no doubt that it is a much more complex task to promote and change attitudes and behavior than it is to market a tangible product or service. Health educators have long been struggling to find effective ways of advancing health messages. The fact remains that even the experts still are not quite sure how behaviors are set and how they can be influenced. One article counts more than 25 different theoretical models to explain health behavior modifications[60]—and that was back in 1976.

Certain types of changes are easier than others to bring about. Marketers usually distinguish among four types of social changes in increasing difficulty: cognitive change, action change, behavioral change, and value change.[61]

Cognitive changes, that is, changes in knowledge, are easier to market since they do not seek to alter any deep-rooted attitudes or behavior. Therein lies the catch, however: contrary to what most practicing health educators seem to think, there appears to be little connection between cognitive change and behavioral change. It is relatively easy to increase the knowledge of a target group but it is far from evident that that will have an impact on behavior.

Although some health educators still hold onto it,[62, 63] their traditional model of linear change from knowledge to attitude to practice (KAP) many times has been proved inadequate and too simplistic.[64]

Even if they are relatively easy to bring about, cognitive changes thus may be of little value when the ultimate aim is an attitude or behavioral change.

Action change refers to attempts at inducing a maximum number of people to take a specific action during a given period. Campaigns for mass immunization, voter turnout, and blood donor recruiting are examples. Action changes are considered more difficult to achieve because the target market has to understand something and then take an action, always at a certain cost of time, effort, energy, etc.

In terms of disease prevention and health promotion, action changes usually involve secondary prevention such as screening programs and early diagnosis of problems (see Chapter 1) and can be divided conceptually according to the amount of activity required by the consumer.[65] Some action changes require a one-time act—mass immunization campaigns and many screening programs. Others call for repeated but noncontinuous acts—annual physical check-ups or pap smears require the periodic repetition of an action.

Behavioral changes involve repeated and continuous acts. Smoking cessation and improved nutritional habits require repeated and continuous behavioral commitment. Behavioral changes are called for most often in efforts at primary prevention (action designed to prevent the occurrence of disease or injury), although tertiary prevention (rehabilitation and prevention of sequelae) also require behavioral changes (for example, after a heart attack).

Not all behavioral changes require the same consumer involvement. A distinction can be made between high-involvement behavioral changes, such as regular exercise and good nutritional habits, in which the consumers usually perceive a direct personal benefit ("feeling better," etc.), and low-involvement activities, such as reduced driving speed, which consumers may perceive as offering more benefits to society than themselves.[66]

Value change refers to attempts at altering deeply rooted beliefs or values toward some object or situation. Efforts to change people's ideas about abortion, about the "appropriate" number of children, about civil rights and race relations are examples of value change. These are the most difficult to market and chances of success may be slim.

Health services managers may (and perhaps should) be more concerned with action and behavioral changes. The various types of action and behavioral changes require different marketing strategies. In some cases, demand for the product or service that the action or behavioral change is aiming at may be negative.[67] In other words, consumers may be avoiding the required change (service). This often is the case with immunization, dental services, sexually transmitted disease treatments, etc. In such situations, sources of resistance must be identified and eliminated or circumvented.

In other cases, demand may be null, consumers being indifferent to the change (service). This may be the case for road safety, periodic health examinations, etc. In such situations, marketers will have to increase the public's perception of the benefits associated with the change.

A third type of situation may arise when the change involves a reduction in the consumption of a product or service for which demand is positive—cigarette smoking and use of alcohol or other drugs. Such situations call for a counter-marketing strategy requiring not only the abandonment of or reduced adherence to an existing behavior but also the subsequent adoption of a new behavior.

The opinion here is that this is a crucial point often forgotten in behavior-modification programs. Emphasis tends to be placed only on the abandonment of harmful behavior while little is said concerning the inevitable subsequent adoption of a new one. Putting more emphasis on this alternative conduct may facilitate the countermarketing of a harmful behavior. This is especially so in the field of primary prevention where specific and direct cause-effect relationships may be lacking and are approximated through risk (or statistical) relationships (see Chapter 1). As Marshall wrote in 1980 concerning smoking-cessation programs:

> Essentially, prevention asks the individual smoker to bet that he will develop lung cancer and advises him to avoid this eventuality by giving up cigarettes. In fact, on the individual level, smoking does not guarantee the eventual occurrence of this disease, and abstinence from smoking does not assure its prevention. The ratio of reward to effort is great, and after years or decades the reward is an abstraction involving a statistical payoff—something bad that might have happened but did not. The modification of life style that is the outcome of successful health education is a "blood, sweat, and tears" approach to prevention. It is not a magic bullet; it is hard work, involving the alteration of old habits and the sustenance of new ones over much of a lifetime.[68]

More emphasis on the benefits of the sustenance of the new behavior, such as increased cardiopulmonary fitness, undoubtedly would increase the effectiveness of the countermarketing.

Marketing: A Misunderstood Process

A second factor that may have contributed to the lack of success of social marketing programs is an incomprehension and misunderstanding of the marketing process itself.[69] The author has insisted on many occasions on the fact that strategic (integrated, modern) marketing is based on and starts with the needs, wants, and desires of the target markets and that product-oriented marketing will be unsuccessful. As a parallel, marketing is not only publicity and advertising; all of the other components of the marketing mix (product, price, place) need to be considered and fitted to the target market.

It seems to the author that many so-called social marketing (and health education) campaigns have consisted of trying to sell a predesigned program, i.e., they have proceeded from a product orientation in which production precedes marketing. Analyses of environment, consumer, etc., have been inadequate or nonexistent. Furthermore, many of these programs have merely been advertising campaigns that gave no consideration to the other elements of the marketing mix.

A strategy based on every dimension of the marketing mix is particularly important in health education aimed at behavioral changes. Behaviors are so complex and deeply rooted, and result from the interaction of so many variables, that a narrow approach to change is doomed to failure. Health education literature has emphasized that behaviors are closely linked to environmental and social variables and that behavior change requires a comprehensive approach.[70, 71, 72, 73] Among other things, this means that a complete marketing process, including a comprehensive marketing mix strategy, is needed.

Preventive health interventions can be broadened to include not only those in which consumers must be active but also in which they can remain passive.[74, 75, 76] Such passive interventions may be of a legal, technological, or economic nature. For example, fluoridation of water and regulation of environmental, chemical, and physical hazards are preventive health measures that do not require active consumer involvement.

Marketing incorporates these passive approaches through consideration of the marketing mix. Effective preventive health interventions consider service characteristics (product), location of service delivery (place), price, and publicity and promotion. For example, a cigarette smoking countermarketing strategy could include the following elements:[77, 78]

Product

- require filters on all cigarettes
- regulate maximum permissible nicotine and tar levels; as was done for gasoline mileage, an average standard can be set so that average sales should be of cigarettes of lower tar and nicotine
- make cigarettes shorter
- sell cigarettes separately or in individual packs only
- print line on each cigarette as "stop line" to avoid the harmful effects of the last part of the cigarette

- force tobacco companies to spend a minimum percentage of their sales dollar on biomedical research aimed at developing better filters
- develop cigarettes made of nontobacco products such as lettuce leaves, etc.
- create other types of cigarette substitutes, mainly stress-reducing techniques and methods

Price

- raise taxes on cigarettes
- reduce health and life insurance premiums for nonsmokers, raise them for smokers
- tax on cigarettes should be incremental on the basis of nicotine and tar levels: more harmful cigarettes should be taxed more and cost more than those low in tar and nicotine

Place

- limit places where cigarettes can be purchased
- limit places where smoking is permitted: not in public places (banks, stores, certain sections of restaurants, etc.), elevators, hospitals, public transportation, etc.

Promotion

- restrict or ban cigarette advertising (no color ads, no pictures, no targeting to "new recruits," etc.)
- multifaceted antismoking advertising and publicity, specifically targeted to different segments and combining many media
- emphasis on the positive benefits of nonsmoking.

This represents a very preliminary outline of what the marketing mix could be if there was a real effort to reduce cigarette smoking. Such a strategy would require legal, technological, economic, and promotional interventions but would have a high probability of reducing the use of cigarettes and their impact on health. However, this outline still is incomplete since it does not include (in the product category) strategies aimed at environmental and social determinants of smoking behavior. Research would be needed before such factors could be identified and understood in such a way as to be manageable operationally, that is, controllable (the marketing mix considers only controllable variables even though the influence of uncontrollable variables may be known and acknowledged).

Promotion: Also Misunderstood

A third factor for the lack of success of social marketing programs may be a misunderstanding of the promotion or communication process. This in fact may be considered as a subcategory of the previous factor.

The promotion component of the marketing mix is a specialized and complex domain, the discussion of which is better left to specialists. There are, however, certain basic principles that should be insisted on.

First, promotion (or communication) is not only advertising and mass media are not the only promotion channels that marketers consider. As Quelch writes:

> Marketers generally agree that although mass media approaches are appropriate for developing consumer awareness in the short term, face-to-face programs such as workplace encounters are more effective (though not always cost effective) in changing behavior in the long term. In designing any communication policy, the marketer commonly considers the effects that may be achievable through the use of a mix of approaches, capitalizing on the strengths of each.[79]

Second, a promotion strategy should result directly from the previous steps of the marketing group, i.e., from analyses of the environments, the competition, the resources, and the markets. It should always be targeted to specific market segments.

Third, there are three basic conditions necessary for the effectiveness of social communication campaigns:[80]

1. Monopolization by the media: no counterpropaganda should be present. This obviously is not the case in most social marketing campaigns, a fact that can explain in part their limited effectiveness.
2. Canalization: there should be present an existing attitudinal base for the feelings (ideas) that the social marketer is trying to communicate. When preexisting attitudes are present, it is much easier to promote an idea since all that is required is their canalization (channeling) in a specific direction.
3. Supplementation: mass media campaigns should be followed (supplemented) with other programs such as face-to-face contacts.

Thus there should be a comprehensive step-down communication process in which the message is passed on and discussed in more familiar terms and surroundings.

Performance Measurement Inadequacies

Social marketing (and health education) campaigns may have been disappointing for yet another reason—inadequate measurement of their impact.[81] The performance of social marketing campaigns is difficult to measure since results essentially are intangible and the relevant time frame wide and long. In addition, social marketers (and particularly health educators) may have unrealistic expectations. In business marketing, companies usually are delighted when a sales increase of 1 percent to 2 percent can be attributed to a marketing campaign.[82] For example, a 1 percent gain is worth millions in sales even for the less popular brands of cigarettes. On the other hand, many health education campaigns have been judged ineffective and disappointing even if 25 percent (and up to 50 percent) of the target markets have modified a behavior.

For example, a study that showed that 34 percent of college students smoked less as a result of antismoking commercials on television, and that 21 percent had stopped smoking completely at least temporarily, concluded that the results were disappointing.[83] Similarly, it was found that after a government publicity campaign, 25 percent of the public had received the entire series of four polio shots and 60 percent at least one.[84] This, too, was considered disappointing.

In Canada, since antismoking campaigns started in the early 1970s, the proportion of regular smokers decreased from 42.8 percent to 34.2 percent (in 1979) while the percentage of nonsmokers increased from 50.2 percent to 60.1 percent. Furthermore, brands low in nicotine and tar attracted a large proportion of smokers between 1977 and 1979. These modifications of the smoking behavior of Canadians occurred even though cigarette companies still were spending dozens of millions of dollars a year on advertising while the government was expending only a fraction of that amount on antismoking promotion.

In the United States, it was estimated that as of 1975, the cumulative effect of persistent antismoking publicity supported by (a few) other public policies had reduced per capita consumption of cigarettes by 20 percent to 30 percent. This was a conservative measure since it ignored the potential health impact that could result from a shift to cigarettes low in tar and nicotine.[85]

It can be said that "the myth of overwhelming advertiser success has exerted a negative effect on health education (and other social marketing efforts) by encouraging the belief that anything short of a success rate approaching 100 percent is unsatisfactory."[86]

In the author's opinion, marketing principles and techniques can and should be used to promote health in conjunction with other education methods. However, the effectiveness of such health marketing depends not only on a thorough understanding of the process but also on the understanding that health (and health-related behaviors) are determined by a wide range of interrelated factors including life style, environment, biology, and medical care organization.

SUMMARY

This chapter examined the contributions of marketing to health services management. Marketing was described as a process complementary to planning that could enrich the managerial task of adapting an organization's services to the needs, wants, and desires of the population.

The marketing approach is essentially similar to the epidemiological approach to health services management in that both promote and call for population-based management. Both of these approaches also can contribute to a more comprehensive understanding of health and its determinants and consequently to more effective management of health services.

Health services managers can use marketing to plan and manage their organization's relationships with other groups such as physicians, employees, suppliers, and community supporters, as well as for health education and promotion.

NOTES

1. Philip Kotler, *Marketing for Nonprofit Organizations,* 2nd ed. (Englewood Cliffs, N.J.: Prentice-Hall, Inc., 1982),

2. Robin E. MacStravic, *Marketing Health Care* (Rockville, Md.: Aspen Systems Corporation, 1977), 302.

3. Robin E. MacStravic, *Marketing by Objectives for Hospitals* (Rockville, Md.: Aspen Systems Corporation, 1980), 280.

4. P.O. Cooper, ed, *Health Care Marketing: Issues and Trends* (Rockville, Md.: Aspen Systems Corporation, 1979), 294.

5. R. Rubright and D. MacDonald, *Marketing Health and Human Services* (Rockville, Md.: Aspen Systems Corporation, 1981), 248.

6. MacStravic, *Marketing Health Care,* 7.

7. J.G. Keith, "Marketing Health Care: What the Recent Literature Is Telling Us," Special 2, *Hospital and Health Services Administration* (1981), 66-94.

8. MacStravic, *Marketing Health Care,* 16.

9. Peter F. Drucker, *Management: Tasks, Responsibilities, Practices* (New York: Harper & Row, Publishers, Inc., 1973), 64-65.

10. Kotler, *Marketing for Nonprofit Organizations,* 7.

11. Ibid., 47.

12. H. Mintzberg, "Organizational Power and Goals: A Skeletal Theory," in *Strategic Management: A New View of Business Policy and Planning,* ed. D.E. Schendel and C.W. Hofer (New York: Little, Brown & Co., 1979), 64-80.

13. MacStravic, *Marketing Health Care.*

14. Kotler, *Marketing for Nonprofit Organizations,* 56.

15. MacStravic, *Marketing Health Care,* 20.

16. Kotler, *Marketing for Nonprofit Organizations,* 108.

17. Philip Kotler, *Marketing Management* (Englewood Cliffs, N.J.: Prentice-Hall, Inc., 1980), ch. 3.

18. Ibid.

19. Ibid.

20. Kotler, *Marketing for Nonprofit Organizations,* 85.

21. Ibid.

22. MacStravic, *Marketing Health Care,* 35-49.

23. Ibid, 22.

24. Rubright and MacDonald, *Marketing Health and Human Services,* 57-74.

25. D. Bell, "Twelve Modes of Prediction: A Preliminary Sorting of Approaches in the Social Sciences," *Daedalus* 93, no. 2 (Spring 1964), 847-868.

26. D.P. Harrison, *Social Forecasting Methodology* (New York: Russell Sage Foundation, 1976).

27. M.F. Arnold, "Tools for Planning," in *Administering Health Systems,* (Chicago: Aldine and Atherton, 1971).

28. D.F. Bergwall, P.H. Reeves, and N.B. Woodside, *Introduction to Health Planning* (Washington, D.C.: Information Resources Press, 1979).

29. P. Lorange, *Corporate Planning* (Englewood Cliffs, N.J.: Prentice-Hall, Inc., 1980), 118-122.

30. Kotler, *Marketing for Nonprofit Organizations,* 85.

31. Rubright and MacDonald, *Marketing Health and Human Services,* 57-114.

32. Kotler, *Marketing for Nonprofit Organizations,* 88-89.

33. D. Finlay, "Geographic Targeting," *American Demographics* (October 1980), 39-41.

34. A.S. Boote, "Mind Over Matter," *American Demographics* (April 1980), 26-29.

35. E.J. Forrest et al., "Psychographic Flesh, Demographic Bones," *American Demographics* (September 1981), 25-27.

36. H. Assael, "Segmenting Markets by Group Purchasing Behavior: An Application of the Aid Technique," *Journal of Marketing Research,* 7 (May 1970), 153-158.

37. Kotler, *Marketing for Nonprofit Organizations,* 240-241.

38. Ibid., 245.

39. P.E. Green and V.R. Rao, *Applied Multidimensional Scaling* (New York: Holt, Rinehart & Winston, Inc., 1972), 292.

40. C. Osgood, G. Suci, and P. Tannenbaum, *The Measurement of Meaning* (Urbana, Ill.: The University of Illinois Press, 1967), 346.

41. J. Snider and C. Osgood, eds, *Semantic Differential Technique: A Sourcebook* (Chicago: Aldine Publishing Co., Inc., 1969), 681.

42. Kotler, *Marketing for Nonprofit Organizations,* 57-58.

43. MacStravic, *Marketing Health Care,* 95-97.

44. Philip Kotler, *Principles of Marketing,* 2nd ed. (Englewood Cliffs, N.J.: Prentice Hall, Inc., 1983), 64.

45. Kotler, *Marketing Management.*

46. MacStravic, *Marketing by Objectives for Hospitals,* ch. 9.

47. Kotler, *Marketing for Nonprofit Organizations,* 93-101.

48. B.D. Henderson, "The Product Portfolio," in *Perspectives on Experience* (Boston: Boston Consulting Group, 1970), 109.

49. Kotler, *Marketing for Nonprofit Organizations,* 95.

50. Ibid., 96-97.

52. Philip Kotler and G. Zaltman, "Social Marketing: An Approach to Planned Social Change," *Journal of Marketing* 35 (July 1971), 3-12.

53. Kotler, *Marketing for Nonprofit Organizations,* 90.

54. K.F.A. Fox and Philip Kotler, "The Marketing of Social Causes: The First Ten Years," *Journal of Marketing* 50 (Fall 1980), 24-33.

55. G.R. Laczniak, R.F. Lusch, and P.E. Murphys, "Social Marketing: Its Ethical Dimensions," *Journal of Marketing* 49 (Spring 1979), 29-36.

56. M. Mushkat, Jr., "Implementing Public Plans: The Case for Social Marketing," *Long Range Planning* 13 (August 1980), 24-29.

57. P.D. Cooper, W.J. Kehoe, and P.E. Murphy, eds., *Marketing and Preventive Health Care: Interdisciplinary and Interorganizational Perspectives* (Chicago, American Marketing Association, 1978), 132.

58. J.A. Quelch, "Marketing Principles and the Future of Preventive Health Care," *Milbank Memorial Fund Quarterly/Health and Society* 58, no. 2 (Spring 1980), 310-347.

59. S. Fine, *The Marketing of Ideas and Social Issues* (Columbus, Ohio: Grid Publishing, Inc. 1981), 240.

60. S. Simonds, "Emerging Challenges in Health Education," *International Journal of Health Education* 19, no. 4 (1976) Special Supplement, 1-18.

61. Kotler, *Marketing for Nonprofit Organizations,* 501-510.

62. M. O'Neill, *Vers une problèmatique de l'éducation sanitaire au Québec.* Master's thesis, Laval University, Quebec, 1976, 289.

63. "La modification des comportements reliés à la santé," *Union Médicale du Canada,* 109 (May 1980): 733-742, (June 1980): 921-928.

64. Simonds, "Emerging Challenges."

65. Quelch, "Marketing Principles," 317.

66. M.L. Rothschild, "Marketing Communications in Nonbusiness Situations; or, Why It's So Hard to Sell Brotherhood Like Soap," *Journal of Marketing* 43, no. 2 (1979), 11-20.

67. D.A. Lussier, "La santé publique: Est-ce possible d'en faire un marketing," *Les Cahiers de Santé Communautaire,* Association pour la Santé Publique du Québec, June 1979, 317.

68. C.C. Marshall, "Prevention and Health Education," in 11th ed., ed. J. M. Last, *Maxcy-Rosenau Public Health and Preventive Medicine* (New York: Appleton-Century-Crofts, Inc., 1980), 1122.

69. Quelch, "Marketing Principles," 325-331.

70. Amitai Etzioni, "Human Beings Are Not Very Easy to Change After All," *Saturday Review,* June 3, 1972, 45-47.

71. O'Neill, "Vers une problèmatique."

72. E.R. Brown and G.E. Margo, "Health Education: Can the Reformers Be Reformed?" *International Journal of Health Services* 8, no. 1 (1978), 3-26.

73. N.D. Richards, "Methods and Effectiveness of Health Education," *Social Science and Medicine* 9 (1975), 141-156.

74. Quelch, "Marketing Principles," 316.

75. J.E. Fielding, "Successes of Prevention," *Milbank Memorial Fund Quarterly/Health and Society* 56 (Summer 1978), 274-302.

76. M. Venkatesan, "Consumer Behavior and Nutrition: Preventive Health Perspectives," in *Advances in Consumer Research,* vol. 5, ed. H.K. Hunt (1978), 518-520.

77. Kotler, *Marketing for Nonprofit Organizations,* 513.

78. G.A. Tocquer and M.A. Zims, "La compagne anti-tabac: Une application de marketing social," *Commerce* (Juillet 1975), 20-24.

79. Quelch, "Marketing Principles," 327-328.

80. Paul F. Lazarsfeld and R.K. Mortar, "Mass Communication, Popular Taste, and Organized Social Action," *Mass Communications* ed. Willard Schramm (Urbana, Ill.: The University of Illinois Press, 1949), 459-480.

81. Quelch, "Marketing Principles," 335-337.

82. Marshall, "Prevention and Health Education," 1122.

83. M. O'Keefe, "The Antismoking Commercials: A Study of Television's Impact on Behavior," *Public Opinion Quarterly* 35 (Summer 1971), 242-248.

84. R. Bauer, "The Obstinate Audience," *American Psychologist* 19 (March 1964), 319-328.

85. K.E. Warner, "The Effects of the Antismoking Campaign on Cigarette Consumption," *American Journal of Public Health* 67, (July 1977) 645-650.

86. Marshall, "Prevention and Health Education," 1123.

Chapter 11

Marketing and Epidemiology: A Case Study

THE PROBLEM: HIGH INFANT MORTALITY

Sunnyvale Civic Hospital is a 400-bed county-owned facility in mythical Ackit County, U.S.A. It is the only hospital in this county, 100 miles from a major metropolitan area. The hospital administrators want to investigate Ackit County's high infant mortality rate. This examination studies how the demographic techniques and the epidemiological analysis of utilization described in earlier chapters could contribute to this investigation and to future marketing of health services.

The first step is to analyze Ackit County's population and its fertility and project the population size and births for the period 1980-1990. Infant deaths for the period 1975-1979 then are analyzed and deaths projected that could be expected if infant mortality rates remained constant.

The study of infant deaths aims at pinpointing high-risk population groups in terms of sociodemographic, geographic, and health services utilization factors. Finally, the results of all these analyses are used to plan an intervention and marketing strategy that can be hospital based.

The question for this hospital is: "Will we need more beds allocated to obstetrical services and do we need to expand our services for high-risk infants?" The county traditionally has had a high infant mortality rate. However, the problem to be addressed is whether the rate will continue and whether the numbers of births in the future will warrant additional or reallocated services. The results of the analysis will provide the hospital administration or manager information needed to help plot the future direction of service development and marketing for the institution.

Ackit County's Population

Table 11-1 shows Ackit County's actual population by age, race, and sex for 1970, 1975, and 1980, from census data. The county clearly has an aging popula-

Table 11-1 Population of Ackit County, 1970, 1975, 1980

By Age, Race, and Sex

Age, Race, Sex	1970	%	1975	%	1980	%
Total	210,650	100%	198,810	100%	185,559	100%
W.M.	77,118		67,073		59,418	
W.F.	79,230		70,120		63,119	
B.M.	25,317		28,432		28,517	
B.F.	28,985		33,185		34,512	
0-4	17,405	8.3	11,985	6.0	11,305	6.1
W.M.	6,513		4,042		3,582	
W.F.	6,206		3,809		3,294	
B.M.	2,337		2,083		2,194	
B.F.	2,349		2,051		2,235	
5-9	19,795	9.4	13,835	7.0	8,439	4.6
W.M.	7,060		4,391		2,475	
W.F.	6,923		4,256		2,361	
B.M.	2,845		2,579		1,785	
B.F.	2,967		2,609		1,818	
10-14	19,805	9.4	17,160	8.6	11,211	6.0
W.M.	7,063		5,758		3,721	
W.F.	6,744		5,524		3,480	
B.M.	2,972		2,837		1,947	
B.F.	3,026		2,041		2,063	
15-19	18,355	8.7	19,015	9.6	16,377	8.8
W.M.	6,588		6,226		5,017	
W.F.	6,599		6,467		5,467	
B.M.	2,557		3,279		3.054	
B.F.	2,611		3,043		2,839	
20-24	19,905	9.4	19,145	9.6	19,800	10.7
W.M.	7,738		6,882		6,829	
W.F.	8,166		7,138		6,984	
B.M.	1,747		2,418		2,827	
B.F.	2,254		2,707		3,106	
25-29	17,920	8.5	17,900	9.0	17,148	9.2
W.M.	7,372		6,512		6,096	
W.F.	6,962		6,597		5,869	
B.M.	1,664		2,288		2,523	
B.F.	1,922		2,503		2,660	
30-34	14,840	7.0	14,400	7.2	14,392	7.8
W.M.	5,641		5,108		4,910	
W.F.	5,438		5,001		5,024	
B.M.	1,753		1,937		1,909	
B.F.	2,008		2,354		2,549	

Table 11-1 continued

Age, Race, Sex	1970	%	1975	%	1980	%
35-39	13,049	6.2	11,925	6.0	11,500	6.2
W.M.	4,921		4,180		3,908	
W.F.	4,801		4,189		4,028	
B.M.	1,554		1,585		1,520	
B.F.	1,773		1,971		1,044	
40-44	13,261	6.3	12,195	6.1	11,089	6.0
W.M.	5,001		4,317		3,785	
W.F.	4,879		4,243		3,869	
B.M.	1,579		1,638		1,472	
B.F.	1,802		1,997		1,963	
45-49	12,657	6.0	12,380	6.2	11,343	6.1
W.M.	4,762		4,462		3,924	
W.F.	4,825		4,508		4,117	
B.M.	1,387		1,568		1,500	
B.F.	1,683		1,842		1,802	
50-54	10,438	5.0	12,175	6.1	11,907	6.4
W.M.	3,773		4,285		4,107	
W.F.	4,128		4,533		4,334	
B.M.	1,098		1,505		1,569	
B.F.	1,439		1,852		1,897	
55-59	10,192	4.8	10,060	5.1	11,713	6.3
W.M.	3,728		3,400		3,945	
W.F.	3,988		3,880		4,354	
B.M.	1,086		1,195		1,508	
B.F.	1,390		1,585		1,906	
60-64	7,818	3.7	9,100	4.6	9,000	4.9
W.M.	2,527		2,815		2,623	
W.F.	3,101		3,181		3,023	
B.M.	944		1,295		1,301	
B.F.	1,246		1,809		2,053	
65-69	6,290	3.0	7,000	3.5	8,134	4.4
W.M.	2,020		2,031		2,343	
W.F.	2,508		2,572		2,755	
B.M.	755		934		1,164	
B.F.	1,007		1,463		1,872	
70-74	5,004	2.4	4,960	2.5	5,590	3.0
W.M.	1,511		1,370		1,450	
W.F.	2,117		1,887		2,040	
B.M.	565		630		714	
B.F.	851		1,073		1,386	

Table 11-1 continued

Age, Race, Sex	1970	%	1975	%	1980	%
75 +	3,876	1.8	5,575	2.8	6,611	3.6
W.M.	974		1,294		1,410	
W.F.	1,861		2,335		2,531	
B.M.	400		661		821	
B.F.	641		1,285		1,849	

W.M.: White Males
W.F.: White Females
B.M.: Black Males
B.F.: Black Females

tion. The proportion under age 20 decreased from 35.8 percent in 1970 to 31.2 percent in 1975 to 25.5 percent in 1980. The proportion of the population in every other age group increased: from 37.4 to 37.9 to 39.9 for the 20-44 group, from 15.8 to 17.4 to 18.8 for the 45-59 group, and from 10.9 to 13.4 to 15.9 for those over 60.

The population is increasingly female and increasingly black, as indicated by the sex and race ratios in Table 11-2. The white population decreased between 1970 and 1980 while the black population increased. This can be explained in part by the fact that (as is discussed later) blacks in that county have a much higher crude birth rate than whites and in part by different outmigration patterns. Whites seem to have left the county (outmigrated) at a much higher rate than blacks.

THE COUNTY'S INFANT MORTALITY RATES

Table 11-3 shows the infant mortality rate for the total, white, and black population of Ackit County for the five-year period 1975-1979.

As shown in Chapter 4, the confidence interval of these rates can be calculated as follows. The 95 percent confidence interval (CI) is given by

$$CI = Rate \pm 1.96 \times SE$$

Where the standard error is

$$SE = \frac{Rate}{\sqrt{Deaths}}$$

For the total infant mortality rate, the standard error is:

$$SE = \frac{19.9}{\sqrt{308}} = 1.13$$

and the confidence limit is:

$$CI = 19.9 \pm (1.96 \times 1.13)$$

upper limit = 22.1
lower limit = 17.7

For the white infant mortality rate, the standard error is:

$$SE = \frac{15.9}{\sqrt{141}} = 1.34$$

and the confidence limit is:

$$CI = 15.9 \pm (1.96 \times 1.34)$$

upper limit = 18.5
lower limit = 13.3

For the black infant mortality rate, the standard error is:

$$SE = \frac{25.0}{167} = 19.3$$

and the confidence interval is:

$$CI = 25.0 \pm (1.96 \times 1.93)$$

upper limit = 28.8
lower limit = 21.1

What do these numbers mean and why is it necessary to calculate their values?
They mean that the health services manager can be 95 percent confident that the infant mortality rate in Ackit County for the five-year period 1975-1979 varies from 17.7 to 22.1 for the total population, from 13.3 to 18.5 for whites, and from 21.2 to 28.8 for blacks.

Table 11-2 Calculation of Sex and Race Ratios

Sex Ratio	1970	1975	1980
Males	77,118 + 25,317 = 102,435	67,037 + 28,432 = 95,505	59,418 + 28,517 = 87,935
Females	79,230 + 28,985 = 108,215	70,120 + 33,185 = 103,305	63,112 + 34,512 = 97,624
Sex ratio: No. of males per 100 females	$\dfrac{102,345}{1,082.15} = 94.7$	$\dfrac{95,505}{1,033.05} = 92.4$	$\dfrac{87,935}{976.24} = 90.1$

Race Ratio	1970	1975	1980
Whites	77,118 + 79,230 = 156,348	67,073 + 70,120 = 137,193	59,418 + 63,112 = 122,530
Blacks	25,317 + 28,985 = 54,302	28,432 + 33,185 = 61,617	28,517 + 34,512 = 63,029
Race ratio: No. of whites per 100 blacks	$\dfrac{156,348}{543.02} = 288$	$\dfrac{137,193}{616.17} = 223$	$\dfrac{122,530}{630.29} = 194$

The rates for the total and for whites are significantly above those for the overall United States population (in 1978, 14.4 for the total population, 12.5 for whites and 24.1 for blacks.[1]) Furthermore, the expected levels for 1990 in the United States are 9.0 for the total population and 12.0 for blacks.[2]

Table 11-3 Infant Deaths, Live Births, and Infant Mortality Rate, 1975-1979

	Infant Deaths	Live Births	Infant Mortality Rate*
Total	308	15,503	19.9
Whites	141	8,837	15.9
Blacks	167	6,666	25.0

*Infant deaths per 1,000 live births.

COUNTY POPULATION PROJECTED TO 1990

Since state (but not county) population projections for 1985 and 1990 are available, the easiest way to project the entire population of the county is through the ratio method (see Chapter 9). If county population projections are available for 1985 and 1990 for the county or other sub-service area then it is obvious population projections are not necessary to compute. For the projection of births (next section) another method of population projection is used (the cohort method) that results in age-specific projections.

The Ackit County's population projection using the ratio method is shown in Table 11-4. The first section (A) is simply a description of Ackit County's proportion of the state population and shows that the county's share has been decreasing but at a slowing rate (i.e., it decreased more between 1970 and 1975 than between 1975 and 1980). This seems to indicate that the outmigration has been slowing and the most probable assumption is that it will continue to slow.

The next section (B) projects the county ratio for 1985 and 1990 as a straight extrapolation of the previous ratios; Ackit County's population is estimated using the projection of the state population. Since it would be useful to know the race and sex breakdown of these 1985 and 1990 projections, Section C (the trends in race and sex ratios, by race) were analyzed. These ratios then were projected (Section D) for 1985 and 1990, again assuming the trends would continue. These projected ratios were used, along with Ackit County's projections from Section B, to project its population by race and sex.

The projections indicate that the total population will continue to decrease until 1985 but then will increase to reach in 1990 the same level as in 1980. This also is true for whites, although they will not quite return to the same level in 1990 as in 1980. The black population will continue to increase, possibly because of different fertility and outmigration rates.

PROJECTION OF BIRTHS IN THE COUNTY

To project births with some validity, it is necessary to use age-specific fertility rates rather than simply crude birth rates since the age distribution of females is changing over time. Consequently, the objective here is to project the 1985 and 1990 female 15-44 population. This can be done using a cohort method in which each female five-year cohort is projected forward five years. Because of age differences in mortality and migration, this projection needs to be adjusted by a growth factor involving the same two age groups for a previous period.

For example, the white female 5-9 population was 2,361 in 1980. If there were no mortality and no migration, this cohort would be expected to be 10 to 14 in 1985, with a population in that group of 2,361. However, this obviously will not be so

Table 11-4 Population, Race, and Sex Projections, Ackit County

The Ratio Method

A. Ackit County's Historical Population Ratio with the State

Year	State Total	Ackit County	Ackit County as a Ratio of State
1970	4,589,600	210,650	.046
1975	4,970,500	198,810	.040
1980	5,151,400	185,559	.036

B. Ratio Projection of Ackit County's Population

Year	State Projection	Ackit County's Ratio	Ackit County Projection
1985	5,466,683	.033	180,401
1990	5,781,968	.032	185,023

C. Ackit County's Historical Race and Sex Ratios

Year	Race Ratio	Sex Ratios	
		Whites	Blacks
1970	288	97.3	87.3
1975	223	95.8	84.9
1980	194	94.1	82.6

D. Ackit County's Projected Population by Race and Sex

Year	Race Ratio	Population by Race	Sex Ratio	Population by Race and Sex
1985	180	White: 115,972	White: 92.6	W.M.: 55,758
				W.F.: 60,214
		Black: 64,429	Black: 80.5	B.M.: 28,734
				B.F.: 35,695
1990	172	White: 117,000	White: 91.2	W.M.: 55,808
				W.F.: 61,192
		Black: 68,023	Black: 78.9	B.M.: 30,000
				B.F.: 38,023

W.M.: White Males
W.F. White Females
B.M.: Black Males
B.F.: Black Females

since some of these females will die between 1980 and 1985, some will outmigrate, and others will inmigrate. The number that will be added or subtracted to the cohort can be estimated by looking at what happened between 1975 and 1980.

Table 11-1 (supra) indicates that the white female population ages 5 to 9 in 1975 was 4,256. Without mortality or migration, there would have been the same number of white females 10 to 14 in 1980; however, the actual figure was only 3,480, producing a net loss of 776, or a net growth of -18.2 percent (i.e., 776/4,256). When this growth rate is applied to the 1980 white female cohort ages 5 to 9, it can be estimated that this bloc will lose 430 (i.e., .182 × 2,361) persons between 1980 and 1985, assuming the same mortality and migration as between 1975 and 1980.

Consequently, the 1985 white female population ages 10 to 14 can be projected by subtracting this loss from the 1980 white female population of 5 to 9. There then will be 1,931 (i.e., 2,361 − 430) white females 10 to 14 years old in 1985. In equation form,

$$
\begin{aligned}
\frac{Population\ 1985}{WF\ 10\text{-}14} &= \frac{Pop.\ 1980}{WF\ 5\text{-}9} + \left[\frac{Pop.\ 1980}{WF\ 5\text{-}9} \right. \\
&\quad \left. \times \frac{(Pop.\ 1980\ 10\text{-}14) - (Pop.\ 1975\ 5\text{-}9)}{(Pop.\ 1975\ 5\text{-}9)} \right] \\
&= 2{,}361 + \left[2{,}361 \times \frac{3{,}480 - 4{,}256}{4{,}256} \right] \\
&= 2{,}361 + [2{,}361 \times (-\ .182)] \\
&= 2{,}361 - 430 = 1{,}931
\end{aligned}
$$

This projection assumes the same growth for each age cohort between 1980 and 1985 as between 1975 and 1980. However, as in the ratio projection of Ackit County's population, the loss (outmigration) seems to be decreasing.

Next, two sets of projections of the female population ages 15 to 44 are developed. Under a first hypothesis, it is assumed that the same migration continues between 1980 and 1990; under a second (more probable) hypothesis, it is assumed that the loss of population is cut by half between 1980 and 1985 and remains at that level between 1985 and 1990. The projection of the female 15-44 population under these two hypotheses is shown in Exhibits 11-1 and 11-2.

Births now can be calculated by using these population projections and the age-specific fertility rates (ASFRs). These rates are calculated using 1975-1980 data and are assumed constant for the period 1980-1990. Table 11-5 shows the calculation of the ASFR and of the projected average annual births for the periods 1980-1985 and 1985-1990. The midpopulation of each of these two periods must be used for the ASFR; the projected age-specific populations are those calculated under the second hypothesis.

The same could be done using the more conservative projections under the first hypothesis. This would lead to a lower number of projected births. It also should be

Exhibit 11-1 Projection of Female Population Ages 15 to 44

Hypothesis 1: Migration Constant

Age Groups		Pop. 1980	Growth Rate		Pop. 1985	Growth Rate	Pop. 1990
White	5-9	2,361	$\frac{3,480-4,256}{4,256} = -.18$		1,931	$-.01$	1,912
	10-14	3,480	$\frac{5,467-5,524}{5,524} = -.01$		3,444	$+.08$	3,720
	15-19	5,467	$\frac{6,984-6,467}{6,467} = +.08$		5,904	$-.178$	4,853
	20-24	6,984	$\frac{5,869-7,138}{7,138} = -.178$		5,742	$-.238$	4,375
	25-29	5,869	$\frac{5,024-6,597}{6,597} = -.238$		4,470	$-.195$	3,598
	30-34	5,042	$\frac{4,028-5,001}{5,001} = -.195$		4,047	$-.076$	3,739
	35-39	4,028	$\frac{3,869-4,189}{4,189} = -.076$		3,720		
	40-44						
Black	5-9	1,818	$\frac{2,036-2,609}{2,609} = -.209$		1,436	$-.066$	1,341
	10-14	2,063	$\frac{2,839-3,041}{3,041} = -.066$		1,926	$+.038$	1,999
	15-19	2,839	$\frac{3,160-3,043}{3,043} = +.038$		2,948	$-.017$	2,898
	20-24	3,160	$\frac{2,660-2,707}{2,707} = -.017$		3,105	$+.018$	3,161
	25-29	2,660	$\frac{2,549-2,503}{2,503} = +.018$		2,709	$-.132$	2,351
	30-34	2,549	$\frac{2,044-2,354}{2,354} = -.132$		2,213	$-.004$	2,204
	35-39	2,044	$\frac{1,963-1,971}{1,971} = -.004$		2,036		
	40-44						

noted that the birth projections are in fact for live births since the age-specific fertility rates are based on live births.

The total fertility rate (TFR) also can be calculated. This indicates the average number of children each woman of the county would have during her lifetime if age-specific fertility rates remain constant. As noted in Chapter 9, the TFR is given by:

$$TFR = \frac{5 \, \Sigma \, ASFR}{1,000}$$

In Ackit County, the TFR for white females is

$$TFR = \frac{5 \times 293.9}{1,000} = 1.47$$

and for black females

$$TFR = \frac{5 \times 488.9}{1,000} = 2.44$$

This means that each white woman of the county would have 1.47 children and each black woman 2.44 if fertility rates remained as they were between 1975 and 1980.

INFANT MORTALITY PROJECTED

Table 11-6 shows the infant deaths that occurred between 1975 and 1980 by age and race of mothers. The age-race rate is calculated simply as the number of infant

Exhibit 11-2 Projection of Female Population Ages 15-44

Hypothesis 2: Decreased Outmigration

Age Groups		Pop. 1980	Growth Rate	Pop. 1985	Growth Rate	Pop. 1990
White	5-9	2,361	$-.18/2 = -.09$			
	10-14	3,480	$-.01/2 = -.005$	2,149	$-.005$	2,138
	15-19	5,467	$+.08/2 = +.04$	3,463	$+.04$	3,602
	20-24	6,984	$-.178/2 = -.089$	5,686	$-.089$	5,180
	25-29	5,869	$-.238/2 = -.119$	6,362	$-.119$	5,605
	30-34	5,024	$-.195/2 = -.0975$	5,171	$-.0975$	4,667
	35-39	4,028	$-.076/2 = -.038$	4,534	$-.038$	4,362
	40-44			3,875		
Black	5-9	1,818	$-.209/2 = -.1045$			
	10-14	2,063	$-.066/2 = -.033$	1,628	$-.033$	1,574
	15-19	2,839	$+.038/2 = +.019$	1,995	$+.019$	2,033
	20-24	3,160	$-.017/2 = -.0085$	2,893	$-.0085$	2,868
	25-29	2,660	$+.018/2 = +.009$	3,133	$+.009$	3,161
	30-34	2,549	$-.132/2 = -.066$	1,381	$-.066$	2,057
	35-39	2,044	$-.044/2 = -.022$	2,381	$-.022$	2,376
	40-44			2,040		

Table 11-5 Projection of Births in Ackit County to 1990

Race	Age Groups	1975-1980				1980-1985		1985-1990	
		No. of births	Avg. annual No. of births	Mid-Year Pop.	ASFR	Mid-Year Pop.	Avg. annual No. of births	Mid-Year Pop.	Avg. annual No. of births
White	15-19	1,096	219.2	6,067	36.1	4,665	168	2,933	106
	20-24	2,593	518.6	7,076	73.3	6,465	474	4,852	356
	25-29	2,940	588	6,306	93.2	6,066	565	5,889	549
	30-34	1,846	369.2	5,010	73.7	5,083	375	5,345	394
	35-39	265	53.0	4,125	12.9	4,230	55	4,587	59
	40-44	97	19.4	4,093	4.7	3,871	18	4,070	19
Black	15-19	1,200	240	2,961	81.1	2,501	203	1,827	148
	20-24	2,799	559.8	2,888	193.8	3,053	592	2,549	494
	25-29	1,800	360	2,566	140.3	2,849	400	3,027	425
	30-34	733	146.6	2,432	60.3	2,603	160	2,875	173
	35-39	101	20.2	2,000	10.1	2,179	22	2,431	25
	40-44	33	6.6	1,983	3.3	1,994	7	2,174	7

Table 11-6 Live Births and Infant Deaths, 1975-1990

Age, Race	1975-1980		
	Infant Deaths	Live Births	Rate
White			
15-19	19	1,096	17.3
20-24	49	2,593	18.9
25-29	40	2,940	13.6
30-34	28	1,846	15.2
35-39	4	265	15.1
40-44	1	97	10.3
Total	141	8,837	15.9
Black			
15-19	40	1,200	33.3
20-24	70	2,799	25.0
25-29	39	1,800	21.7
30-34	16	733	21.8
35-39	2	101	19.8
40-44	0	33	—
Total	167	6,666	25.0
Total			
15-19	59	2,296	25.7
20-24	119	5,392	22.1
25-29	79	4,740	16.7
30-34	44	2,579	17.1
35-39	6	366	16.4
40-44	1	130	7.7
Total	308	15,503	19.9

Age, Race	1980-1985	
	Projected Births	Projected Deaths
White		
15-19	840	15
20-24	2,370	45
25-29	2,825	38
30-34	1,875	29
35-39	275	4
40-44	90	1
Total	8,275	132
Black		
15-19	1,015	35
20-24	2,960	75
25-29	2,000	43
30-34	800	17

Table 11-6 continued

Age, Race	1980-1985	
	Projected Births	Projected Deaths
Black		
35-39	110	2
40-44	35	1
Total	6,920	173
Total		
15-19	1,855	50
20-24	5,330	120
25-29	4,825	81
30-34	2,675	46
35-39	385	6
40-44	125	2
Total	15,195	305

Age, Race	1985-1990	
	Projected Births	Projected Deaths
White		
15-19	530	9
20-24	1,780	35
25-29	2,745	37
30-34	1,970	30
35-39	295	5
40-44	95	1
Total	7,415	117
Black		
15-19	740	25
20-24	2,470	63
25-29	2,125	47
30-34	865	19
35-39	125	3
40-44	35	1
Total	6,360	158
Total		
15-19	1,270	34
20-24	4,250	98
25-29	4,870	84
30-34	2,835	49
35-39	420	8
40-44	130	2
Total	13,775	275

deaths per 1,000 live births. Using the projected births calculated previously, it also is possible to project the number of infant deaths that could be expected if age-race rates remained constant.

In Ackit County, the infant mortality rate varies from a low of 10.3 in white mothers ages 40 to 44 to a high of 33.3 in black mothers under 20. The few births and deaths to mothers under 15 have been added to the 15-19 groups. Among white mothers, the rate is higher in the 20-24 group, followed by those 15-19 and 30-39. All of these rates are lower than for black mothers, whose rates decrease with age, ranging from 33.3 among teenagers to 19.8 in the 35-39 group.

However, since the population is aging, it can be seen that there will be fewer births at younger ages and more at older ones. Assuming constant fertility and infant mortality rates, it is projected that there will be a 40 percent reduction in the number of births and infant deaths to black teenage mothers and a 50 percent reduction among white teenagers.

From the data in Table 11-6, it seems certain that the high-risk groups for infant mortality and, consequently, the ones that should be targeted for a reduction in infant mortality in Ackit County are the younger whites and blacks, particularly the teenagers. High-risk groups can be pinpointed further by analyzing infant deaths by other sociodemographic and geographic variables.

It would be interesting to analyze infant deaths in relation to such factors as mothers' life style (cigarette smoking, nutrition, stress, exercise, use of alcohol and drugs, etc.) and environmental variables (occupation, housing, leisure, etc.). However, this would necessitate a special survey. If the analysis is limited to variables readily available from birth and death certificates, factors include maternal education and marital status, father's race and education, prenatal care, birth weight, weeks of gestation, result of mother's last pregnancy, and geographical area of residence. Other information could include complications of pregnancy and cause of death.

INFANT MORTALITY: A RETROSPECTIVE ANALYSIS

Analysis such as this of infant mortality can be done by hospital managers following the principles of a retrospective (case-control) epidemiological study (Chapter 1). To perform such a study using only simple data from birth and death certificates, a control group must be selected first. The study group is the 308 women who had an infant death between 1975 and 1980. The control group is women of similar age, race, and education who had a baby during this period but no infant death.

These two groups could be matched on any variables other than age, race, and education, but these three probably would suffice for the managers' purposes. This matched control group can be selected from a listing of all the births that occurred between 1975 and 1980 in Ackit County. For every woman in the study group, a control can be found. The analysis then would consist simply of comparing the study and control groups on the other variables. For variables used in matching, the study group should be compared with the overall population of women who had a child between 1975 and 1980.

Tables 11-7 through 11-12 show the results of such a study for Ackit County. The data show that there is a greater proportion of unwed mothers in the study group than in the control group (Table 11-9). The prenatal care information from the birth certificates (Tables 11-8 and 11-9) indicates that the study and control groups differed only slightly and that the study mothers apparently were receiving early prenatal care: 58.8 percent of them initiated care in the first trimester compared to 65.7 percent of the controls.

Although the study group had an average of only 7.6 visits compared to 10.4 for the controls, this may be explained in part by the fact that 64.2 percent of the study infants were premature (Table 11-13), thus causing the study mothers to have less of an opportunity to seek care. On the whole, prenatal care of the study groups seems adequate in terms of quantity and time of initiation.

The study group data on birth weight and weeks of gestation (Tables 11-10 and 11-11) provide the most obvious explanations of the infant deaths. The association between a short duration of pregnancy and low birth weight is well established, as is the relationship between low birth weight and a greatly elevated risk of infant mortality, congenital malformations, and other physical and neurological impairments.[3, 4, 5, 6] The mean study group birth weight of 5.8 pounds was just over the low birth weight standard of 5.5 pounds (2,500 grams), which is not surprising considering the fact that two-thirds of the study infants were premature.

Data on the results of mothers' last pregnancies (Table 11-12) indicate that those in the study group tended to be at high risk in terms of their history of prematurity and spontaneous abortions, especially compared to the controls. This points out the necessity of eliciting a complete history from the woman as soon as pregnancy is discovered and preparing for a referral to a high-risk center for delivery.

In addition to all these variables, the geographical distribution of births and deaths could be analyzed by service area. It could be found, for example (Table 11-13) that although only 15 percent of the live births were to mothers who lived in service area 02, 36 percent of infant deaths occurred to those mothers.

IMPLICATIONS FOR ACTION

These demographic and epidemiological analyses point to several conclusions and recommendations for action. The population of Ackit County is aging, increasingly female, and increasingly black. Probably as a consequence of very high outmigration (particularly of whites), the county's population has been

Table 11-7 Marital Status of Mothers

Marital Status	Study Group (Percent)	Control Group (Percent)
Married	85.1*	89.9
Unmarried	14.9	10.1
Unknown	(1.7)	(1.8)
Totals	100.0	100.0

*These are adjusted percentages, i.e., percentages calculated without the "unknowns."

Table 11-8 Month Prenatal Care Began

Month of Pregnancy	Study Group (Percent)	Control Group (Percent)
1	11.4	14.3
2	34.2	37.1
3	13.2	14.3
4	12.3	8.6
5	5.3	3.8
6	2.6	5.7
7	1.8	5.7
8	2.6	1.9
9	1.8	5.7
None	3.5	5.7
Unknown	(1.7)	(5.4)
Totals	100.0	100.0
Mean	3.7 Months	3.0 Months

Table 11-9 Total Number of Prenatal Visits

Number of Prenatal Visits	Study Group (Percent)	Control Group (Percent)
1 - 4	26.9	8.5
5 - 9	30.1	18.1
10 - 13	28.0	42.6
14 - 19	9.7	21.3
20 +	1.1	3.2
None	4.3	.3
Totals	100.0	100.0
Mean	7.6	10.4

Table 11-10 Birth Weight of Infants

Birth Weight (Pounds)	Study Group (Percent)	Control Group (Percent)
Less than 1	9.2	0.0
1.0 - 1.9	25.7	0.0
2.0 - 2.9	16.5	0.0
3.0 - 3.9	2.8	0.0
4.0 - 4.9	7.3	1.8
5.0 - 5.9	6.5	10.9
6.0 - 6.9	12.0	30.0
7.0 - 7.9	8.2	33.7
8.0 - 8.9	7.3	21.0
9.0 - 9.9	3.7	2.7
10.0 and over	0.9	0.0
Unknown	(6.0)	(0.9)
Totals	100.0	100.0
Mean Birth Weight	5.8 Lbs.	7.2 Lbs.

Table 11-11 Weeks of Gestation at Delivery

Weeks	Study Group (Percent)	Control Group (Percent)
15-19	5.3	0.0
20-27	31.6	0.0
28-31	14.7	0.0
32-35	8.4	6.4
36	4.2	2.1
37-39	10.5	28.7
40	8.4	23.4
41-42	11.6	28.6
More than 42	6.3	10.6
Unknown	(18.1)	(15.3)
Totals	100.0	100.0
Mean	31.9	39.9

Table 11-12 Result of Mothers' Last Pregnancy

Result	Study Group (Percent)	Control Group (Percent)
No previous pregnancy	1.5	25.3
Full term	57.6	67.5
Premature	13.6	2.4
Spontaneous abortion	19.7	3.6
Induced abortion	6.1	1.2
Dead, full term	1.5	0.0
Unknown	(43.1)	(25.2)
Totals	100.0	100.0

Table 11-13 Live Births and Infant Deaths

By Geographical Area

Service Area	Live Births (Percent)	Infant Deaths (Percent)
01	23	16
02	15	36
03	37	26
04	25	22
Totals	100	100

decreasing but it is projected that this trend eventually will taper off so that between 1985 and 1990, it will increase again.

Infant mortality rates for the total and white populations are significantly above the average for the United States; the rates for blacks, although not significantly higher than the national average, also present a serious problem.

As a consequence of the aging of the population, the number of births can be expected to decrease through 1990. However, the drop will be associated mostly with whites.

The analyses point to high-risk groups for infant mortality in this county. The high proportion of black, teenage, and unwed mothers among those having infant deaths makes these women particularly at high risk for infant mortality and especially suited for maternal health care and preventive programs involving health education and counseling.

The high frequency of low birth weight and premature infants in the study group, and the established association of these characteristics with less educated, teen-aged black mothers, indicates the need for intervention to prevent infant deaths. This intervention may take the following forms:

• Family planning programs, with emphasis on counseling teenagers on con-traceptive use and follow-up, and the availability of abortion in the case of unwanted pregnancies, should be accessible. This is a major market that institutions and hospitals can capture. Furthermore, efforts in this area would promote preventive strategies. However, any needs that would arise would be most likely to be purchased from the hospital by the client. The push by the United States Department of Health and Human Services to inform parents of teenagers' contraceptive use (later prohibited by the United States Supreme Court) made the burden greater at local and state levels as well as increasing the probability that teenagers would avoid family planning services. Research indicates little evidence for the prevention of a first unwanted teenage preg-nancy; instead, the emphasis is on closely following the pregnancy and administering special treatment and referral to a tertiary center for delivery.

However, good evidence exists for prevention of the second unwanted teenage pregnancy, either through contraception or follow-up abortion.[7]

- Health education with emphasis on sex education in the schools should begin in the very early years of adolescence (seventh and eighth grades) when sexual experimentation begins and before unwanted pregnancies occur. Hospitals could develop a market for these services through a special program to address this issue.

- Parent or adult education is an important component in preventing teenage pregnancy, low birth weight, and infant deaths. The parents in the community must be exposed to the facts concerning the high incidence of teenage pregnancy, and especially the high-risk factors and consequences, e.g., infant deaths, so that they may better accept rather than oppose sex education in schools and in family planning programs. The prevention of these events is a most critical area that hospitals could pursue.

- Early prenatal care programs should be readily available and accessible to pregnant teenagers and should emphasize their special problems. These programs should provide treatment and counseling in nutrition and other life style/environmental factors such as smoking and alcohol, and should include mental health counseling and parenting programs. The bottom line for hospitals—particularly Sunnyvale Civic—should be a wellness center for the growth of healthy babies and well mothers. Health services managers can apply the concept of marketing and other factors to this population in an ambulatory setting.

Prenatal care data seem to indicate that the study group, overall, had adequate care in terms of quantity and time of initiation. In light of the data on weeks of gestation and previous pregnancies, prenatal care programs must emphasize elicitation of complete histories, readily available high-risk program care, and especially tertiary center delivery for these women with past or present problems. Community outreach and other prenatal health care marketing programs should be initiated and should emphasize the characteristics of a high-risk pregnancy and the availability of special help for these women.

SUMMARY

Special efforts should be made by Sunnyvale Civic Hospital in Ackit County to prevent teenage pregnancies and to reach the black population and the women in service area 02. The projection of births and deaths can serve as a sound basis for forecasting and allocating resources to tackle the infant mortality problem and to develop preventive medical centers to evaluate and monitor the progress that could be accomplished.

For example, between 1985 and 1990, the hospital can expect 13,775 live births and an additional 275 pregnancies that, if infant mortality rates remained constant, would lead to infant deaths. If a standard of 14 prenatal visits is followed, there would be a need of 196,700 prenatal visits ([13,775 + 275] × 14). The targeting of teenagers and blacks would necessitate 98,798 visits ([530 + 9 + 6,360 + 158] × 14). The planning for delivery and postnatal services, as well as family planning, sex education, and high-risk pregnancies services could proceed on the same basis.

Thus Sunnyvale Civic needs to consider the future need for high-risk newborn care services in concert with the prevention programs just discussed. It is fairly clear that the hospital does not need increased obstetrical services as the birthrate will not be increasing. Again, preventive services appear to be the most practical marketing strategy.

The marketing of services from the hospital's perspective must meld the concept of preventive medicine with the need for care and treatment. The demographic, epidemiological, and utilization analysis of the problems in Ackit County reflect a major need for Sunnyvale Civic Hospital to embark on a significantly new approach to the marketing and delivery of its services.

The county is changing demographically, epidemiologically, and in its utilization of services. The hospital therefore must keep pace with the change.

Although this is an isolated example, the concepts and strategies can be applied quite easily in most areas of the country.

NOTES

1. U.S. Public Health Service, *Health, United States, 1981* (Washington, D.C.: U.S. Department of Health and Human Services, National Center for Health Statistics, 1981), 113.

2. U.S. Public Health Service, *Health, United States, 1980* (Washington, D.C.: U.S. Department of Health and Human Services, National Center for Health Statistics, 1980), 309.

3. Joel C. Kleinman, "Trends and Variations in Birth Weight," in *Health, United States, 1981* (Washington, D.C.: U.S. Department of Health and Human Services, Public Health Service, National Center for Health Statistics, 1981), 7-13.

4. National Center for Health Statistics, "A Study of Infant Mortality from Linked Records by Birth Weight, Period of Gestation, and Other Variables," U.S. Department of Health, Education, and Welfare, Health Services and Mental Health Administration, *Vital and Health Statistics*, Series 20-No. 12 (DHEW Publication No. [HSM] 72-1055). (Washington, D.C.: U.S. Government Printing Office, May 1972), 90.

5. National Center for Health Statistics, "Factors Associated with Low Birth Weight," U.S. Department of Health, Education, and Welfare, Public Health Service, *Vital and Health Statistics*, Series 21-No. 37 (DHEW Publication No. [PHS] 80-1915). (Washington, D.C.: U.S. Government Printing Office, April 1980), 37.

6. D.M. Reed and F.J. Stanley, eds., *The Epidemiology of Prematurity* (Baltimore: Urban and Schwarzenberg, 1977), 370.

7. Health and Welfare, Canada, *Periodic Health Examination Monograph*, Report of a Task Force to the Conference of Deputy Ministers of Health (Spitzer Report) (Ottawa: 1980), 194.

Chapter 12

Epidemiology and Environmental Health

THE ENVIRONMENT'S INFLUENCE ON HEALTH

As noted in Chapter 2, the relationship between man's environment and the occurrence of health and disease has long been acknowledged (at least ever since Hippocrates). Both the traditional epidemiological model of disease causation (agent-host-environment) and the health field concept model (human biology, environment, life style, and health care organization) provide for this environmental influence on health. This chapter discusses the environment and its influences on health, the contributions of epidemiology to environmental health, and the implications for health care providers and managers.

In the health field concept model adopted in this book as the epidemiological framework for health, the environment is one of four broad elements influencing health and disease causation. In this context, the environment can be defined as including "all those matters related to health which are external to the human body and over which the individual has little or no control".[1]

It is this notion of little or no control that separates environmental factors from life style factors. For this reason, such items as smoking, alcohol, and use of seat belts were classified previously (perhaps arbitrarily) as personal life style factors (Chapter 5). With this understanding, the following quotation from Lalonde gives a good overview of what is meant by environmental factors influencing health and disease:

> Individuals cannot, by themselves, ensure that foods, drugs, cosmetics, devices, water supply, etc., are safe and uncontaminated; that the health hazards of air, water, and noise pollution are controlled; that the spread of communicable diseases is prevented; that effective garbage and sewage disposal is carried out; and that the social environment, including the rapid changes in it, do not have harmful effects on health.[2]

For purposes here, a distinction is drawn between the physical and the socio-psychological environments. In both of these, many different material and social factors may constitute health risks or health hazards—physical, chemical, biological, or social. Exhibit 12-1 lists the various environmental components and health hazards.

This classification is somewhat arbitrary and the listing is incomplete. However, it provides an adequate framework for examining the influences of the environment on health and disease. Before doing so, it should be pointed out that although the relationship between selected environmental components and factors, and health and disease, is discussed independently, many environmentally induced diseases such as cancer, coronary heart disease, and chronic obstructive lung disease have a multifactorial origin,[3] i.e., several factors may be necessary to induce disease manifestations. The interaction of these multiple factors may lead to a wide variety of disease manifestations.

THE PHYSICAL ENVIRONMENT

The first four components of the physical environment (Exhibit 12-1) can be considered as life support systems[4] essential for human life. Air, water, soil, and food are the fundamental prerequisites of life and of health. The physical components of the environment also include the climate and noise and radiation levels.

The deleterious effects of the life support systems (air, water, soil, food) on health may come from either chemical or biological hazards. The harmful effects

Exhibit 12-1 Environmental Components and Health Hazards

Components		Health Hazards	
Physical:	air	Physical:	heat and cold
	water		radiation
	soil		noise
	food		
	climate and weather	Chemical:	metals
	noise level		chemical substances
	radiation level		
		Biological:	microorganisms
Social:	work		flora and fauna
	transport		
	leisure	Social:	culture/customs
	housing		interpersonal relations
	family and community		social and political structure
			housing factors

of the climate involve thermal exposures (heat and cold). Radiation and noise also may constitute hazards. These are discussed in detail in specialized texts.[5,6,7,8,9]

Air

An individual ordinarily inhales approximately 30 pounds of air a day. This air is made up of several gases, chemicals, and particulates. The best-known air pollutants are carbon monoxide (CO), then sulfur oxides (SO_2, SO_3), the hydrocarbons, the nitrogen oxides (N_2O, NO, NO_2, N_2O_5), and the particulates (soot, fly ash, other industrial emissions, and volcanic debris).

Carbon monoxide, which stems mainly from vehicle engines, accounts for about half the total weight of air pollutants in the United States. Vehicle emissions have been reduced significantly since the 1975 regulations requiring new cars to be equipped with exhaust catalytic converters (which convert carbon monoxide to carbon dioxide, a less harmful gas). Carbon monoxide emissions in the nation dropped from 81.3 million tons per year in 1973 to 69.7 million tons in 1979.[10] Sulfur oxides account for 15 percent of the air pollutants and are produced by coal and oil combustion in power plants and by refineries and smelters. Hydrocarbons (also 15 percent) derive from vehicle engines, natural gas combustion, refineries, and volatile solvent plants. Nitrogen oxides (10 percent of the weight of air pollutants) also are produced by vehicle engines and by some industries. Particulates (13 percent) appear from industries, incinerators, heating sources, and vehicle engines.

Although these air pollutants are the ones most often associated with disease incidence, this is primarily because they are in fact the ones for which measurement methods have been developed.[11] Other inert or noxious gases or trace metals such as cadmium, lead, arsenic, beryllium, vanadium, and fluorine are accumulating in the atmosphere but less is known about them and their health consequences.

Air pollution quite understandably is associated most with respiratory system diseases. As can be seen in Table 12-1, diseases of other systems (circulatory, digestive, and sensorial) as well as general well-being and mortality also are associated with air pollutants. (This table is limited to community air pollution; occupational and domestic air hazards are discussed later.)

The relationship between episodes of air stagnation-pollution and acute episodes of aggravated pulmonary disease has been well demonstrated.[12] The most striking incident occurred in London in December 1952 when a temperature inversion combined with fog and no air movement to result in sharply increased levels of sulfur dioxide, hydrocarbon, carbon monoxide, and particulates. Throughout the area, hospitalizations for pulmonary complications soared. Some 4,000 additional deaths resulted from the incident.[13] The very young and the very old with preexistent chronic pulmonary disease were particularly affected.

Table 12-1 Definite and Possible Health Effects of Community Air Pollution

Agent, Pollutant, or Source	Definite Effect	Possible Effect
Sulfur dioxide (effects of sulfur oxides may be caused by sulfur, sulfur trioxide, sulfuric acid, or sulfate salts)	1. Aggravation of asthma and chronic bronchitis 2. Impairment of pulmonary function 3. Sensory irritation	
Sulfur oxides and particulate matter from combustion sources	4. Short-term increase in mortality 5. Short-term increase in morbidity 6. Aggravation of bronchitis and cardiovascular disease 7. Contributory role in etiology of chronic bronchitis and emphysema 8. Contributory role to respiratory disease in children	
		9. Contributory role in etiology of lung cancer
Particulate matter (not otherwise specified)		10. Increase in chronic respiratory disease
Oxidants	11. Aggravation of emphysema, asthma, and bronchitis 12. Impairment of lung function in patients with bronchitis-emphysema 13. Eye and respiratory irritation and impairment in performance of student athletes	
		14. Increased probability of motor vehicle accidents

Table 12-1 continued

Agent, Pollutant, or Source	Definite Effect	Possible Effect
Ozone	15. Impairment of lung function	
		16. Acceleration of aging, possibly because of lipid peroxidation and related processes
Carbon monoxide	17. Impairment of exercise tolerance in patients with cardiovascular disease	
		18. Increased general mortality and coronary mortality rates
		19. Impairment of central nervous system function
		20. Causal factor in atherosclerosis
Nitrogen dioxide		21. Factor in pulmonary emphysema
		22. Impairment of lung defenses such as mast cells and macrophages or altered lung function
Lead	23. Increased storage in body	
		24. Impairment of hemoglobin and porphyrin synthesis
Hydrogen sulfide	25. Increased mortality from acute exposures	
	26. A cause of sensory irritation	
Mercaptans		27. Headache, nausea, and sinus affections

Table 12-1 continued

Agent, Pollutant, or Source	Definite Effect	Possible Effect
Asbestos	28. Production of pleural calcification 29. Malignant mesothelioma, asbestosis	
		30. Contributor to chronic pulmonary disease (asbestos and lung cancer)
Organophosphorus pesticides	31. Acute fatal poisoning 32. Acute illness 33. Impaired cholinesterase activity	
Other odorus compounds		34. Headache and sinus affections
Beryllium	35. Berylliosis with pulmonary impairment	
Airborne microorganisms	36. Airborne infections	

Source: Adapted from "Statistics Needed for Determining the Effects of the Environment on Health," *Vital and Health Statistics,* ser. 4, no. 20; U.S. Department of Health, Education, and Welfare, Public Health Service, Health Resources Administration (DHEW Publication No. [HRA] 77-1457) (Washington, D.C.: U.S. Government Printing Office, July 1977).

The relationship between air pollution and the incidence of chronic respiratory disease is less well demonstrated, although several studies have reported that the irritant action of air pollutants may lead to asthma, chronic bronchitis, and pulmonary emphysema.[14,15] Certain groups such as infants and children,[16] and smokers,[17] are regarded as particularly vulnerable.

Air pollution also has been implicated as a contributor to diseases of the heart and blood vessels, sensory irritations, headaches, nausea, poisoning, etc. It has been shown that it increases susceptibility to viruses, including flu.[18]

A 1979 study estimates that a 50 percent reduction in sulfates and suspended particulates in urban areas could help produce at least a 4.7 percent decrease in the total mortality rate.[19] This in turn could lead to an increase in life expectancy at birth of approximately eight-tenths of one year (almost ten months).

Water and Food

The effects of water and food on the incidence of disease are examined jointly since the major sources that contaminate them are the same chemical and biological health hazards. (The influence of nutrition on health was considered a life style factor and was examined as such in Chapter 5.)

Table 12-2 lists the major food and water contaminants and their health effects. Biological contaminants include bacteria, viruses, and protozoa and metazoa. The contamination of water by such microorganisms was once the source of much morbidity and mortality (as in the London cholera epidemic discussed in Chapter 7). Although this has been much reduced by filtration and chlorination of drinking water, occasional contamination still occurs when sewage disposal and water protection mechanisms are disrupted. It is estimated that 5 percent of the population is affected yearly by diseases related to the contamination of foods by microorganisms.[20]

Both water and food also can be contaminated by chemical substances, including industrial and agricultural wastes involving such chemical substances as pesticides, arsenic, nitrites, cyanides, copper, cadmium, lead, mercury, borates, chromium, sulfates, phosphates, and fluorides. All of these have been associated with the incidence of disease.

For example, the level of nitrites in drinking water has been convincingly associated with the prevalence, and mortality from, hypertension.[21] The same may be true for cadmium.[22] There also is growing concern that the increasing radioactive debris that can be found in both food[23] and water[24] and that results mostly from the use of atomic energy may have serious long-term health effects.

A study of exposure to radium in Iowa and Illinois shows a significantly higher death rate from bone cancer in an exposed group than in a control population.[25] The radioactivity of drinking water also has been associated with cardiovascular diseases and, in particular, with hypertensive ailments.[26] It also should be noted that increasingly large amounts of radioactive wastes for which appropriate long-term disposal methods have yet to be found eventually will enter the waterways and alimentary chain, with possible terrifying health effects.

Although the subject of controversy, some current practices in food processing may constitute long-term health hazards. Several food additives whose long-term effects on health are unknown are used frequently. The addition of antibiotics to poultry, hogs, and cattle feed may induce the development of resistant strains of microorganisms. Residues of antibiotics often are found in milk and may accumulate in the flesh of livestock, with undesirable effects on the health of humans.

The "softness" of drinking water (mainly its calcium content) has been linked to heart diseases [27,28,29] and to infant mortality.[30]

Soil

Soil is considered one of the support systems necessary and essential for human life. The geochemical composition of soil and its relationship to the occurrence of

Table 12-2 Definite and Possible Health Effects of Food and Water
Contaminants

Agent, Pollutant, or Source	Definite Effect	Possible Effect
Bacteria	1. Epidemic and endemic gastrointestinal infections (typhoid, cholera, shigellosis, salmonellosis, leptospirosis, etc.)	
		2. Secondary interaction with malnutrition and with nitrates in water
Viruses	3. Epidemic hepatitis and other viral infections	
		4. Eye and skin inflammation from swimming
Protozoa and metazoa	5. Amoebiasis, schistosomiasis, hydatidosis, and other parasitic infections	
Metals	6. Lead poisoning 7. Mercury poisoning (through food chains) 8. Cadmium poisoning (through food chains) 9. Arsenic poisoning 10. Chromium poisoning	
		11. Epidemic nephropathy 12. "Blackfoot" disease
Nitrates	13. Methemoglobinemia (with bacterial interactions)	
Water "softness" factor		14. Increase in cardiovascular disease
Sulfates and/or phosphates	15. Gastrointestinal hypermotility	
Fluorides	16. Fluorosis of teeth when in excess	

Source: Reprinted from "Statistics Needed for Determining the Effects of the Environment on Health," *Vital and Health Statistics,* ser. 4, no. 20, U.S. Department of Health, Education, and Welfare, Public Health Service, Health Resources Administration, DHEW Publication No. (HRA) 77-1457 (Washington, D.C.: U.S. Government Printing Office, July 1977).

some diseases has some importance; however it is mainly its role as a reservoir of pollutants that may be deleterious to health.

As with air and water, the health hazards in soil may be either of biological or physiochemical origin. Table 12-3 lists possible and definite health effects of land pollutants. These include pathogenic microorganisms from human or animal excreta, other infectious agents that may proliferate because of unusual sewage disposal and treatment, chemical elements from industrial and automotive wastes, radioactive wastes, and pesticides.

Naturally occurring chemicals in soil may be associated with the incidence of some diseases, particularly hypertensive ones and some types of cancer. Although evidence is not yet conclusive, a correlation between soil characteristics and the incidence of diseases does exist. It has been shown that cancers of the stomach and breast are more frequent where soils have equable moisture at all seasons, that stomach cancer is more frequent where there are high levels of organic matter, zinc, cobalt, and chromium, and that esophageal cancer is geographically associated with geological type and with severe soil impoverishment.[31] Overall mortality rates also are associated with sedimentary and volcanic rocks[32] and with low levels of many trace elements.[33] Trace metals in soil are associated with the proliferation and spread of infectious agents.[34]

Table 12-3 Definite and Possible Health Effects of Land Pollution

Agent, Pollutant, or Source	Definite Effect	Possible Effect
Human excreta	1. Schistosomiasis, taeniasis hookworm, and other infections	
Sewage		2. Typhus, plague, leptospirosis, and other infectious diseases
Industrial and radioactive waste	3. Storage and effects from toxic metals and other substances through food chains	
Pesticides—lead arsenate	4. Increased storage of heavy metals in smokers of tobacco grown on treated areas	

Source: Reprinted from "Statistics Needed for Determining the Effects of the Environment on Health," *Vital and Health Statistics,* ser. 4, no. 20, DHEW Publ. No. HRS 77-1457. Hyattsville, MD., July 1977. U.S. Department of Health, Education, and Welfare, Public Health Service, Health Resources Administration, DHEW Publication No. (HRA) 77-1457 (Washington, D.C.: U.S. Government Printing Office, July 1977).

Climate and Weather

Pathological biometeorology is the science that studies the influence of weather and climate on the various physiological and pathological phenomena associated with human diseases, their period of outbreak, intensity, and geographical distribution.[35] The literature reports many relationships between climate/weather and health, from the obvious effects of thermal exposures (heat and cold) to the intriguing seasonal variations in birth weight and birth rates.

The physiological reaction to changes in weather and climate is mediated by the endocrine system—the hypothalamus and, consequently, the pituitary gland. Meteorological stimuli have been shown to influence a wide range of physiological processes,[36] including the level and production of hemoglobin, leukocytes, thrombocytes, eosinophils, serum proteins, etc. Diastolic blood pressure is higher in winter but general metabolism decreases sharply in that period.

Diseases whose incidence is thought to be associated with weather and climate are called meteorotropic. These may be classified into four major groups:[37]

1. diseases resulting from disturbances of the natural biological rhythms (short- and or long-term, i.e., seasonal, disturbances)
2. diseases caused by thermal stresses (and consequently by hypothalamic disturbances)
3. diseases stemming from ultraviolet solar radiation
4. diseases that are infectious.

The incidence of infectious diseases shows clear seasonal variations, mostly caused by the influence of temperature and humidity on the proliferation and propagation of infectious agents. The incidence of many respiratory conditions (asthma, bronchitis, rhinitis), of some rheumatic diseases (particularly rheumatoid arthritis), of heart diseases (myocardial infarction and angina pectoris), and of cerebrovascular accidents has been associated with moderate thermal stresses. Excessive thermal stresses may lead to heatstroke, edema, syncope, sweat gland disorders, and frostbite. Table 12-4 presents possible and definite effects of various thermal exposures.

A last point worth mentioning is the emergence of pharmacological biometeorology, i.e., the study of the influence of weather and climate on the effect of drugs. It has been shown that drugs may have varying pharmacological effects because weather influences membrane permeability and speed of absorption at the cellular level.[38]

Noise Level

Primarily because of urbanization, industrialization, higher population density, and transportation, noise is becoming an increasing problem and noise pollution may be legitimately considered as an environmental health hazard.

Table 12-4 Definite and Possible Effects of Thermal Exposure

Thermal Stress	Definite Effects	Possible Effects
Cold damp	1. Excess mortality from respiratory disease and fatal exposure	
		2. Contribution to excess mortality and morbidity from other causes
	3. Excess morbidity from respiratory and related diseases and morbidity from exposure	
		4. Rheumatism
Cold dry	5. Mortality from frostbite and exposure	
		6. Impaired lung function
	7. Morbidity from frostbite and respiratory disease	
Hot dry	8. Heatstroke mortality	
	9. Excess mortality attributed to other causes	
	10. Morbidity from heatstroke and from other causes	
	11. Impaired function; aggravation of renal and circulatory diseases	
Hot damp	12. Increase in skin affections	
		13. Increase in prevalence of infectious agents and vectors
	14. Heat-exhaustion mortality	
	15. Excess mortality from other causes	
	16. Heat-related morbidity	
	17. Impaired vigor and circulatory function	
	18. Aggravation of renal and circulatory disease	

Source: Reprinted from "Statistics Needed for Determining the Effects of the Environment on Health," *Vital and Health Statistics,* ser. 4, no. 20; U.S. Department of Health, Education, and Welfare, Public Health Service, Health Resources Administration, DHEW Publication No. (HRA) 77-1457 (Washington, D.C.: U.S. Government Printing Office, July 1977).

Noise can be deleterious to health in two main ways:[39] (1) it can damage the ear and cause a loss of hearing and (2) it can influence a number of other physiological functions. The damage noise does to hearing depends mainly on both its intensity and the duration of exposure.[40] There are wide individual variations in susceptibility to hearing loss from noise.[41]

Noise can cause stress and therefore can be held responsible in part for a wide variety of stress-induced morbidities. More specifically, noise seems to influence the release of many pituitary gland hormones through its stimulation of the autonomic nervous system.[42] In such cases, the time pattern of noise (continuous or impulsive) is more important than its intensity—impulsive (interrupted) noise being more damaging (i.e., having a more stimulating effect on the autonomic nervous system) than continuous noise. It also has been reported that high-intensity noise (for example, from aircraft) could aggravate or even cause mental illness.[43]

Noise pollution is most prevalent in industrial/work settings and most noise-induced health damage can be associated with occupation. As noted earlier, however, noise also is produced almost continously by traffic, aircraft, railways, construction, etc. Studies indicate that urban noise may lead to a steady diminution of hearing throughout life[44] (in addition to normal aging-related hearing loss).

Radiation Level

The last component of the physical environment discussed here is the radiation level. Sources of radiation may either be natural or man-made. The impact of radiation on health depends on the duration of exposure, the amount of absorption by the person, and the type or, more specifically, its wavelength. The most hazardous emissions are those with small wavelengths, including ionizing and ultraviolet radiation. Other nonionizing radiations include visible light, infrared, microwave, and radio frequency, and as a general rule are much less hazardous to health.

Both ionizing and untraviolet radiations are both naturally present in the environment and are man-made. Natural sources of ionizing radiations include terrestrial radiation, that is, emanating from such radioactive elements as thorium, uranium, and radium that are present in the soil and in the earth's crust, as well as cosmic radiation, which is from space. Man-made ionizing radiations are produced by such activities as nuclear explosions (detonation of nuclear devices), nuclear power, medical and dental radiography, and occupational exposure. Ultraviolet radiations may come from the sun or be man-made. Many persons such as aircraft workers, construction workers, food irradiators, foundry workers, etc.,[45] can be exposed to ultraviolet radiation.

Table 12-5 lists possible and definite health effects of radiations. Ultraviolet radiation from sunlight primarily affects the skin and the eye. In addition to the

Table 12-5 Definite and Possible Health Effects of Radiation

Source	Definite Effects	Possible Effects
Natural sunlight	1. Fatalities from acute exposure 2. Morbidity due to "burn" 3. Skin cancer 4. Interaction with drugs in susceptible individuals	5. Increase in malignant melanoma
Diagnostic x-ray	6. Skin cancer and other skin changes	7. Contributing factors to leukemia 8. Alteration in fecundity
Therapeutic radiation	9. Skin cancer 10. Increase in leukemia	11. Increase in other cancers 12. Acceleration of aging 13. Mutagenesis
Industrial use of radiation and mining of radioactive ores	14. Acute accidental deaths 15. Radiation morbidity 16. Uranium nephritis 17. Lung cancer in cigarette-smoking miners	18. Increase in adjacent community morbidity or mortality
Nuclear power and reprocessing plants		19. Increase in cancer incidence 20. Community disaster 21. Alteration in human genetic material
Microwaves		22. Tissue damage

Source: Reprinted from "Statistics Needed for Determining the Effects of the Environment on Health," *Vital and Health Statistics,* ser. 4, no. 20; U.S. Department of Health, Education, and Welfare, Public Health Service, Health Resources Administration, DHEW Publication No. (HRA) 77-1457 (Washington, D.C.: U.S. Government Printing Office, 1977).

obvious sunburns, sunlight has been shown conclusively to promote skin cancer. As of 1980 there were more than 300,000 skin cancer cases reported annually in the United States and there is concern that the potential depletion of the atmosphere's ozone layer, which partially filters the ultraviolet sun rays, may cause an increase in skin cancer rates.[46] Ultraviolet radiation also affects the eye and can lead to keratitis inflammation of the cornea and to conjunctivitis.[47]

Ionizing radiation has carcinogenic properties and it is known that virtually all types of cancer are capable of being induced by radiation.[48] In addition, ionizing radiation is thought to have the potential to induce genetic damage by modifying the chromosomal structure and increasing the gene mutation rate.[49]

Although this obviously is not the place to settle the controversies over nuclear armament and nuclear power, both of those definitely can be considered environmental health hazards. Nobody can question the carcinogenic and genetic effects of the use and testing of nuclear weapons. As for nuclear power plants, even day-to-day operations can produce slight leakage of various radioactive materials.

Although studies of the health effects of such "planned" pollution have not reported any significant results, nothing is known of the possible impact of the gradual (and rapidly expanding) accumulation of radioactive materials in the environment. Unplanned releases of radioactivity, such as already have occurred on several occasions, could have serious health effects, including stress-related morbidity.

A study of the health-related economic costs of the Three-Mile Island accident concludes that for a ten-month period within a five-mile ring the total was about $5.2 million.[50] This does not include any consideration of possible long-term impact on morbidity and mortality.

THE SOCIAL ENVIRONMENT

The components of the social environment are work, transport, leisure, housing, and the family and community. Except in the case of the family and community where health risks are of a social nature, the deleterious effects on health of these components can come from physical, chemical, biological, or social sources.

Work

Since work occupies such a large part of modern life, it is not surprising that it can have a tremendous influence on people's health. Occupational health may be defined as the branch of public or community health concerned with all job-related factors potentially affecting worker (and, secondarily, community) health.[51] Health hazards in the work environment can either be material (physical, chemical biological, or mechanical), or psychosocial.

As is the case with other environmental health problems, occupational hazards are acute or chronic (temporarily or continually present) and their effects may be immediate or delayed. There can be either direct cause-effect relationships (as in the case of physical injuries such as asbestos and lung disease) or indirect relationships (as in the case of boredom or stress leading to alienation or injury, or toxic exposure aggravating existing health conditions).[52]

Occupational health has been the subject of so much research and has become such a specialized discipline that it obviously is much beyond the scope of this book to discuss individually all of the hazards that have been shown or are thought to influence workers' health. Figure 12-1 lists work environment hazards affecting health and social well-being and Table 12-6 lists physical and chemical health hazards in the job environment, their health effects, and the types of employees affected.

The physical and chemical health hazards have been studied extensively. It is estimated that at least 10 percent of male cancers are related to such occupational hazards,[53] and this is a conservative estimate based only on direct evidence. A researcher of the International Agency for Cancer Research of the World Health Organization states that "there is good circumstantial evidence that 80 to 90 percent of all cancers are dependent, directly or indirectly, on environmental factors . . . and at least 90 percent of these factors are chemical in nature".[54]

Since much of the exposure to carcinogenic chemical and physical agents takes place in the work environment, and since there might be a synergistic action between different occupational agents and other types of environmental agents,[55] the proportion of cancer that may result, directly or indirectly, from exposures on the job probably is much larger than 10 percent. Chemical occupational hazards also contribute significantly to chronic obstructive pulmonary disease (mainly bronchitis and pulmonary emphysema).[56]

Biological agents such as viruses, bacterias, and parasites may constitute important hazards to the health of workers such as farmers, veterinarians, butchers, grain handlers, etc. Hospital employees often are exposed to such agents, leading to respiratory, skin, or other infections.

Mechanical hazards include all physical arrangements that may present opportunities for accidents. This is the domain of what is known as occupational or industrial safety and traditionally has been the best-known part of work health, perhaps because it is the one in which direct cause-effect relationships are the most evident. In 1977, the direct and indirect costs of occupational accidents in the United States were estimated at more than $20 billion.[57]

The impact of occupational psychosocial factors on workers' health is less well understood. Strike rates, accident rates, and absenteeism are influenced substantially by the psychosocial climate and morale in the work environment.[58] Psychosocial working conditions may lead to both detrimental life style behaviors (e.g., increased use of alcohol, drugs, or tranquilizers) and undue stress, indirectly leading to peptic ulcers, mental illness, coronary heart disease, etc.[59]

Other psychosocial factors include shift work (evenings and nights). Workers who must rotate shifts have more sleeping problems and use more sleeping pills, report more stomachaches, and have a higher incidence of ulcers than those on regular schedules.[60] The level of physical activity required by the job also may

Figure 12-1 Work Environment Hazards Affecting Health and Social
Well-Being

WORK ENVIRONMENT/CONDITIONS

PHYSICAL			
Mechanical/ Biomechanical	*Physical*	*Chemical*	*Biological*

WORK SITE DESIGN
 	
Fundamental features for comfort, productivity and safety:
● layout and traffic flow
● lighting
● sound (level and type)
● temperature, humidity and ventilation
● mobility/basic activity
● etc.
 	
PROCESS AND EQUIPMENT DESIGN (functional and safety)
 	
TASK FUNCTIONS (person-job fit)
	MOLECULAR/ KINETIC PROPERTIES
	● barometric pressure
	● thermal
	● mechanical vibration
	● air vibration (noise, ultra sound and infrasound)
	● acceleration— linear and angular
	● electricity
	● magnetism
	NONIONIZING RADIATION
	● light (visible, ultraviolet [UV] and infrared [IR])
	  −conventional
	  −coherent (laser)
	● microwave and radio
	IONIZING RADIATION
	● x-ray and gamma radiation
	● radioactive substances and emitted particles
		Elements and compounds (inorganic and organic)
		● gas
		● liquid
		● solid
		● dusts
		● fumes
		● vapours
			Sources of infection, infestation and certain allergies
			● plants
			● organisms
			● materials (dusts, spaces, etc.)
			● animals
			● organisms
			● micro (bacteria, virus, etc.)
			● visible
			  −trauma infestations
			● materials
			● toxins
			● venoms, etc.

WORK ENVIRONMENT/CONDITIONS

PSYCHOSOCIAL		
Nature of Occupation[1]	*Nature of Organization*[2]	
	Social Structure[3]	*Social Cohesion*[4]
Identifying features: • knowledge and technique • occupational standing (skill type) • flexibility • societal responsibility • social isolation • self-perceived status	JOB CHARACTERISTICS • job status • job design • person-job/role fit • complexity of work • skills required • workload • role ambiguity • potential role conflict • responsibility for work of others ORGANIZATION CHARACTERISTICS • degree of hierarchy • organization design • formal/informal • degree of relevance • authority conflict • built-in mechanisms for: promotion and mobility retraining and education, health promotion, etc. • management style	JOB CHARACTERISTICS • group harmony • job commitment • decision-making participation • job satisfaction • job security • resource availability (manpower, materials) CONDITIONS AT WORK • job-related • wages and benefits • job content and context • esthetics and housekeeping, etc. • associated conditions • parking, cafeteria • recreation/social clubs, programs etc. • family activities • self-help groups, etc.

These factors determine: 1. *performance* conditions for work (comfort, productivity, and satisfaction)
2. *potentially hazardous* conditions to health and social adjustment arising out of work

1. Nature of Occupation: distinctive occupational elements brought to work world.
2. Nature of Organization: distinctive work arrangements organized for productivity.
3. Social Structure: patterns of working relationships.
4. Social Cohesion: integration of social bonds.

Source: Adapted from *Occupational Health in Canada—Current Status* with permission of Dept. of Health and Welfare, Ottawa, Ontario, Canada, June 1977.

Table 12-6 Physical and Chemical Occupational Health Hazards

Agent, Pollutant, or Source	Disease, Effect, Illness, or Injury	Types of Workers Affected
Acrylonitrile	Lung cancer, colon cancer	Manufacturing of apparel, carpeting, blankets, draperies, synthetic furs, and hair wigs.
4-aminobiphenyl	Bladder cancer	Chemicals.
Anesthetic gases	Miscarriages, birth defects, decreased alertness, increased reaction time, reticuloendothelial cancer, lymphoid cancer.	Physician-anesthetists, nurse-anesthetists, other operating room personnel.
Arsenic	Poorly differentiated epidermoid bronchogenic carcinoma, skin cancer, scrotal cancer, cancer of the lymphatic system, hemangiosarcoma of the liver.	Metallurgical industries, sheep-dip, pesticide production, copper smelters, children living near copper smelters, people living where arsenical insecticide was sprayed, vineyards, insecticide makers and sprayers, tanners, (gold) miners.
Asbestos	Asbestosis (pneumoconiosis), cancer of lung, GI tract, larynx, mesothelioma	Asbestos factory, textile, relatives of asbestos workers, people who live near asbestos factories, rubber tire manufacturing, miners, insulation, shipyards.
Auramine	Bladder cancer	Dyestuffs manufacturers, rubber, textile dyers, paint manufacturers.
Benzene	Aplastic or hypoplastic anemia, leukemia	Rubber tire manufacturing, painters, shoe manufacturing, rubber cement, glue and varnish, distillers, shoemakers, plastics, chemicals.
Benzidine	Bladder cancer, pancreatic cancer	Dyeworkers, chemicals.
Beryllium	Berylliosis (pneumoconiosis)	Beryllium, electronics, missile parts.
Bis-chloromethyl ether (BCME)	Bronchogenic cancer	In plants producing anion-exchange resins (chemicals).

Agent, Pollutant, or Source	Disease, Effect, Illness, or Injury	Types of Workers Affected
Cadmium	Lung cancer, prostatic cancer	Cadmium production, metallurgical, electroplating industry, chemicals, jewelry, nuclear, pigments.
Carbon disulfide	EKG changes, hypertension, neurological abnormalities, decreased sperm counts, menstrual disorders, increased spontaneous abortions.	Rayon manufacturers, textiles, paint industry.
Carbon monoxide	Neurological and behavioral disturbances	Miners, iron and steel industry, gas plants, tunnels.
Carbon tetrachloride	Liver and kidney damage	Plastics, dry cleaners.
Chloromethyl methyl ether (CMME)	Lung cancer	Chemicals, plants producing ion exchange resins.
Chloroprene	Central nervous system depression, lung, liver, kidney injuries, lung and skin cancer, miscarriages.	Rubber-producing plants.
Chromium	Bronchogenic cancer	Chromate-producing industry, acetylene and aniline, bleachers, glass, pottery, pigment, linoleum.
Coal dust	Pneumoconiosis	Miners, gashouse stokers and producers.
Coal tar pitch volatiles	Lung cancer, scrotal cancer	Steel industry, aluminum potroom, foundries.
Coke oven emissions	Lung cancer, kidney cancer	Steel industry, coke plants, children born of female steel industry workers.
Cold temperatures	Chilblains, erythrocyanosis, immersion foot, frostbite, general hypothermia.	Farmworkers, sailors, fishermen, telephone line-persons.
Cotton dust	Byssinosis ("brown lung disease")	Textiles.

Table 12-6 continued

Agent, Pollutant, or Source	Disease, Effect, Illness, or Injury	Types of Workers Affected
Decaborane	Neurological and behavioral disturbances	
Dibromo-3-chloropropane	Sterility, impotence	Pesticide production workers/applicators.
Hair spray	Chronic lung disease	Hairdressers.
Heat	Decreased alertness, decreased psychomotor coordination.	Steel, railroads, foundries.
Hematite	Lung cancer	Miners.
Inadequate lighting	Eye strain, fatigue, headache, eye pain, lachrymation, congestion around the cornea, "miner's nystagmus."	Miners, offices.
Kepone	Weakness, tremors, numbness, tingling, blurred vision, temporary memory loss, loss of balance.	Kepone (insecticide) plants, agriculture.
Lead	Miscarriage, birth defects; defects in hearing, eye-hand coordination; anemia, acute encephalopathy, "lead colic" (abdominal pain), decreased male fertility, decreased muscular strength and endurance, end stage renal disease, wrist drop, hostility, depression, anxiety.	Lead production, lead battery plants, smelters, firing range attendants, welders, solderers.
Leptophos	Weakness, tremors, numbness, tingling, blurred vision, temporary memory loss, loss of balance.	Insecticide production, agriculture.

Agent, Pollutant, or Source	Disease, Effect, Illness, or Injury	Types of Workers Affected
Manganese	Neurological and behavioral disturbances	Steel, ceramic makers, electric arc welders, battery makers, drug makers, food additive makers, foundries, glass makers, match, paint, and varnish makers, ink makers, water treaters.
Mercury	Nephrosis, pneumonitis, bronchitis, chest pain, shortness of breath, coughing, neurological and behavioral disturbances.	Dental assistants, dental hygienists, chemicals.
Methyl butyl ketone	Peripheral neuropathy	Solvents, varnish and stain makers, wax makers, adhesive makers, dope (glue), explosives, garage mechanics, celluloid makers, dyemakers, oil and lacquer processors, shoemakers.
2-naphthylamine	Bladder cancer, pancreatic cancer	Dyeworkers, rubber tire manufacturing, chemicals, coal gas manufacturing, nickel refiners, copper smelters, electrolysis.
Noise	Headaches, hearing losses	Factories, construction, textiles.
Radiation	Cancer of paranasal and mastoid sinuses, cancer of the: skin, pancreas, brain, stomach, breast, salivary glands, thyroid, GI organs, bronchus, lymphoid tissue; leukemia, multiple myeloma.	Uranium miners, radiologists, radiographers, luminous dial painters.
Silica	Silicosis (pneumoconiosis)	Workers in mines and quarries, steel, iron foundries, glass, ceramics.

Table 12-6 continued

Agent, Pollutant, or Source	Disease, Effect, Illness, or Injury	Types of Workers Affected
Thorium dioxide	Angiosarcoma of the liver	Chemicals, steel, ceramic makers, incandescent lamp makers, nuclear reactors, gas mantle makers, metal refiners, vacuum tube makers.
Tin	Neurological and behavioral disturbances	Aluminum and steel, welders, solderers.
Toluene diisocyanate (TDI)	Pulmonary sensitization	Adhesives, isocyanate resins, organic chemical synthesizers, insulation, paint sprayers, lacquer, polyurethane makers, rubber, textile processors, wire coating.
Trichloroethylene	Neurological and behavioral disturbances	Operating room personnel.
Ultraviolet radiation	Conjunctivitis, keratitis, skin cancer	Farmers, sailors, arc welders.
Vinyl chloride	Angiosarcoma of the liver, chromosome aberrations, cancer of the lung, brain, lymphatic and hematopoietic systems, gall bladder, and liver; lymphoma, miscarriages, birth defects.	Plastics, vinyl chloride polymerization plants, pregnant women living in communities near PVC plants.
Polybrominated biphenyls (decabromobiphenyl) Polybrominated biphenyl oxides (decabromobiphenyl oxide)	Hypothyroidism	Chemical plants where PBB and PBBO are manufactured.

Source: Adapted from *Costs of Environment-Related Health Effects: A Plan for Continuing Study* by permission of the Institute of Medicine, National Academy Press, © January 1981.

constitute a health hazard. White-collar workers whose jobs do not include physical activity may be at greater risk of coronary heart disease.

Unemployment also may constitute an important health hazard. Evidence is accumulating that the unemployed experience a higher incidence of health problems because of stress associated with the loss of a job as well as because of feelings of inadequacy.[61,62,63,64]

Transport

Transport is an element of the social environment that, directly and indirectly, can affect health status and therefore should be considered an environmental health concern. As Chapter 11 noted, motor vehicle accidents are a major cause of death and in fact are the leading fatality cause for individuals under 30 years of age.

In the United States, there are approximately 50,000 deaths a year from motor vehicle accidents, 150,000 permanently disabling injuries, and more than 4.5 million injuries. Both the death and injury rates are higher for males than for females and are higher in rural areas than urban. They also are higher among single, divorced, and separated persons than among married individuals. Forty-five percent of all fatal motor vehicle accidents involve at least two motor vehicles, 34 percent a single vehicle, and 17.6 percent pedestrians.[65] Per mile traveled, motorcyclists are seven times more likely to die in a crash than are car or truck occupants.

Also as stated earlier, about half of fatally injured car drivers and, perhaps more surprisingly, pedestrians are intoxicated by alcohol.[66] About 35 percent of motorcycle deaths involve alcohol and 36 percent of fatally injured truck drivers are intoxicated.[67] Contrary to popular misconception, intoxicated drivers usually are problem drinkers or alcoholics rather than social drinkers.

The second motor vehicle accident risk factor is youth. Both the accident ratio and fatal accident rates are 75 percent higher among drivers under 25 than among the whole driving population. Inexperience and higher use of alcohol and other drugs seem to explain this. Accident and fatal accident rates also are higher among the older population because of decreased vision, hearing, mobility, and higher prevalence of health problems such as cardiovascular conditions, diabetes, etc.[68] Older drivers in good health have the same accident rates as other adults (30-59).[69]

From 5 of 13 percent of all accidents are caused by vehicle factors, 35 percent of which are related to tires and wheels, 21 percent to the communication system (lights, vision), and 28 percent to brakes.[70] It is not known what proportion of accidents results from vehicle design and road features (surface, lighting, curvature, slope, etc.).

As for preventive measures, it has been shown numerous times that compulsory use of seat belts can reduce the death rate in motor vehicle accidents. The lowering of the maximum speed limit in the United States in 1973 resulted in an immediate

16 percent reduction in the number of motor vehicle deaths. There is no doubt that if intoxicated drivers could be kept off the road, the accident rate would go down dramatically. Improved street lighting at night significantly reduces accidents.[71] Training in defensive driving also may prove beneficial.

Per mile traveled, planes and trains are much safer than roads. In the United States, there are about two deaths of car occupants per 100 million passenger miles as compared to 0.3 by certified carrier airlines. However, other forms of air travel (general aviation) are much more dangerous, with 18 deaths per 100 million miles.

The death rate per mile traveled may not be an optimal way of comparing the relative risks of different modes of transportation: measured that way, walking is the most dangerous, with almost 50 deaths per 100 million miles traveled. It should be noted that alcohol again is a major factor in general aviation crashes but not in certified carrier crashes. Studies show that 24 percent of general aviation crashes involve alcohol, with 13 percent of the pilots severely intoxicated.[72]

Rail travel is even safer than certified carrier air travel.[73] Furthermore, two-thirds of the deaths are grade crossing fatalities, with alcohol again a major factor—30 percent of car drivers and 64 percent of pedestrians age 15 and over who died after collisions with trains were intoxicated.[74] No statistics are available on the use of alcohol by train drivers.

Transport also indirectly influences the population's health status through environment pollution. Cars are the main air polluters and major contributors to noise pollution. Airplanes also are a major source of noise pollution and supersonic air travel may be affecting the atmospheric ozone layer that, as noted, protects Earth against ultraviolet radiations. Airplane travel also has been implicated in transporting infectious diseases.[75]

Leisure

Leisure, a third component of the social environment, may be defined as including the activities people voluntarily engage in after having fulfilled or being relieved from their familial, occupational, and social obligations. Leisure may have both positive and negative effects on health.

On the positive side, it can increase individuals' ability to cope with stress and stressful events by creating social networks that bring together persons with common interests. Evidence is accumulating that both every-day support and crisis support that can be provided by such networks may influence health status positively. This in turn may help reduce the incidence of stress-related health problems such as coronary heart disease, peptic ulcers, mental problems, etc. Since much leisure in America involves physical activity, it also can be a positive influence by promoting healthy life style behaviors through an increased fitness level.

On the negative side, leisure, of course, can lead to detrimental life styles and to injuries. It also can have detrimental health effects by leading to such behaviors as physical inactivity (for example, watching television too much) or use of alcohol (with all its health consequences). Leisure injuries are common. Bicycling, swimming, skiing, boating, use of snowmobiles, football, hockey, etc., all can lead to injuries, fortunately not too serious in most cases.

Housing

Housing may well be one of the most complex elements of the environment as to its relationship with health. The place where people live is so intricately linked with economics, social conditions, education, customs, and traditions that it is difficult to assess its influence on health accurately and fully. The housing environment may well combine synergistically with other factors to produce serious health effects such as mental illness.

Overcrowding has long been known to increase the incidence of infectious diseases such as rheumatic fever, nephritis, and tuberculosis as well as infestation with lice, fleas, bedbugs, and scabies.[76] Many physical housing environment characteristics are related to health. The American Public Health Association's Recommended Housing Maintenance and Occupancy Ordinance[77] include such factors as location (not near swamps or landfills, for example), structure, fire safety, basic equipment (sinks, refrigerators, stove, toilets, etc.), standards for light, ventilation, heat, plumbing fixtures, and protection against flies, mosquitoes, other pests, and rodents.

Table 12-7 summarizes some of these housing health hazards and their definite and possible health effects. It should be noted that home injuries, including falls, poisonings, burns, and suffocation are common, causing about 3.6 million disabling injuries and 24,000 deaths annually in the United States.[78]

Family and Community

The last element included in the social environment is the family and the community. The social milieu in which individuals live undoubtedly can influence their health status. However it would be a major task to try to untangle the specific effects the family and the community can exert on people's health. Such family-related factors as marital status and number of children already have been noted as associated with the incidence of need for health services. Sexual life also is associated with health, both directly through the incidence of venereal disease and some types of cancer (breast, uterus), and indirectly through satisfaction and fulfillment. Family factors influence children's cognitive and affective development and can have direct physical health consequences through spouse and child abuse.

Table 12-7 Definite and Possible Health Effects of Housing Hazards

Agent, Pollutant, or Source	Definite Effect	Possible Effect
Heating, cooking, and refrigeration	1. Acute fatalities from carbon monoxide, fires and explosions, and discarded refrigerators	
		2. Increase in diseases of the respiratory tract in infants
Fumes and dust	3. Acute illness from fumes	
	4. Aggravation of asthma	
		5. Increase in chronic respiratory disease
Crowding	6. Spread of acute and contribution to chronic disease morbidity and mortality	
Structural factors (including electrical wiring, stoves, and thin walls)	7. Accidental fatality	
	8. Accidental injury	
	9. Morbidity and mortality from lack of protection from heat or cold	
	10. Morbidity and mortality due to fire or explosion	
Paints and solvents	11. Childhood lead-poisoning fatalities, associated mental impairment, and anemia	
	12. Renal and hepatic toxicity	
	13. Fatalities	
Household equipment and supplies (including pesticides)	14. Fatalities from fire and injury	
	15. Morbidity from fire and injury	
	16. Fatalities from poisoning	
	17. Morbidity from poisoning	
Toys, beads, and painted objects	18. Mortality and morbidity	

Table 12-7 continued

Agent, Pollutant, or Source	Definite Effect	Possible Effect
Urban design	19. Increased accident risks	
		20. Contribution to mental illness
Formaldehyde from insulation	21. Eye and respiratory tract irritation	

Source: Adapted from "Statistics Needed for Determining the Effects of the Environment on Health," *Vital and Health Statistics,* ser. 4, no. 20; U.S. Department of Health, Education, and Welfare, Public Health Service, Health Resources Administration, DHEW Publication No. (HRA) 77-1457 (Washington, D.C.: U.S. Government Printing Office, July 1977).

The community to which individuals belong can contribute to health, not only through its social networks and social support but also through its culture, traditions, and religion—all of which are associated with physical and mental status and with health care utilization. Violence and its associated injuries also can be a factor in community life.

This examination of the different elements of the environment and their influences on health demonstrates that although the effects of some environmental hazards are well documented, it often is difficult to isolate the effects of specific ones. Many diseases associated with environmental components actually have a multifactorial origin. Furthermore, environmental factors can act as intervening variables, either predisposing individuals to the deleterious effects of other health determinants, or stimulating such causes.

This discussion is far from exhaustive, notably in relation to occupational health and the other components of the social environment. However, it is sufficient to demonstrate the importance of the environment and the wide range of factors that should be considered as part of environmental health.

THE CONTRIBUTIONS OF EPIDEMIOLOGY

Epidemiology contributes to environmental health in four main ways:[79] in the discovery of new etiological factors, in helping monitor changes and trends in the impact of known etiological factors, in managing programs in this field, and in serving as the basis of environmental health programs. Epidemiologists also can contribute to environmental health by communicating with nonepidemiologists.

Identifying Etiological Factors

Epidemiology contributes first to environmental health by helping to identify, along with laboratory-based sciences, new etiological factors. All epidemiological methods can and have been used for that purpose.[80] Surveys, simple descriptive and prospective studies, and case control all have contributed to the identification of environmental health hazards. However, their use in the identification of causal environmental factors presents several difficulties.[81]

Inadequate measurements of the level of toxic contaminants, variable dose-response relationships and individual susceptibility, multiplicity of exposures, multifactorial origins of many environment-related diseases, and difficulty in defining precisely both numerators (number of disease cases that were exposed to the environmental factor) and denominators (population at risk) all combine to make the epidemiological demonstration of cause-effect relationships especially difficult.

It has been suggested that the improvement of data collection of environmental exposures, the sharpening of the study of combined exposures, and better integration of experimental and epidemiological evidence might enhance the contributions of epidemiology to the discovery of new environmental health hazards.[82] It might be added that a widening of the interests of epidemiology to include investigations of the impact of other environmental (notably social) health hazards also would be beneficial.

Monitoring Trends and Changes

Epidemiology's second contribution is the monitoring of trends and changes in the impact on health of known environmental hazards. Since it already is known that such factors as described in the first section of this chapter are associated with health status and the incidence of specific problems, it would be advisable to undertake systematic rather than occasional descriptive epidemiological analysis of mortality and incidence of health problems in relation to these factors.

Management Programs

Epidemiology also can be used in the management of environmental health programs. In this regard, the contributions of epidemiology are the same as in the management of health services in general (Chapter 3). Most notably, epidemiology can be used for planning the environmental health program, determining priorities among competing problems, choosing among alternative programs, and evaluating the approach's impact on health outcomes.[83] Such a use of epidemiology need not be restricted to governments and public agencies. For example, every organization should monitor the health of its employees and their exposure to known hazards and take appropriate corrective actions.

Communication of Information

Epidemiology's fourth contribution is through communication of knowledge about environmental health hazards to nonepidemiologists. Epidemiologists must communicate with other scientists, both to avoid superficiality and blunder[84] and to increase the role that their data can play in explaining the etiology of diseases. Epidemiologists also must communicate with the general public to contribute to its development of a soundly informed opinion on environmental health hazards. Epidemiologists should not forget that it may only be through pressures from the general public that governmental policies may change, notably when strong economic interests also are at stake, as is often the case with environmental issues.

Primary Prevention: The Common Denominator

The common denominator or common target of the four types of contributions of epidemiology is primary prevention,[85] i.e., the removal or control of environmental health hazards. Since environmental factors theoretically can be manipulated, such primary prevention through environmental health may be one of the most effective strategies to improve the population's status.

IMPLICATIONS FOR HEALTH CARE PROVIDERS, ORGANIZATIONS

It should be clear by now that the environment can influence the population's health in significant ways. Consequently, an awareness and understanding of environmental factors should permeate the delivery of health services at all levels. This has implications for all health care providers, from large hospitals to individual practitioners. Although the following discussion is centered on hospitals, much of it can be applied to any other health care organizations and providers.

The discussion covers four main ways in which hospitals should be involved in environmental health and the role of epidemiology in each. These contributions result from four distinct hospital roles: (1) as responsible for its constituency; (2) as a health care provider; (3) as responsible for patient safety; and (4) as employer.

Responsibility for a Constituency

In addition to the major aspect of self-responsibility for health, a recurring theme in this book is the responsibility that the hospital (and any other provider) must assume for the status of its constituency, including its environmental health. This can be done in several ways.

The hospital (and its health services manager specifically) should be involved first in an environmental health assessment to determine the specific hazards to which its constituency is exposed. This can be done rather simply by using the first section of this chapter as a guide: Are there any unusual sources of air, water, or noise pollution? What kind of industries could present special problems? What of disposal of wastes? What is the housing situation?

The analysis of problems (Chapter 4) and of health services utilization (Chapter 8) next should incorporate consideration of environmental health hazards. Are any of the health problems identified possibly related to environmental factors? Do mortality and incidence of specific health problems vary according to location, housing, occupation, etc.?

Health services utilization can be analyzed in the same way according to exposure to environmental hazards (notably occupational). The discovery of disease or injury clusters in a particular subgroup of the constituency should lead to a detailed environmental survey and appropriate referrals and consultations with specialized agencies such as the state health department, environmental protection agencies, occupational health offices, etc.

The hospital could offer its services to the industries in its constituency for the identification and monitoring of occupational health hazards as well as for instituting specific environmental health programs. Injuries and illnesses of employees could be analyzed and monitored.

All of these involve the use of epidemiological principles and methods.

In addition to their involvement in such activities because of the major importance of the environment to health, hospitals may find this constitutes good public relations and effective marketing of their other services. For example, it might be very cost effective for a hospital to offer its services to industries even if only on a break-even basis since it will increase the facility's profile in the constituency and could generate added clientele.

The Hospital as a Health Care Provider

The second implication for the hospital is that, as a health care provider, it must consider the possible impact of environmental factors on its patients. In other words, comprehensive health care must include consideration of environmental health hazards.

The hospital may set up training courses for appropriate staff (physicians, nurses, program coordinators, etc.) in recognition of injuries and illnesses with possible environmental etiology. The institution also should have an official policy that each clinical case history include an occupational history. Recurring problems (notably injuries) should be assessed as to possible environmental (and occupational) factors. Patient and public health education campaigns could be set up, and in the case of patients with environmentally induced problems, counseling and education to prevent recurrence should be arranged.

Patient Safety

The hospital has a duty, both legal and ethical, to provide for patients' safety. This includes sanitation and protection from injuries. This responsibility is much better known, and acknowledged, than the first two. Minimum functional safety and sanitation standards are required for hospital accreditation. These standards have been published in a self-evaluation form.[86] Several practical guides also have been published.[87,88,89] It is sufficient to note here that most patient injuries result from falls, with electrical shocks and explosions as other major causes.

One topic not often discussed in safety textbooks is nosocomial infections, i.e., infections developed during a stay in hospital or resulting from microorganisms acquired there.[90] Nosocomial infections have always been a problem in hospitals and indeed were one of the major causes of death in the nineteenth century's facilities.[91] Even today, it is estimated that from 3 to 14 percent of patients develop infections while in the hospital.[92,93,94,95]

There are several reasons for the high incidence of hospital infections.[96,97] The concentration of microorganisms, patients' decreased resistance, the use of corticosteroids and immunosuppressive therapies, as well as medical and nursing therapeutic and diagnostic procedures, including catheters, inhalation, and surgery all are obvious factors. It has been shown repeatedly that nosocomial infections significantly increase cost of treatment. Most studies have attributed these greater costs to longer length of stay, [98,99] but increased need for professional services, mainly nursing care, also has been cited.[100]

Here again, the use of epidemiological principles and methods is essential in the identification of patient safety problems (through analysis of incidence), in monitoring, and in setting and evaluating control programs.

The Hospital as an Employer

The fourth way in which environmental health is of importance to hospitals is related to the employees. The delivery of health care is a particularly personnel-intensive industry and hospitals often are the largest employers in the town or county.

In the United States, hospitals are expected to comply with the general requirements of the Occupational Safety and Health Act (OSHA).[101] Most occupational injuries in hospitals result from falls and improper lifting of heavy objects (including patients). Others are caused by electricity, moving machinery, and improper use of all types of tools and equipment including handling of explosive gas and flammables. Cuts, bruises, and puncture wounds from blades, needles, and broken glass are common and can lead to such diseases as viral hepatitis (type B).

Many environmental hazards also are specific to, or at least more frequent in, hospitals.[102] Chemical agents are common, particularly in patient care areas, laboratories, pharmacies, operating rooms, etc. Many skin conditions can result from contact with drugs, detergents, and antiseptics. Ethylene oxyde, a widely used sterilant, is very toxic.[103] Hexachlorophene is associated with increased incidence of birth defects in the offspring of nurses who repeatedly washed their hands with detergents containing this substance. Formalin, used for sterilization in renal dialysis units, has induced asthma in nurses working in those units.

Anesthetic gases can lead to congenital abnormalities, spontaneous abortions, hepatic disease, renal disease, central nervous system damage, and cancer.[104,105] Female anesthetists and operating room personnel and wives of male anesthetists have a much higher incidence of spantaneous abortion.[106] Infections from medical wastes and from patients can be a serious problem. Ionizing radiation could pose long-term health hazards. Drug abuse in professional employees with ready access to medications is much higher than in the general population. Finally, many hospital employees work on rotating shifts, which can pose distinct health hazards.[107]

Hospitals also can use epidemiological methods to analyze employees' medical records and identify high-incidence health problems. This function can be delegated to the employee health service where personnel trained in basic epidemiological methods and occupational health can set up, as needed, monitoring systems and employee wellness programs.[108] An effective occupational health program can lead to better management-employee relations, reduced absenteeism, better morale, and a healthier, more productive work force.

SUMMARY

This chapter first reviewed the components of the environment and their possible effects on health, then the contributions of epidemiology to environmental health, and ways in which hospitals and health care providers are concerned with environmental health issues.

Many environmental health hazards are not yet fully understood. There is little doubt, however, that the environment is an important determinant of health status. Health services managers therefore can and should use epidemiological principles and methods in promoting environmental health and in preventing environmentally induced diseases and injuries.

NOTES

1. M. Lalonde, *A New Perspective on the Health of Canadians* (Ottawa: National Health and Welfare, 1974), 32.

2. Ibid.

3. D.H.K. Lee and Philip Kotin, *Multiple Factors in the Causation of Environmentally Induced Disease* (New York: Academic Press, Inc., 1972), 225.

4. G.M. Howe, "The Environment, Its Influences and Hazards to Health," in *Environmental Medicine*, (2nd ed), ed. G.M. Howe and J. A. Loraine (London: William Heinemann Medical Books, 1980), 1-8.

5. J.M. Last, ed., *Maxcy-Rosenau Public Health and Preventive Medicine*, 11th ed. (New York: Appleton-Century-Crofts, Inc., 1980), 1926.

6. Howe and Loraine, *Environmental Medicine*.

7. W. Hobson, ed., *The Theory and Practice of Public Health*, 5th ed. (Oxford, England: Oxford University Press, 1979), 75.

8. Lee and Kotin, *Multiple Factors*.

9. E.P. Eckholm, *The Picture of Health: Environmental Sources of Disease* (New York: W.W. Norton & Co., Inc., 1977), 256.

10. M.A. Mehlman, M. Norvell, and N. Dwyer, "Toxic Gases and Fumes," in Last, *Maxcy-Rosenau*, 756.

11. T.C. King, "Environmental Health: Effluence, Affluence, and Influence," in *The Challenges of Community Medicine*, ed. R.L. Kent (New York: Springer Publishing Co., Inc. 1974), 237-259.

12. Ibid.

13. National Air Pollution Control Administration, *Danger in the Air* (Washington, D.C.: Department of Health, Education, and Welfare, May 1970).

14. L.C. Neri et al., "Chronic Obstructive Pulmonary Disease in Two Cities of Contrasting Air Quality," *Canadian Medical Association Journal* 113 (1975): 1043-1046.

15. B.Q. Hafen, ed., *Man, Health, and Environment* (Minneapolis: Burgess Publishing Company, 1972), 65-66.

16. P.F. Wehrle, et al., "Pediatric Aspects of Air Pollution," *Pediatrics* 46 (1970): 637-639.

17. J.R. Goldsmith, "Effects of Air Pollution on Human Health," in *Air Pollution and Its Effects*, ed. A.C. Stern (New York: Academic Press, Inc., 1968), 547-615.

18. Hafen, *Man, Health, and Environment*, 61.

19. E.P. Seskin and L.B. Lave, "The Air Pollution-Health Relationship: Data Opportunities and Data Needs," in *The Public Health Conference on Records and Statistics* (U.S. Department & Health, Education, and Welfare, Public Health Service, DHEW Publication No. [PHS] 79-1214, August 1979), 289-295.

20. D.F. Newton, *Elements of Environmental Health* (Columbus, Ohio: The Charles E. Merrill Publishing Co., Inc., 1974).

21. W.E. Morton, "Hypertension and Drinking Water Constituents in Colorado," *American Journal of Public Health* 61 (1971): 1371-1378.

22. R. Masironi, "Trace Elements and Cardiovascular Diseases," *Notes-WHO*, 1969, 305-12.

23. C.W. Kruse, "Sanitary Control of Food," in Last, *Maxcy-Rosenau*, 875-919.

24. King, "Environmental Health," 254.

25. N.J. Petersen, et al., "An Epidemiologic Approach to Low-Level Radium 226 Exposure," *Public Health Reports* 81, no. 9 (1966): 805-814.

26. R. Masironi, "Cardiovascular Mortality in Relation to Radioactivity and Hardness of Local Water Supplies in the U.S.A.," *Bulletin of the WHO*, 43 (1970): 687-697.

27. H.A. Schroeder et al., "Relation Between Mortality from Cardiovascular Disease and Treated Water Supplies," *Journal of the American Medical Association* 172, no. 17 (1960): 1902-08.

28. H.A. Schroeder et al., "Cardiovascular Mortality, Municipal Water and Corrosion," *Archives of Environmental Health* 28 (1974): 303-11.

29. M.D. Crawford et al., "Hardness of Drinking Water and Cardiovascular Disease," *Proceedings of the Nutrition Society* 31 (1972): 345-353.

30. M.D. Crawford et al., "Infant Mortality and Hardness of Local Water Supplies," *The Lancet* (1972): 988-992.

31. R.W. Armstrong, "Is There a Particular Kind of Soil or Geologic Environment That Predisposes to Cancer?" in "Geochemical Environment in Relation to Health and Disease," ed. H.C. Hobbs and H.L.Cannon, *Annals of the New York Academy of Science,* 199 (June 28, 1972), 240.

32. C.J. Pfeiffer et al., "An Epidemiological Analysis of Mortality and Gastric Cancer in Newfoundland," *Canadian Medical Association Journal* 108 (1973): 1374-1380.

33. H.I. Sauer, "Geographic Patterns in the Risk of Dying and Associated Factors," in Vital and Health Statistics, ser. 3, no. 18, U.S. Department of Health and Human Services, Public Health Service (DHHS Publication No. [PHS] 80-1402, September 1980), 44.

34. E.O. Weinberg, "Infectious Diseases Influenced by Trace Element Environment," in Hobbs and Cannon, *Geochemical Environment,* 241.

35. S.W. Tromp, *Medical Biometeorology* (Amsterdam: Elsevier Publications, 1963).

36. S.W. Tromp, "The Relationship of Weather and Climate to Health and Disease," in *Environmental Medicine* 2nd. ed., ed. G.M. Howe and J.A. Loraine (London: William Heinemann Medical Books, 1980), 73.

37. Ibid., 82.

38. Ibid., 100.

39. A.R. Moller, "Noise as a Health Hazard," in Last, *Maxcy-Roseneau,* 790-799.

40. A. Archer and D. Christie, "Noise in Relation to Health," in Hobson, *Theory and Practice,* 122-129.

41. Moller, "Noise as a Health Hazard," 790.

42. Ibid., 798.

43. U.S. Public Health Service, "Statistics Needed for Determining the Effects of the Environment on Health," *Vital and Health Statistics,* ser. 4, no. 20, U.S. Department of Health, Education, and Welfare, Health Resources Administration (DHEW Publication No. [HRA] 77-1457). (Washington, D.C.: U.S. Government Printing Office, July 1977), 28.

44. Archer and Christie, "Noise in Relation to Health," 124.

45. R.D.E. Rumsey, "Radiation and Health Hazards," in *Environmental Medicine,* 1st ed., G.M. Howe and J.A. Loraine (London: William Heinemann Medical Books, 1973), 27-28.

46. A.L. Frank, "Nonionizing Radiation," in Last, *Maxcy-Rosenau,* 779.

47. E. Eckholm, *The Picture of Health: Environmental Sources of Disease* (New York: W.W. Norton & Co., 1977), 102.

48. Frank, "Nonionizing Radiation," 779.

49. Rumsey, "Radiation and Health Hazards," 34.

50. T.W. Hu, "Health-Related Economic Costs of the Three-Mile Island Accident," in *New Challenges for Vital and Health Records,* Proceedings of the 18th National Meeting of the Public Health Conference on Records and Statistics, U.S. Department of Health and Human Services, Public Health Service (DHHS Publication No. [PHS] 81-1214) (Washington, D.C.: U.S. Government Printing Office, December 1980), 181-186.

51. Canada National Health and Welfare, *Occupational Health in Canada-Current Status* (Ottawa: June 1977), 4.

52. Ibid.

53. U.S. Public Health Service, "Statistics Needed," 9.

54. J. Higginson, Address to a conference in Lyons, France, in *Canada Health and Welfare,* 10-11.

55. A.M. Lilienfeld, "Cancer," in Last, *Maxcy-Rosenau*, 1156.

56. S. Milham, Jr., *Occupational Mortality in Washington State, 1950-1971*. NIOSH, Washington State Department of Social and Health Services, Publ. No. (NIOSH) 76-175 (Washington, D.C.: U.S. Government Printing Office, 1977).

57. U.S. Public Health Service, *Health, United States, 1980*, U.S. Department of Health and Human Services, DHHS Publication No. [PHS] 81-1232 (Washington, D.C.: U.S. Government Printing Office, December 1980), 289.

58. J. Surry, *Industrial Accident Research: A Human Engineering Appraisal*. Labour Safety Council, Ontario Ministry of Labour, June 1972. Canada Health and Welfare, 9.

59. H. Selye, *Stress in Health and Disease* (Boston: Butterworths, 1976), 725-895.

60. M.L. Simond, "Conditions de travail et santé des travailleurs: Le cas du régime notatif de travail," *Environnement et Santé: Elements d'une Problematique Québecoise*, ed. R. Pompalar (Quebec: Ministèrè des Affaires Sociales, Juillet 1980), 133.

61. R. Bunn, "Unemployment, Morbidity and Mortality," *The Lancet* (April 1979): 923-924.

62. S. Cobb, "Physiologic Changes in Men Whose Jobs Were Abolished," *Journal of Psychosomatic Research* 18 (1974): 245-258.

63. S. Gore, "The Effect of Social Support in Moderating the Health Consequences of Unemployment," *Journal of Health and Social Behavior* 19 (June 1978): 157-165.

64. S.V. Kasl, S. Gore, and S. Cobb, "The Experience of Losing a Job: Repeated Changes in Health, Symptoms, and Illness Behavior," *Psychosomatic Medicine* 37 (1975): 116-122.

65. J.A. Waller, "Injury as a Public Health Problem," in Last, *Maxcy-Rosenau*, 1557.

66. Ibid., 1556.

67. Ibid., 1563.

68. Ibid., 1559.

69. J.A. Waller, "Cardiovascular Disease, Aging, and Traffic Accidents," *Journal of Chronic Diseases* 20 (1965): 615-620.

70. S.T. McDonald and R.A. Romberg, "Driver/Vehicle Characteristics Related to Accident Vehicle Condition and Causation and an Assessment of Indiana PMVI Effectiveness," *Proceedings of the American Association for Automotive Medicine*, 22nd conference, 1978, 98-111, quoted in Waller, "Injury as a Public Health Problem," 1561.

71. J.P. Bull, "Accidents and Their Prevention," in Hobson *Theory and Practice*, 423.

72. Waller, "Injury as a Public Health Problem," 1565.

73. Bull, "Accidents and Their Prevention," 423.

74. Waller, "Injury as a Public Health Problem," 1566.

75. World Health Organization, *Risques pour la santé du fait de l' environment* (Geneva: 1972), 161.

76. J.M. Last, "Housing and Health," in Last, *Maxcy-Rosenau*, 869.

77. American Public Health Association, *Recommended Housing Maintenance and Occupancy Ordinance 1969* (Washington, D.C.: U.S. Public Health Service Publication No. 1935, 1969).

78. Waller, "Injury as a Public Health Problem," 1568.

79. R. Saracci, "Epidemiological Strategies and Environmental Factors," *International Journal of Epidemiology* 7, no. 2 (1978): 101-111.

80. Irving J. Selikoff, "Scientific Basis for Control of Environmental Health Hazards," in Last, *Maxcy-Rosenau*, 529-542.

81. P.E. Sartwell and J.M. Last, "Epidemiology," in Last, *Maxcy-Rosenau*, 58-60.

82. Saracci, "Epidemiological Strategies," 101-104.

83. J.M. Lance, "The Role of Epidemiology in Planning and Evaluation of Health and Safety Programs." Paper presented at 2nd International Symposium in Epidemiology in Occupational Health, Montreal, August 23-25, 1982, 25.

84. Saracci, "Epidemiological Strategies," 106.

85. Ibid., 108.

86. Joint Commission on Accreditation of Hospitals, *Hospital Self-Evaluation Form for Safety and Sanitation* (Chicago: Author, 1977).

87. American Hospital Association and National Safety Council, *Safety Guide for Health Care Institutions* (Chicago: Authors, 1972), 238.

88. A.M. Pascal, *Hospital Security and Safety* (Rockville, Md.: Aspen Systems Corporation, 1977), 159.

89. R.G. Bond, G.S. Michaelson, and R.L. De Roos, *Environmental Health and Safety in Health Care Facilities* (New York: Macmillan Publishing Co., Inc., 1973), 368.

90. P.S. Brachman, "Epidemiology of Nosocomial Infections," in *Hospital Infections,* ed. J.V. Bennett and P.S. Brachman (Boston: Little, Brown & Co., 1979).

91. R.F. Bridgman, "The Control of Infection in Hospital," in Hobson, *Theory and Practice,* 687.

92. American Hospital Association, *Infection Control in the Hospital* (Chicago: Author, 1979), 3.

93. W.E. Scheekler, "Nosocomial Infections in a Community Hospital," *Archives of Internal Medicine* 138, (1978): 1792-1794.

94. R.W. Haley et al., "Extra Charges and Prolongation of Stay Attributable to Nosocomial Infections," *The American Journal of Medicine* 70 (January 1981): 51-58.

95. R.W. Haley et al., "Nosocomial Infections in U.S. Hospitals, 1975-1976," *The American Journal of Medicine* 70 (April 1981): 947-959.

96. H.D. Riley, Jr., "Hospital-Acquired Infections," *Southern Medical Journal* 70, no. 11 (1977): 1265-1266.

97. R. Thoburn et al., "Infections Acquired by Hospitalized Patients: An Analysis of the Overall Problem," *Archives of Internal Medicine* 121, no. 1 (1968): 1-10.

98. Haley et al., "Extra Charges."

99. J. Freeman et al., "Adverse Effects of Nosocomial Infection," *The Journal of Infectious Diseases* 140, no. 5 (1979): 732-740.

100. D. Larouche, *Évaluation du coût de l'infection nosocaniale.* (Master's thesis, Université de Montréal, 1982), 114.

101. The Catholic Hospital Association, *OSHA and the Hospital Manager* (St. Louis: 1975), 19.

102. M.F. Foley and M.A. Babbitz, "Hospitals Neglecting the Need For Employee Health Programs," *Occupational Health and Safety,* June 1980, 46-48.

103. G. Runnells, "Guidelines to Assist Hospitals in the Use of Ethylene Oxide," *Hospitals* 52 (May 1, 1978): 119-122.

104. B.E. Dahlgren, "Hepatic and Renal Effects of Low Concentrations of Methoxyflurane in Exposed Delivery Ward Personnel," *Journal of Occupational Medicine* 22, no. 12 (December 1980): 817-819.

105. Medical News, "Escaping Anesthetic Gases May Affect Neurophysiological Functions," *Journal of the American Medical Association* 240 (1978): 1939.

106. National Institute for Occupational Safety and Health, *Criteria for a Recommended Standard: Occupational Exposure to Waste Anesthetic Gases and Vapors,* U.S. Department of Health, Education, and Welfare, Public Health Service (DHEW Publication No. [PHS] 77-140). (Washington, D.C.: U.S. Government Printing Office, 1977).

107. National Institute for Occupational Safety and Health, *Health Consequences of Shift Work,* U.S. Department of Health, Education, and Welfare, Public Health Service (DHEW Publication No. [PHS] 78-154). (Washington, D.C.: U.S. Government Printing Office, 1978).

108. J. Thomas, *Promoting Health in the Work Setting* (Madison, Wis.: The Institute for Health Planning, 1981), 18.

Chapter 13

Epidemiology's Future in Health Management

HEALTH SERVICES MANAGEMENT AND DELIVERY

The American health care system undoubtedly will be the subject of much discussion and concern in the coming years. Although it is not the purpose here to discuss future health policy options, it is a fact that rising costs of providing care are leading inevitably to changes. Whether inspired by promarket or progovernment intervention philosophies, the changes have an impact on every health care provider and institution.

This final chapter discusses the role of health services management in the delivery of care, then summarizes the contributions of epidemiology to major trends, issues, and problems facing the system.

It is the author's contention and the raison d'être of this book that many of the problems facing the health care system in the United States, as well as in Canada and most other countries, including the developing nations, can be attenuated through better and more effective management.

Evaluation of management practices obviously is a difficult task since assessment of its outcome should be based on the improvement of the health status of the population. A list of criteria has been proposed to serve as proxy (indirect) indicators of successful management of health services.[1] From a review of the literature, a list of features of a "good" health care system, and therefore of successful management, has been developed. It includes the following characteristics:

- It is comprehensive.
- It has no serious barrier to care.
- It aims at continuity of care for individuals and families.
- Its care is effective and appropriate.

- Its care is efficient, i.e., it conserves resources and uses appropriate personnel and technology.
- Its total population is involved so that care is available both for those who are ill and for those who are vulnerable and at risk.
- Its care is a part of community responsibility and involvement.
- Its care uses traditional as well as new therapeutic practices and ideas.
- It takes its place with other priority development systems in the community.
- It generates accurate and useful information and respects its confidentiality.
- It has built-in mechanisms for evaluation and innovation.
- It promotes advances in knowledge for everyone about health promotion and disease prevention and cure.

Conversely, unsuccessful management includes the following characteristics:

- It isolates health from other aspects of national development.
- It lacks clear and logical priorities.
- It has inadequate community involvement.
- It provides irrelevant training of health personnel.
- It has inadequate resources or utilizes them poorly.
- Its costs of care are rising.
- It restricts the use of primary health workers.
- It lacks planning capability.
- It relies on old-fashioned cure-oriented, nonecological approaches.
- It is overcentralized and has a variety of technical weaknesses.

Successful management of health services thus should be conducive to accessible, continuous, and high-quality care; services provided should be geared to the needs, wants, and desires of the population; it should be compatible and integrated with community characteristics (including culture); care should be comprehensive (from preventive to superspecialization); and care should proceed from a holistic or ecological understanding of health and its determinants. In other words, successful management necessitates an epidemiological approach.

In a study aimed at examining "new and more effective means to cope with the broader issues of health for the 1980s" around the world, Evans concludes that there is a pressing need for an epidemiological approach to the management of health services:

> The most pressing problem in the broader field of health in both industrialized and developing countries is more effective management of

health services at all levels. Management in this context involves the evaluation of resources and successful implementation of programs that depend on a human services organization.[2]

The contributions of health services managers to resolving the major problems confronting the system is limited by two main factors.[3] First, managers have been putting (and have been trained to put) the emphasis on their institution and not on the health needs of the population. Second, they have concentrated their attention on the support or hotel functions of their facility and have been reluctant to intervene in the health service functions where large savings might be possible.

> This reluctance to intervene is not due to lack of recognition of the problems: it is due to the conflict between institutional and health interests and the uncertainty that the administrator's leadership will be sustained in the face of the opposition from those adversely affected, particularly the medical staff. There is increasing recognition from those in practice in the field that familiarity with epidemiological methods and a more critical approach to review of evidence are invaluable tools for rational decision making in administration and for objective communication with the health professions.[4]

Managers will have to assume an important role in solving health and health care delivery problems, a role that will be facilitated by the adoption of epidemiology:

- as a tool to better equate resources and services with the population's health needs
- as a framework for a more global (holistic, ecological) understanding of health and its determinants;
- as a guide to the development and provision of comprehensive services
- as an objective basis for communication between management and health professionals
- as a method for reconciling organizational interests (including not for profit) with the population's health interests.

EPIDEMIOLOGY AND TRENDS AND ISSUES IN CARE

The contributions of epidemiology to health services management can be summarized by examining some current trends and issues facing the health care system. Some of these are specific to health care while others are global trends affecting the whole of American society. In both cases, they will have deep impact on the delivery of health care in coming years and health services managers must get them in place now. As Naisbitt writes, "trends, like horses, are easier to ride in the direction they are already going. When you make a decision that is compatible with the overarching trend, the trend helps you along."[5]

Evolution of Disease Patterns

As noted in Chapter 1, there has been a definite shift in disease patterns from the infectious to the chronic. At the beginning of the 20th century, the major killers were infectious diseases, and the impact of the health care system was felt through such factors as improved nutrition, housing, sanitary conditions (water, sewage, etc.), immunization, and general socioeconomic improvements. Chronic diseases, mainly cardiovascular and cerebrovascular, and cancer thus become the major problems. The health care system was reoriented toward diagnosis and care of those conditions, with most interventions being highly dependent on and centered on technology.

The incidence of chronic diseases in the United States has showed definite patterns.[6] Life expectancy at birth for males has increased from 67.1 years in 1970 to 69.5 in 1978 and for females from 74.7 to 77.2. Infant mortality rates have shown a sharp decrease from 20.0 per 1,000 live births in 1970 to 13.0 in 1979. Age-adjusted death rates (all causes) have decreased from 714.3 deaths per 100,000 population in 1970 to 588.8 in 1979. Most of this results from large drops in heart disease and stroke mortality (from 253.6 to 207.7 and from 66.3 to 45.3, respectively).

Overall death rates from cancer have risen slightly because of a large increase in lung cancer (particularly in women) and to higher cancer mortality for those over 50. However, overall cancer mortality for those under 50 has declined, as have deaths from several specific types including the uterus and the digestive system. Death rates from influenza and pneumonia also fell between 1970 and 1978 (from 22.1 to 15.4), tuberculosis (from 2.2 to 1.0), cirrhosis of the liver (from 14.7 to 12.5), and diabetes (from 14.1 to 10.4).

An interesting statistic is that death rates among young people rose in the late 1970s, mostly because of an increase in accidental deaths between 1975 and 1978. The motor vehicle accident death rate decreased between 1970 and 1975 (from 27.4 to 21.3), then turned up (to 23.4). Suicide death rates increased slightly while homicide rates advanced from 6.2 in 1965 to 9.6 in 1978.

It is difficult to predict whether these trends will continue through the 1980s and 1990s. However, there still is such a wide variation between sexes, races, and geographical areas (see Chapters 5 and 6) that overall death rates are bound to continue their decline if efforts are made to reach these high-risk, high-incidence groups.

For example, infant mortality rates still are twice as high in the black population as in the white. Among whites in 1978 they ranged from a low of 10.4 in Maine to a high of 14.4 in Colorado. Among blacks (where numbers are large enough to provide reliable estimates), the rates range from 18.4 in Arizona to 29.5 in the District of Columbia and 30.5 in Rhode Island.

These are but a few examples of wide variations in disease patterns. There also are tremendous variations among states and even among local areas. Only the use of epidemiological methods to better focus health services on the needs of local populations can make further improvements possible.

It should be clear that the epidemiological approach advocated here necessitates high flexibility in the allocation of health care resources. Resources should be assigned at the local level, where the problems are. Much of public health financing still is done on a broad program basis that does not consider local variations in disease patterns. This can only lead to ineffective and irrelevant programs.

Some other trends in disease patterns are important. As noted in earlier chapters, the nation's population is aging rapidly. If the trends toward lower death rates and higher life expectancy continue, there soon will be a large elderly population faced with multiple chronic health problems and functional impairments. Emphasis will have to be placed more on improving the quality of life of this population than on merely adding years to life. Health personnel will have to be trained in the disciplines of geriatrics and gerontology. Chronic care beds will have to be provided and support services such as day hospitals, meals-on-wheels, and house-keeping services, will have to be developed or expanded.

More generally, the health care system will have to get more involved in the identification and treatment of social and environmental pathology. As Evans points out, a third stage of the evolution of disease patterns (after the infectious and the chronic) may already be under way in industralized countries:[7] environmental exposures and changes in social conditions (in the family, community, and workplace) may represent the greatest future health risks.

A Widening Conception of Health

A second important trend, closely related to the preceding one, is the widening conceptualization of health and its determinants. As discussed in Chapter 1, there has been a progressive but definite shift in the understanding of health from a single-cause, single-effect germ (or agent) theory of disease to a multifactorial model that regards health as influenced by four fields: human biology, environment, life style, and health care organization.

This conceptualization of health has deep implications for the delivery of services in the 1980s and 1990s. As noted, more attention will have to be given to social and environmental determinants of health, including occupational factors.

Individual providers will have to widen their consideration and investigation of problems to include social and environmental determinants. Health information systems maintained by public agencies as well as epidemiological analyses by health care organizations need to include population-based data on environmental hazards. Life style factors should be considered and more data about health-related behaviors such as cigarette smoking, obesity, and alcohol and drug use need to be collected.[8]

Emphasis on life style has become a major trend in society, with concerns about nutrition, physical fitness, and well-being spreading throughout the population. The health care industry should find disease prevention and health promotion a promising opportunity for development.

A noteworthy indicator of such a trend is that in 1981, for the first time, *Hospitals,* the journal of the American Hospital Association (AHA), included in its annual "administrative reviews" a section on health promotion.[9] The AHA also established a Center for Health Promotion that provides assistance to hospitals in developing and implementing such programs. Finally, a 1980 analysis of the changing role of hospitals and their options for the future contained an appeal that they get into health promotion:

> Wellness is here; health promotion is in the forefront. In communities large or small, who has the best resources to develop a wellness or a health promotion program? Where are the facilities? Where is the manpower to establish the programs other than in the hospitals? Health system agencies could do it, and county health departments could do it, but basically, hospitals have the best resources to make these programs work. The community leadership in health promotion and wellness is in the same place as illness and disease care: the hospitals.[10]

It is evident that the health care industry is getting into health promotion and wellness at least partly out of self-interest.[11] There is a danger that disease prevention and health promotion services may simply be added to the health care arsenal and become professionalized and medicalized without really affecting other traditional services.

The importance of the reconceptualization of health is that all problems should be considered within an expanded framework as resulting from a wide range of factors including environmental and life style issues. Disease prevention and health promotion should permeate all levels and types of health services rather than merely being added as separate entities.

From Institutional Help to Self-Help

In his book describing ten "megatrends" transforming American society,[12] Naisbitt reports on a general thrust toward more self-reliance in everything from food and housing to education and health care. He describes how after the Great Depression, people relied more and more on institutions to provide for their basic needs. In the 1960s however, they came to realize that these institutions had failed them and that they really could trust only themselves. During the 1970s, they began to grow more self-sufficient and to help each other and themselves. Naisbitt describes self-help as follows:

> Self-help has always been part of American life. In the 1970s it again became a movement that cut across institutions, disciplines, geographic areas, and political ideologies. Self-help means community groups acting to prevent crime, to strengthen neighborhoods, to salvage food for the elderly, and to rebuild homes, without government assistance or at least with local control over government help.

> Medically, self-help is taking responsibility for health habits, environment, and life style, and is demanding to be treated holistically. It is asking to be treated as a whole person—body, mind, and emotions—by medical practitioners.

> It is people reclaiming personal control over the mysteries of life and death from the medical establishment through the hospices movement, natural childbirth, home births, and an increase in midwives and birthing centers where whole families participate in the birth experience in a homelike, low-technology setting.

> Self-help is the blossoming of America's entrepreneurial movement, which rejects large corporations in favor of self-employment and small business.[13]

This trend toward more self-help is reinforced by what Naisbitt describes as a shift from forced technology to high-tech/high touch. Too much medical technology has led patients to seek and adopt more humane and controllable alternatives. This rejection of technology has produced, for example, birthing centers and other birth alternatives, as well as hospices for the care of the terminally ill.

The trend also has led to the formation of an increasing number of self-help community groups to help individuals deal with such problems as retirement, widowhood, alcohol and drug abuse, weight control, mental illness, child and spouse abuse, divorce, etc.[14] This development is interesting since a growing body of literature seems to indicate that social networks may be associated positively with health status (as discussed earlier). Such self-help groups may fill a void left by the demise of the nuclear family.[15]

Increasing Participation and Decentralization

A fourth major trend affecting health care management is the decentralization of decision making to the local level. This is clearly evident in politics, where more and more power is being transferred from the federal level to state and local governments. This may be a consequence of an even more fundamental trend toward increased public participation in decision making. This "ethic of participation" is based on the principle that people whose lives are affected by a decision ought to be part of the process of arriving at that conclusion.[16]

These two trends also are included in Naisbitt's ten megatrends. He describes how decentralization of political power does not result from delegation of power from the federal to the local level but from "initiatives taken by the state or neighborhood in the absence of an effective top-down solution."[17] It is a grass-roots trend that could be difficult to reverse by a simple change of policy of the federal government.[18]

The epidemiological approach to health services management is essentially decentralized. It calls for matching services to local health needs and requires decentralized decision making. The epidemiological approach as promoted here also is consistent with participatory management. Successful identification of local needs is facilitated by consumers' decisions in the identification process. As pointed out in Chapter 10, the public also wants an image of the organization as an all-important element of effective population-based management.

Many organizations, including hospitals, may be afraid to adopt such a participatory approach. However, this trend may become so strong that there may be little choice. Failure to include consumers in the corporate decision-making process can lead to a "virulent new strain of militant consumer action."[19] Involvement of consumers also can only increase organizational effectiveness in achieving its own goals. As Naisbitt comments:

> In reality, producers should be eager . . . to engage consumers as early in the production process as possible. I do not think it an oversimplification to state that producers can only become more successful by learning how better to satisfy consumers. . . . Perhaps corporations are simply scared because they do not understand participatory democracy. It does not mean consumers will make corporate decisions. Remember, being part of the process doesn't mean controlling its outcome.[20]

Increasing Use of Information Systems

Society is changing from an industrial to an information society. Some 13 percent of the labor force is engaged in manufacturing industries; more than 60 percent can be considered as working in information occupations.[21] Computers are prevalent and will become even more so.

Although hospitals and other health care organizations may once have lagged behind other industries in the use of computerized information systems, they since have widely adopted such devices to support patient care and administrative activities.[22] As the director of the National Center for Health Services Research writes in a report on computer applications in health care:

> We know that computers can be gainfully used and will be accepted in some of the more obvious health applications at the institutional level, such as hospital information systems and ambulatory medical record systems. What lies ahead is to extend and expand this research experience in two directions. One direction is to explore the ways of aggregating the health service information available from computers at the institutional level and making it available at the planning and resource allocation level. The other direction is to utilize the extensive clinical data bases that are becoming available as a result of computerization to improve the medical care process.[23]

Health services managers will find that comprehensive information systems represent a prime opportunity for an epidemiological approach, including the daily availability of data on utilization and morbidity. The regional aggregation of data plus analysis of the constituency's health needs and services utilization could become a routine operation.

Two points should be noted. First, the availability of information obviously should lead to its increased use. Many hospitals and other health care organizations already have computerized information systems (mainly admissions and discharges) but put such data to little use. Second, health services managers should plan information systems to include comprehensive data. The epidemiological approach, based on the health field model, involves the inclusion of social, environmental, and life style data in the information routinely collected.

Reaching Equilibrium between Costs and Goals

Health care expenditures in the United States have been rising to where in 1981 they accounted for 9.8 percent of the gross national product (GNP). Since 1965, price increases (i.e., inflation) have accounted for 58 percent of the growth in health care spending.[24] A third of the increase between 1965 and 1981 was related to increased consumption of health care, the remaining 9 percent to population growth. In the 1980s and 1990s, the changing age distribution of the population can be expected to increase health care expenditures since per capita personal health care utilization is much higher in the elderly.

Much progress toward cost containment has been achieved in recent years and pressure will continue on health services managers to reduce expenditures. It is essential that they realize that cost containment is not an objective in itself but rather a constraint within which objectives should be pursued.[25] The objectives of any health care system are the delivery of accessible, continuous, comprehensive, and high-quality services equitably for all segments of the population. Cost containment is but one of several constraints (including professional, governmental, and corporate interests) affecting the pursuit of these goals.

As seen throughout this book, inequities do remain in the delivery of health services in the United States.[26] Epidemiology can help reduce those inequities by allowing health services managers to allocate scarce resources (i.e., in a cost containment context) where the health problems are greatest.

Another issue regarding rising health care costs is the use of medical technology. It is a rather delicate question to assess to what extent abuse of technology is responsible for increasing expenditures.[27, 28, 29] However, there is no doubt that there is a growing need for better evaluation and management of technological innovations.[30] In addition to providing formal methods for education in the new technologies, epidemiology can help by guiding health services managers in deciding whether a given innovation is appropriate to the needs of their organizations' constituency, taking into account their highest priority health problems and the availability of the technology in other facilities.

Trends toward deregulation, increased competition, and multi-institutional arrangements also are issues. These all have been suggested, jointly or independently, as possible solutions to rising health care expenditures. This trend is likely to continue for some years.

Once again, epidemiology can help health services managers adapt to these trends. Deregulation and increased competition call for a market-oriented attitude that (as seen in Chapter 10) is consistent with and strengthened by the adoption of an epidemiological approach. Epidemiology represents an effective management tool for adapting to increased competition. Multi-institutional arrangements represent a good opportunity for the use of epidemiology. As the president of a corporation overseeing five hospitals and several related organizations stated:

> The planning aspect, which I think is neglected when it's left up to a hospital administrator, can be tackled more effectively [in a corporate, multi-institutional arrangement]. Instead of going from crisis to crisis, you can start doing long-range, strategic planning. You can examine the needs of the market you are serving.[31]

Although health care costs represent a real problem and concern for health services managers, they should not overshadow the pursuit of the goals and objectives of the health care system. Their impact can be attenuated in part by the use of epidemiological principles and methods, since epidemiology can lead to improved management, mainly by providing a guide to focus resources where the greatest need exists.

SUMMARY

Although it is difficult to evaluate management practices and to agree on what good management of health services is, there is no doubt that an epidemiological orientation is a component.

As a tool to better equate scarce resources with the population's health needs, as a framework for a more global understanding and conceptualization of health and its determinants, as a guide to the development and delivery of comprehensive services, as an objective basis of communication between management and health professionals, and as a method for reconciling organizational interests with those of the population, epidemiology is a requirement for the modern management of health services.

This will become even more so in coming years as the trends toward self-help, a widening conception of health, increased participation and decentralization, and expenditure containment put more pressure on health services managers and necessitate more effective management.

"The most reliable way to anticipate the future is to understand the present."[32] This is what can be epidemiology's main contribution to the management of health services. With the help of epidemiology, the so-called crisis in health care delivery can present sound opportunities to achieve health system, organizational, and professional objectives.

NOTES

1. World Health Organization, "The Role of WHO in Training in Public Health and Health Programme Management, Including the Use of Country Health Programming," Unpublished background working document for Executive Board, December 7, 1978, 17.

2. J.R. Evans, *Measurement and Management in Medicine and Health Services: Training Needs and Opportunities* (New York: The Rockefeller Foundation, October 1981): 11.

3. Ibid., 32-33.

4. Ibid., 33.

5. J. Naisbitt, *Megatrends—Ten New Directions Transforming Our Lives* (New York: Warner Books, Inc., 1982), 9.

6. U.S. Public Health Service, *Health, United States, 1981* (Washington, D.C.: Department of Health and Human Services, National Center for Health Statistics), 191.

7. Evans, *Measurement and Management,* 10.

8. L. Breslow, "The Challenge to Health Statistics in the Eighties," *Public Health Reports* 96, no. 3 (May-June 1981): 231-237.

9. R. Behrens et al., "Health Promotion—Past Year Saw Large Increase in Number of Hospital Programs," *Hospitals* 55, no. 7 (April 1, 1981): 105-110.

10. H.S. Strait, "Wellness," in *The Changing Role of the Hospital,* ed. Minnesota Hospital Association (Chicago: American Hospital Association, 1980): 141.

11. R. Evans, "A New Perspective on the 'New Perspective,'" *Journal of Health Politics, Policy, and Law* 7, no. 2 (Summer 1982): 325-344.

12. Naisbitt, *Megatrends,* 131-157.

13. Ibid., 133.

14. Ibid., 150.

15. Alvin Toffler, *The Third Wave* (New York: Bantam Books, Inc., 1980), 214.

16. Naisbitt, *Megatrends,* 159.

17. Ibid., 112.

18. Ibid., 163.

19. Ibid., 177.

20. Ibid., 178-179.

21. Ibid., 14.

22. G.A. Mecklenburg, "Types and Uses of Hospital Information Systems Expand," *Hospitals* 55, no. 7 (April 1, 1981): 112-119.

23. National Center for Health Services Research, *Computer Applications in Health Care* U.S. Department of Health and Human Services, Public Health Service (DHHS Publication No. [PHS] 80-3251, June 1980), iii.

24. U.S. Public Health Service, *Health, United States, 1981,* 81-82.

25. G. Rosenthal, "Controlling the Cost of Health Care," in *Economics and Health Care* (a Milbank Reader #1), ed. J.B. McKinlay (Cambridge, Mass.: The MIT Press, 1981), 203-226.

26. L. Wyszewianski and A. Donabedian, "Equity in the Distribution of Quality of Care," *Medical Care* 19, no. 12 (1981), Supplement, 28-56.

27. U.S. Public Health Service, *Medical Technology: The Culprit Behind Health Care Costs?* Proceedings of the Sun Valley Forum on National Health, U.S. Department of Health, Education, and Welfare (DHEW Publication No. [PHS] 79-3216), Washington, D.C.: U.S. Government Printing Office, 306.

28. Office of Technology Assessment, *The Implications of Cost-Effectiveness Analysis of Medical Technology.* Washington: OTA-H-126, 1980.

29. K.E. Warner, "Effects of Hospital Cost Containment on the Development and Use of Medical Technology," *Milbank Memorial Fund Quarterly/Health and Society* 56, no. 2 (Summer 1978): 187-211.

30. G.B. Devey, "Technology: Focus on Management Grows in Face of High Costs," *Hospitals* 55, (April 1, 1981): 169-173.

31. Stephen M. Morris, quoted in C.M. Ewell, "Changes in Hospital Management Demand 'Specialist' Administrator," *Modern Healthcare* 12, no. 3 (March 1982): 90.

32. Naisbitt, *Megatrends,* 2.

Index

I.D.
demography
234

[handwritten margin note: Health field dimensions — envir. lifestyle biol. H.care system]